DISCLAIMER

Every effort has been made to ensure the accuracy of this text, and that the best information available has been used. However, palliativedrugs.com Ltd neither represents nor guarantees that the practices described herein will, if followed, ensure safe and effective patient care. The recommendations contained in this book reflect the editors' judgement regarding the state of general knowledge and practice in the field as of the date of publication. Information in a book of this type can never be all-inclusive, and therefore will not cover every eventuality.

Thus, those who use this book must make their own determinations regarding specific safe and appropriate patient-care practices, taking into account the personnel, equipment, and practices available at the hospital or other facility at which they are located. Neither palliativedrugs.com Ltd nor the editors can be held responsible for any liability incurred as a consequence of the use or application of any of the contents of this book. Mention of specific product brands does not imply endorsement.

Particularly when prescribing a drug for the first time, a doctor (or other independent prescriber) should study the contents of the manufacturer's Summary of Product Characteristics (SPC), paying particular attention to indications, contra-indications, cautions, drug interactions, and undesirable effects.

EDITORIAL STAFF

Editors-in-Chief

Robert Twycross DM, FRCP
Emeritus Clinical Reader in Palliative Medicine, Oxford University

Andrew Wilcock DM, FRCP
Macmillan Clinical Reader in Palliative Medicine and Medical Oncology, Nottingham University
Honorary Consultant Physician, Hayward House, Nottingham University Hospitals NHS Trust

Palliativedrugs.com Editorial team

Claire Stark Toller MA, MA, MRCP
Consultant in Palliative Medicine, Countess Mountbatten House, University Hospital Southampton NHS Foundation Trust

Paul Howard BMedSci, MRCP
Consultant in Palliative Medicine, Earl Mountbatten House, Isle of Wight NHS Trust

Sarah Charlesworth BPharm, DipClinPharm, MRPharmS
Specialist Pharmacist, Palliative Care Information and Website Management, Hayward House, Nottingham University Hospitals NHS Trust

Sarah Keeling
Publishing Office Manager, Palliativedrugs.com Ltd, Hayward House, Nottingham University Hospitals NHS Trust

Editorial board

Stephen Barclay MD, FRCGP
Clinical Senior Lecturer in General Practice and Palliative Care, Cambridge University
General Practitioner, Cornford House Surgery, Cambridge
Honorary Consultant in Palliative Medicine, Arthur Rank Hospice, Cambridge

Sarah-Louise Hamlyn MRCGP
Palliative Care Fellow, Hayward House, Nottingham University Hospitals NHS Trust
General Practitioner, Cripps Health Centre, Nottingham University

Daniel Knights MA MBBChir
> Academic Foundation Doctor, Newcastle University and Newcastle upon Tyne Hospitals NHS Foundation Trust

Iain Lawrie MMed, FRCP, MRCGP
> Consultant in Palliative Medicine, The Pennine Acute Hospitals NHS Trust
> Honorary Clinical Senior Lecturer in Palliative Medicine, Manchester University

Paul Paes MSc, MMedEd, FRCP
> Consultant in Palliative Medicine, Northumbria Healthcare NHS Foundation Trust
> Honorary Clinical Senior Lecturer in Palliative Medicine, Newcastle University

Amelia Stockley MSc, MRCPCH
> Consultant in Palliative Medicine, Helen & Douglas House, Oxford

Jason Ward MMed, FHEA, MRCGP
> Clinical Senior Lecturer in Palliative Medicine, Leeds University
> Honorary Consultant in Palliative Medicine, St Gemma's Hospice, Leeds

Phil Wilkins MSc, MRCP
> Consultant in Palliative Medicine, Priscilla Bacon Centre for Specialist Palliative Care and Norwich and Norfolk and Norwich University NHS Foundation Trust
> Honorary Clinical Senior Lecturer, University of East Anglia

CONTENTS

Contents

Appendices

Indexes

PREFACE

Over two decades, *Introducing Palliative Care (IPC)* has been used by medical students, doctors, nurses, and other health professionals in the UK and beyond. It has been translated into several other European languages, and a special economy edition has been available in Africa and India since 2003.

This fifth edition (*IPC5*) represents a major step in the book's evolution as it moves from single authorship to a collaborative project which has seen the palliativedrugs.com Editorial team work with eight new contributors. All have an interest in education, with many undertaking leading educational roles in their respective medical schools. Seven are members of the Association for Palliative Medicine of Great Britain and Ireland (APM) *Undergraduate Medical Education Special Interest Forum*.

We are grateful for their important contributions. Because of their involvement, *IPC5* contains more topics than previous editions and in greater detail. Although medically oriented, there is much of use to both undergraduates and recently graduated health professionals of various disciplines, particularly those engaged in providing palliative care in a generalist setting.

IPC5 covers the requirements of the APM 2014 *Recommended curriculum for undergraduate medical education* (Appendix 1). It is thus a key resource for medical students which will also serve them well as junior hospital doctors and general practitioners.

Although the clinical focus is on advanced cancer, the general principles and most of the details are equally applicable to patients dying from other progressive disorders.

Readers may spot the influence of two other key texts by palliativedrugs.com: *Symptom Management in Advanced Cancer* (Twycross, Wilcock, Stark Toller), which ceased publication in 2015, and the *Palliative Care Formulary (PCF)*. The latter has enabled the section on drugs in *IPC* to expand into the *The Essential Palliative Care Formulary*.

We acknowledge with thanks the help of past and present colleagues, and specific advice provided by Emma Heckford, Andrew Hughes, Vaughan Keeley, Kacey Leader, and Bridget Taylor.

We are grateful to Sarah Keeling for co-ordinating production, John Shaw for assistance in copy-editing and to Karen Isaac for secretarial support.

Robert Twycross
Andrew Wilcock
Editors-in-Chief
March 2016

     www.palliativedrugs.com

IPC AND BEYOND

Medical, nursing and other students

The content of *IPC* covers the essential aspects of palliative care, which will enable you to care for dying patients in the future.

IPC is *not* a book to be read all at once. Chapter 1 sets the scene and should be read first. The rest of *Part 1* covers a range of basic topics from ethical aspects through to bereavement support.

Part 2 comprises eight chapters relating to symptom management. Chapter 7 covers general principles and their application in the management of pain and should be read first. The remaining chapters 8–14 deal with a range of other symptoms, grouped together according to system or circumstance.

These can be read as required when you encounter patients with various issues. However, we advise you not to get bogged down by details about drug regimens – save those for when you are qualified and looking after someone with a particular problem.

Part 3 contains three chapters relating to the palliative care needs of children.

Part 4, The Essential Palliative Care Formulary, contains invaluable information about many of the drugs used in palliative care. Use this as a reference book when you are qualified and dealing with specific situations.

General information

As a primer, references have been purposely limited. For those wishing to delve deeper, suggestions are made in *Further reading* at the end of most chapters.

The Oxford Textbook of Palliative Medicine (5th edition, 2015; ISBN: 978-0-199-65609-7) and The Oxford Textbook of Palliative Care for Children (2nd edition 2012; ISBN: 978-0-199-59510-5) are recommended as larger standard reference textbooks.

References are completely absent in the *The Essential Palliative Care Formulary*. If necessary, the reader should refer to the latest edition of *PCF* (www.palliativedrugs.com) for such information.

In palliative care, many drugs are used beyond (off-label) and without Marketing Authorization. This has implications for the prescriber, and is discussed comprehensively in the *PCF*.

IPC includes a number of *Quick Clinical Guides*. To enhance user-friendliness, most are limited to no more than two pages.

Of the many other resources which exist, one of particular note for teachers and students alike is the e-learning resource for *End-of-life care for all* (*e-ELCA*). This provides over 150 interactive sessions covering many topics. It is accessed via the NHS Health Education England e-Learning for Healthcare website, www.e-lfh.org.uk/programmes/end-of-life-care/

ABBREVIATIONS

Abbreviations used in IPC for the times of drug administration

Times	UK	Latin
Twice per day	b.d.	*bis die*
Three times per day	t.d.s.	*ter die sumendus*
Four times per day	q.d.s.	*quarta die sumendus*
Every 4 hours etc.	q4h	*quaque quarta hora*
Rescue medication (as needed/required)	p.r.n.	*pro re nata*
Give immediately	stat	

General

GMC	General Medical Council
IMCA	Independent Mental Capacity Advocate
MCA	Medicines Control Agency (UK)
MHRA	Medicines and Healthcare products Regulatory Agency
NICE	National Institute for Health and Care Excellence
UK	United Kingdom
USA	United States of America
WHO	World Health Organisation

Medical

ACE	angiotensin-converting enzyme
ACP	advance care planning
AD	assisted dying
ADH	antidiuretic hormone (vasopressin)
ADRT	advance decision to refuse treatment
ALS	amytrophic lateral sclerosis (motor neurone disease)
APPT	activated partial thromboplastin time
AS	assisted suicide
β_2	beta 2 adrenergic (receptor)
BMI	body mass index
BNP	brain natriuretic peptide
BP	blood pressure
CBT	cognitive behavioural therapy
CHF	congestive heart failure
CNS	central nervous system
COPD	chronic obstructive pulmonary disease
COX	cyclo-oxygenase; alternative, prostaglandin synthase
CPR	cardiopulmonary resuscitation
CRP	C-reactive protein
CT	computed tomography
CTZ	chemoreceptor trigger zone
CVS	cardiovasculare system
δ	delta-opioid (receptor)
D_2	dopamine type 2 (receptor)

DIC	disseminated intravascular coagulation
DNACPR	do not attempt cardiopulmonary resuscitation
DoLS	deprivation of liberty safeguards
DVT	deep vein thrombosis
ECG (EKG)	electrocardiogram
EEG	electro-encephalograph
EOL	end of life
EOLC	end-of-life-care
FBC	full blood count
FEV_1	forced expiratory volume in 1 second
GABA	gamma-aminobutyric acid
GI	gastro-intestinal
Hb	haemoglobin
HIV	human immunodeficiency virus
H_1, H_2	histamine type 1, type 2 (receptor)
HLA	human leucocyte antigen
IL	interleukin
IL	interleukin
ITU	intensive therapy unit
IVCO	inferior vena cava obstruction
IVF	in vitro fertilisation
LDH	lactate dehydrogenase
LFTs	liver function tests
LMWH	low molecular weight heparin
LPA	lasting power of attorney
MAOI	mono-amine oxidase inhibitor
MARI	mono-amine re-uptake inhibitor
MCCD	medical certificate of cause of death
MND	motor neurone disease (amytrophic lateral sclerosis)
MRI	magnetic resonance imaging
MSCC	malignant spinal cord compression
μ	mu-opioid (receptor)
NCSE	non-convulsive status epilepticus
NDRI	noradrenaline (norepinephrine) and dopamine re-uptake inhibitor
NMDA	N-methyl D-aspartate
NMS	neuroleptic (antipsychotic) malignant syndrome
NRI	noradrenaline (norepinephrine) re-uptake inhibitor
NSAID	non-steroidal anti-inflammatory drug
OIH	opioid-induced hyperalgesia
PAS	physician-assisted dying
PG	prostaglandin
PPI	proton pump inhibitor
PT	prothrombin time
RCT	randomized controlled trial
RPR	relevant person's representative
SaO_2	oxygen saturation
SCLC	small-cell lung cancer

SIADH	syndrome of inappropriate ADH secretion
SNRI	serotonin and noradrenaline (norepinephrine) re-uptake inhibitor
SRE	skeletal-related events
SSRI	selective serotonin re-uptake inhibitor
SVC	superior vena cava
SVCO	superior vena cava obstruction
TCA	tricyclic antidepressant
TNF	tumor necrosis factor
UVB	ultraviolet B
WBC	white blood cell

Drug administration

a.c.	ante cibum (before food)
CIVI	continuous intravenous infusion
CSCI	continuous subcutaneous infusion
e/c	enteric-coated (gastroresistant)
IM	intramuscular
IT	intrathecal
IV	intravenous
IVI	intravenous infusion
m/r	modified-release; alternatives, controlled-release, extended-release, pro-longed-release, slow-release, sustained-release
OTC	over the counter (i.e. can be obtained without a prescription)
PO	per os, by mouth
PR	per rectum
SC	subcutaneous
SL	sublingual
TD	transdermal
TM	transmucosal
vial	sterile container with a rubber bung containing either a single or multiple doses (cf. amp)
WFI	water for injections

Units

cm	centimetre(s)
Gy	Gray(s), a measure of radiation
h	hour(s)
Hg	mercury
kg	kilogram(s)
L	litre(s)
mg	milligram(s)
mL	millilitre(s)
mm	millimetre(s)
mmol	millimole(s)
min	minute(s)
sec	second(s)

1. SCOPE OF PALLIATIVE CARE

DEFINITIONS

Palliative care is the *active total care* of patients with an incurable progressive life-threatening condition, and their families, by a multiprofessional team. Palliative care extends far beyond physical care, as is emphasized in the definition from the World Health Organization (Box A). The word 'palliative' is derived from the Latin word 'pallium' meaning 'a cloak'. Thus in palliative care, symptoms are 'cloaked' with treatments whose primary aim is to promote comfort.

Box A WHO definition of palliative care[1]

Palliative care is an approach that improves the quality of life of patients and their families facing the problems associated with life-threatening illness, through the prevention and relief of suffering by means of early identification and impeccable assessment and treatment of pain and other problems, physical, psychosocial and spiritual.

Palliative care:
- provides relief from pain and other distressing symptoms
- affirms life and regards dying as a normal process
- intends neither to hasten nor postpone death
- integrates the psychological and spiritual aspects of patient care
- offers a support system to help patients live as actively as possible until death
- offers a support system to help the family cope during the patient's illness and in their own bereavement
- uses a team approach to address the needs of patients and their families, including bereavement counselling, if indicated
- will enhance quality of life, and may also positively influence the course of illness
- is applicable early in the course of illness, in conjunction with other therapies that are intended to prolong life, such as chemotherapy or radiation therapy, and includes those investigations needed to better understand and manage distressing clinical complications.

Patients can live for many years with an incurable, progressive but ultimately fatal condition, and the need for palliative care is not defined by a set time limit. Nonetheless, most patients referred to specialist palliative care services will be in their last 6–12 months of life, and increasingly the term 'end-of-life care' is applied to the care of patients within this time frame. 'Terminal care' is now generally restricted to the care of patients when it becomes clear that they are going to die in the next few weeks or days.

'Supportive care' is an umbrella term used to describe the provision of all aspects of care from pre-diagnosis to bereavement, whether physical or non-physical, and curative or palliative in intent.[2] It is also used more narrowly to describe measures to combat the undesirable effects of disease-modifying treatment.[3]

In paediatric palliative care (see p.287), the terms 'life-limiting condition' and life-threatening condition' are used. A life-limiting condition is defined as a condition for which there is no reasonable hope of cure and from which a child (or young adult) will die. A life-threatening condition is one for which curative treatment may be feasible but can fail, such as cancer.[4]

Palliative care is a form of care in which the patient's physical, psychological, social and spiritual needs are regarded as equally important, and which emphasizes the inextricable link between them. This is well illustrated by the concept of *total pain*, initially proposed by Cicely Saunders, which emphasizes that a patient's suffering can relate to any or all of the four dimensions (Figure 1).

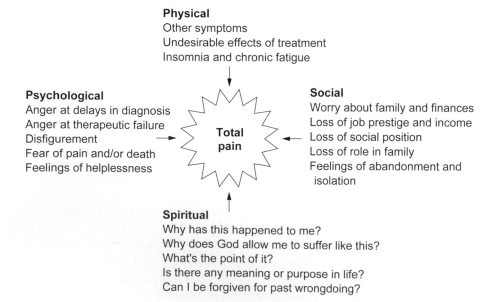

Figure 1 The four dimensions of total pain

A 'listening ear', notably that of a doctor or other health professional, is just as necessary as the right drugs, *either alone is not enough*. For example, anxiety about family finances can increase the severity of a patient's pain-related distress. If so, optimal benefit will result from the provision of financial advice and support, not just the progressive increase in analgesic dose (see p.81).

QUALITY OF LIFE

'Quality of life is what a person says it is.'

Palliative care is about quality of life, and includes rehabilitation. It seeks to help patients achieve and maintain their maximum potential physically, psychologically, socially and spiritually, however limited these may have become as a result of disease progression.

Quality of life relates to an individual's overall subjective satisfaction with life, and is influenced by all aspects of personhood.[5] In essence, there is good quality of life when the aspirations of an individual are matched and fulfilled by present experience.

There is poor quality of life when there is a wide divergence between aspirations and present experience.[6] To improve quality of life, it is necessary to narrow the gap between aspirations and what is possible (Figure 2). Palliative care aims to do this.

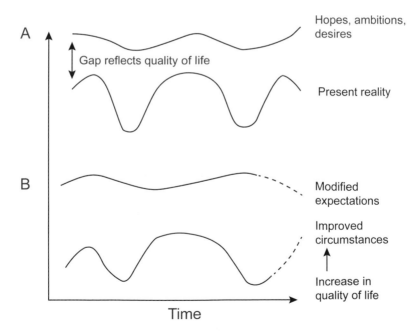

Figure 2 A representation of the gap between reality and hopes (A); an improvement in quality of life reflects either a reduction in expectations or a change in present reality (B).[6]

Thus, a tetraplegic ex-gymnastics instructor is able to say, 'The quality of life is excellent, though to see me you wouldn't believe it. I've come to terms with my loss and discovered the powers of my mind'. And a 30-year-old man dying of disseminated osteosarcoma complicated by paraplegia comments, 'The last year of my life has been the best'.

DEVELOPMENT OF PALLIATIVE CARE

Palliative care is a relatively new concept in modern medicine. In its early stages, it was synonymous with 'hospice care'. (Historically, hospices were 'houses of rest and entertainment for pilgrims, travellers, or strangers'.) In the mid–late 19th century, hospices in Dublin and London were set up by nuns to offer care to the 'dying poor'. However, there was relatively little medical input. Other similar establishments opened during the middle years of the 20th century.

In the late 1950s, Cicely Saunders, a recently qualified doctor and research fellow in pharmacology went to St Joseph's Hospice in East London to study pain in dying cancer patients, and to provide the necessary medical input. Having previously worked as a nurse and then a social worker, Saunders had resolved to dedicate her life's work to improving the care of the dying. Motivated by her Christian faith, she went on to found St Christopher's Hospice in South London in 1967. She was a passionate advocate of 'efficient loving care' for dying patients, and she is universally recognized as the founder of the modern palliative care.[7]

Palliative care is now a well-established element of healthcare provision, with over 8,000 hospice and palliative care programmes in more than 100 countries. In the UK, palliative care has been a medical specialty since 1987, with specialist services available in hospitals, hospices and the community. There is increasing recognition of the importance of generalist and other health professionals providing high quality palliative care within their own care settings and specialties.

In 2014, the World Health Assembly adopted a landmark resolution emphasizing the importance of palliative care as an ethical responsibility of healthcare, and called for both individual countries and the WHO to take action to improve provision globally.

CURRENT CHALLENGES IN PALLIATIVE CARE

Annually worldwide:
- 54 million people die (all causes)
- 30 million die from progressive organ failure or other degenerative diseases
- 8.5 million die from cancer
- 1.5 million die from HIV/AIDS.

With technological advances in public health and healthcare provision, life expectancy is increasing rapidly in many parts of the world. Globally currently almost 1 in 10 people are over 60; by 2050, this proportion will have risen to 1 in 5. An ageing population brings with it a rise in chronic conditions and multiple co-morbidities, and an increased need for palliative care.[8]

At its inception, palliative care had a strong focus on cancer, particularly in younger patients. In recent years, the importance of other chronic progressive conditions, such as cardiorespiratory disease and dementia, has been increasingly recognized. However, with less predictable disease trajectories, access for non-cancer patients to palliative care services is still relatively poor.

In the UK, end-of-life care has been subject to damaging media coverage, with controversy about the way in which the *Liverpool Care Pathway for the Dying Patient* was sometimes implemented. A subsequent report highlighted the need for care to be more than an unthinking 'tick-box' exercise but, instead, based on adequate training and sensitive communication with patients and families.[9,10] New NICE guidelines stress the need for an individualized approach and the need for frequent review, at least on a daily basis.[11]

Coping with uncertainty at the end of life is a key challenge for health professionals, patients and families. It has inevitable ethical implications (see p.13) as well as impacting on communication strategies (see p.35).

In many countries, more deeply ingrained barriers remain, such as limited access to strong opioid analgesics (because of overly restrictive governmental control on narcotic drugs) and 'opiophobia' (fear of opioids) among many clinicians. In many developing countries, healthcare is massively underfunded and unable to provide basic preventive and curative treatments, and certainly not palliative care.

WHO IS A 'PALLIATIVE PATIENT'?

Often, there is *not* a clear-cut division between disease-modifying therapy and palliative care (Figure 3). However, once disease-modifying treatments are no longer available or appropriate, the primary focus will shift to palliative care.

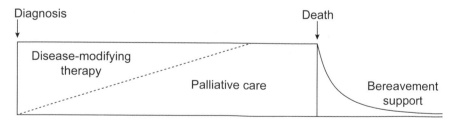

Figure 3 The relationship between disease-modifying therapy and palliative care in a patient with an incurable progressive condition.

Clinicians' estimates of prognosis in cancer can be very inaccurate, and are commonly over-optimistic. In non-cancer patients, in whom the illness trajectory is less predictable, prognosis is even harder to estimate. Different groups of patients have different trajectories of functional decline towards death (Figure 4).

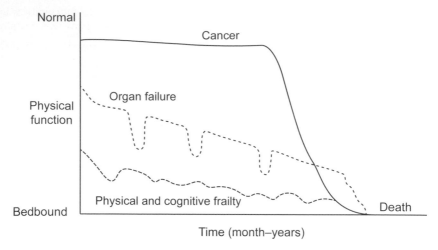

Figure 4 Disparate trajectories in progressive conditions.

Cancer deaths tend to follow a fairly predictable course, with a long period of relatively good physical function, followed by a steady, rapid and progressive decline towards death.

In contrast, deaths from organ failure (heart, lung, liver) tend to follow a course of progressive decline with unpredictable acute exacerbations. In many cases, the patient makes a good recovery from each exacerbation, but there will ultimately be an episode from which they will not recover, and they may die fairly rapidly. It is very difficult to foresee which exacerbation will be the final blow.

Chronic frailty associated with dementia, degenerative neurological disease or old age is even more unpredictable with a prolonged progressive decline in physical and mental function. Thus, when talking with patients and their families about the future, it is important to communicate the uncertainty surrounding prognosis (see p.42).

WHO PROVIDES PALLIATIVE CARE?

Teamwork and partnership are central to palliative care: between different members of the multiprofessional team, and between clinicians and patients and their families.

Teamwork

'Together Everyone Achieves More'

A climate of mutual respect and trust where hierarchy is minimized and each individual is empowered to provide the best possible care is fundamental. Because there is an overlap of roles, co-ordination is an important part of teamwork.

Conflict inevitably erupts from time to time in a team of highly motivated, skilled professionals. One of the challenges of teamwork is how to handle conflict constructively and creatively.

Most palliative care is delivered by doctors and nurses who are not specialists in palliative care. With the growing needs of an ageing population, it is neither possible nor appropriate for all palliative care to be provided by specialists. Thus, all health and social care professionals need to be equipped with appropriate skills in order to provide good palliative care (Table 1), with specialist services involved for the more difficult and complex cases.

Table 1 Roles of health professionals in providing palliative care

Role	Description
General Practitioner	Co-ordinates care in the community, ensuring all appropriate professionals are involved. Normally the lead doctor for patients at home or in residential and nursing homes. On average, a GP in the UK will have 20 patient deaths per year: five from cancer, six from organ failure, seven from chronic frailty and two from sudden death.
Hospital Consultant	Consultants in specialties such Oncology, Chest Medicine, Cardiology or Care of the Elderly usually remain in overall charge of a patient's specialist care when inpatients or in outpatient clinics. They may transfer patients directly to a palliative care service but, more commonly, will discharge them back to the GP to provide continuing care.
Palliative Medicine Consultant	Generally involved only in more complex cases. Responsible for a patient's care when admitted to a palliative care unit/hospice. In the community or hospital, they generally provide an advisory service, with ultimate responsibility for the patient's care remaining with the GP or other hospital consultant.
Non-consultant grade doctors (e.g. junior doctors, staff grade, associate specialists)	Provide palliative care in all settings in various ways with the support of a consultant/GP, e.g. co-ordinating the day-to-day care of inpatients and optimization of their medical management, review of patients in outpatients, day care, GP clinics and at home. In hospital, a junior doctor is likely to be the first to be called to see dying patients out of hours, and to confirm death.
Inpatient Nurse	In hospital or care home, the nurses and healthcare assistants provide the physical care and administer drugs. In hospices and other clinical areas where dying patients are cared for regularly, nurses become confident in administering 'as needed' drugs.
District Nurse	Provides regular nursing care in the community; available 24/7 in most areas of the UK. Will regularly visit a patient to monitor physical symptoms and nursing needs, provide nursing care, arrange equipment in the home such as a hospital bed, arrange overnight nursing care and administer drugs such as morphine by injection or syringe driver.

continued

Table 1. Contd.

Role	Description
Macmillan Nurse/ Clinical Nurse Specialist in Palliative Care	Specialist nurses whose role is to provide information and advice regarding the patient's care and condition, and provide emotional support to patients and families. Do not provide hands-on nursing care and are generally not available 'out-of-hours'.
Marie Curie Nurse and Hospice at Home service	Nurses or Healthcare Assistants who provide hands-on nursing care in the home, often co-ordinated by the patient's District Nurse. They aim to support a patient to remain in their own home for as long as possible, frequently staying with patients for several hours overnight.
Home Carer	Community-based carers (Social Services or agency) attend to a patient's hygiene, toileting, eating and drinking needs, and support the family. They may get to know the patient very well, and thus may identify subtle changes in their condition.
Physiotherapist and Occupational Therapist	Maximizes a patient's functional ability for as long as possible, either through exercises or home modifications. May also advise in the non-drug management of symptoms such as breathlessness or anxiety.
Social Worker	Responsible for advising on and arranging community care packages, including home carers and access to care homes. Provide advice on the financial aspects of care, and the availability of grants.
Chaplain/Religious leader	Spiritual care practitioners are particularly helpful for patients who have a religious faith. Also helpful for the non-religious who have existential questions they would like to talk through in a non-religious framework.
Complementary Therapist	Complementary therapies may be available, particularly in hospices. Relaxation techniques are often used in the management of anxiety and insomnia.
Volunteers	Although not health professionals, volunteers are an integral part of most palliative care services, providing 'added value' as a result of their own life experiences and skills. They help with a wide range of tasks, including serving food and drink, co-ordinating activities for patients, and being an additional listening ear for patients and families. They also form an important link with the wider community.

Partnership

Palliative care is based on partnership between the multiprofessional team and the patient and family. Consultations should be seen as a meeting of experts: patients are the experts about how they feel and the overall impact of the illness, and health professionals are the experts in diagnosis and management. Partnership emphasises equality rather than hierarchy, and requires mutual respect (Box B).

Box B Partnership with the patient	
Be courteous and polite	Explain
Listen	Agree priorities and goals
Don't be condescending	Discuss treatment options
Be honest	Accept treatment refusal

PLACE OF CARE

In recent years, significant emphasis has been placed on the patient's preferred place of care and preferred place of death. Although the majority of the *general public* say they would prefer to die in their own home, among *patients* there is a wide range of preferences, many of whom are undecided or view issues such as symptom management as a greater priority than the place of their care and death.[12]

It is important that patients and their families are aware of all the options, how to access them urgently if necessary, and be assured that they have not failed should they change their minds about remaining at home.

The most common place of death in the UK is still the acute hospital. This discrepancy between preferred and actual place of death has been one of the drivers behind Advance Care Planning, where people record their wishes before becoming seriously ill, e.g. to avoid unwanted emergency hospital admissions (see p.268).

Home

High quality care at home is often possible, particularly if social networks are strong and family members are able to be closely involved. A good support network is essential: ready access to medical and nursing care at all times of day and night, access to specialist advice when needed, and equipment or adjustments to the home speedily available.

Planning for the last days of life is particularly important, in which possible outcomes are discussed sensitively, and family and carers are appropriately prepared. A 'Just-in-case' set of drugs enables health professionals to administer drugs rapidly should distressing symptoms develop (see p.273). Well co-ordinated teamwork among the various professionals involved is vital to avoid a succession of disjointed visits (very tiring for the patient) and ensuring continuity of care.

Despite initially expressing a wish to be cared for at home, many patients and families change their minds as the illness progresses, with preference for home care declining over time.[13] Caring is far more demanding than most people imagine, and exhaustion is an ever-present threat.

Hospice day care

Hospices often also provide day care 1–2 days per week for patients in the community. This may be for a limited period of time because of restrictions on numbers. It is very beneficial for patients who are socially isolated or whose family need some respite. Day care patients often receive complementary and relaxation therapies alongside more traditional medical and nursing care, enabling them to remain in their own homes for longer.

Nursing or residential care homes

These provide a significant amount of palliative care, particularly for patients with chronic frailty and dementia. Care homes look after people on a long-term basis, in a constant environment; they become familiar with the staff, who get to know their preferences. The nurses can also become expert at detecting troubling symptoms, and involving other health professionals when appropriate.

Hospice/palliative care unit

Hospices are centres of excellence providing specialist palliative care. The majority of patients have a cancer diagnosis, reflecting their historical focus. They typically receive considerable amounts of charitable funding (sometimes well over 50% of their running costs), and often provide various additional services such as complementary therapies.

The number of hospice beds in the UK is limited and allocation of this scarce resource is a challenge. Inpatient beds are generally reserved for patients with complex physical, psychological, social or spiritual needs which cannot be met elsewhere. Average duration of stay is 10–14 days, typically with the aim of improving symptom control. About half will die at the hospice, with the remainder discharged back to their own home or to a care home.

Hospital

Patients approaching the end of life are often admitted to hospital when crises arise, and many never recover sufficiently to be discharged before their death. Early in a patient's disease process it may be entirely appropriate for them to be admitted to hospital, particularly if they are still receiving curative treatment. However, the busy environment of a hospital ward is less appropriate for patients near the end of their lives. Often, staff looking after acutely ill patients do not have sufficient time also to care adequately for the rapidly changing needs of dying patients.

CONCLUSION

Over the past 50 years, palliative care has developed into an important clinical specialty, but is also fundamental to the role of all health professionals, regardless of specialty. On average, in their first year post-qualification, a UK F1 doctor will care for around 40 dying patients. It is thus vital that they have a good understanding of palliative care.

Further, over half of all medical graduates become GPs, who have a central role in the care of the 40% of UK patients who die at home or in care homes. With only one chance to get it right, caring for dying patients is both hugely challenging and hugely rewarding.

Clinical, pharmacological, communication and team-working skills are crucial. As one family member wrote to a junior doctor:

'We will never forget the calm and reassuring way that you looked after mum in her last few days. Your quiet confidence that you would keep it comfortable for her, and that you knew where to get advice, made our painful loss so much easier to bear. Thank you.'

REFERENCES

1   WHO (2002) *National Cancer Control Programmes. Policies and managerial guidelines (2e)*. World Health Organization, Geneva.
2   National Council for Hospice and Specialist Palliative Care Services (2002) *Definitions of Supportive and Palliative Care Briefing paper 11*. London.
3   Senn H-J and Glaus A (2002) Supportive care in cancer - 15 years thereafter. *Supportive Care in Cancer*. **10:** 8–12.
4   Association for Childrens Palliative Care (2011) *A care pathway to support extubation within a children's palliative care framework*. www.togetherforshortlives.org.uk/professionals/resources/2433_the_extubation_care_pathway_2010
5   Cohen S and Mount B (1992) Quality of life in terminal illness: defining and measuring subjective well-being in the dying. *Journal of Palliative Care*. **8:** 40–45.
6   Calman KC (1984) Quality of life in cancer patients - an hypothesis. *Journal of Medical Ethics*. **10:** 124–127.
7   Boulay du S (2007) *Cicely Saunders: the founder of the modern hospice movement*. Society for Promoting Christian Knowledge, London.
8   Murtagh FE *et al.* (2014) How many people need palliative care? A study developing and comparing methods for population-based estimates. *Palliative Medicine*. **28:** 49–58.
9   Neuberger J (2013) *More care, less pathway: a review of the Liverpool Care Pathway*. Department of Health, London.
10 Leadership Alliance for the Care of Dying People (2014) One chance to get it right. Improving people's experience of care in the last few days and hours of life. www.gov.uk/government/uploads/system/uploads/attachment_data/file/323188/One_chance_to_get_it_right.pdf
11 NICE (2015) *Care of dying adults in the last days of life*. www.nice.org.uk/guidance/ng31
12 Hoare S (2015) Do patients want to die at home? A systematic review of the UK literature, focused on missing preferences for place of death. *PLoS ONE*. **10:** e0142723.
13 Munday D *et al.* (2009) Exploring preferences for place of death with terminally ill patients: qualitative study of experiences of general practitioners and community nurses in England. *British Medical Journal*. **338:** b2391.

2. ETHICAL ASPECTS

ETHICAL DECISION-MAKING

All clinical care includes making decisions, and sometimes these are ethically challenging because the choices to be made have significant consequences for the patient, health professionals, or society generally.

Cardinal principles

In relation to medical care, the same cardinal principles apply in all specialties and settings, namely:

- autonomy (self-determination)
- beneficence (do good)
- non-maleficence (minimize harm)
- justice (fair use of available resources).[1]

Ethically the four cardinal principles have equal weighting and are underpinned by the general professional values of respect for human life, protecting the health of patients, and treating patients with respect and dignity.[2] Towards the end of life, respect for life is combined with an acceptance of the ultimate inevitability of death.[3] Thus, in practice, there are three dichotomies which need to be held in balance:

- the potential benefits of treatment versus the potential risks and burdens
- striving to preserve life but, when the burdens of life-sustaining treatments outweigh the potential benefits, withdrawing or withholding such treatments and providing comfort in dying
- individual needs versus the needs of society.

'Clinical integrity' is another way of applying the cardinal principles. The term emphasizes the importance of respecting a patient's values, needs and wishes, and the integration of the best available care or treatment with a desire to bring genuine benefit to a person in a way that is fair to everyone involved.[4]

Clinical integrity implies being up to date in all aspects of care, recognizing one's limitations and, when necessary, seeking help from others to improve care. Clinical integrity needs to be paired with personal integrity in relation to character and consistency. Maintaining clinical integrity will help you navigate your way through most of the challenges which will inevitably come your way in end-of-life care.

There is also need for a sense of urgency – just as much in palliative care as in acute care. This aspect of applied ethics is encapsulated in what has been called the Emancipation Principle of palliative care:

> Spare no scientific or clinical effort to free dying persons from twisting and racking pain that invades, dominates, and shrivels their consciousness, that leaves them no psychic or mental space for the things they want to think and say and do before they die.[5]

Partnership

When considering autonomy, the recent focus has generally been on the patient, partly because of a revolt against medical paternalism. However, a more nuanced interpretation embraces the autonomy of both patient and professional.[6] Thus, in practice, shared ('principled') autonomy means *partnership between patient and professional*. Both are experts: the patient in relation to the impact of the illness on their life and family, and the professional in relation to clinical evaluation and treatment options.

Thus, autonomy does *not* mean simply doing whatever a patient requests, as this is an abdication of one's professional role. When there is persistent disagreement and a doctor still believes a certain treatment is inappropriate, they should iterate their reasoning and assist the patient in obtaining a second opinion.[2]

Conversely, in the UK and many other countries, a person is not legally obliged to accept a clinician's treatment recommendation, even if refusal results in earlier death.[7,8]

However, most patients want partnership, and are generally happy to accept professional advice. Consequently, doctors have a legal obligation to discuss treatment options and their implications with patients, taking their values and wishes into account, and to obtain informed consent.

Without consent, a doctor risks being found guilty of assault.[9] Likewise, ignoring the views of patients can lead to breaches of the law.[10] Good communication is crucial to avoid misunderstanding (see p.35).

Capacity

Capacity is about the ability of a patient to make a particular decision. It should be presumed that people have capacity unless there is a suspicion of cognitive impairment. Severe depression, delirium (acute confusional state) or dementia are common causes of a loss of capacity.

In the UK, there are four components to having capacity; these are the ability to:
- understand what decision needs to be made and why
- understand the likely consequences of making or not making the decision
- understand, retain, use and weigh up the information relevant to the decision
- communicate their decision (by talking, using sign language or any other means).[11]

People may have capacity to make some decisions and not others. Loss of capacity is decision-specific and may be temporary. If a patient lacks capacity for a particular decision, a health professional's legal obligation is to make a decision in the person's best interests following a clear set of principles (see p.263), including the involvement of anyone who holds legal authority for the patient or any legally binding decisions:

- judgements should be non-discriminatory; not based on age, appearance or condition
- all relevant circumstances pertinent to the individual should be considered in the context of the decision being made
- consideration should be made to delaying a decision if capacity may be regained in the future
- individuals lacking capacity should participate in decision making as much as they are able
- if decisions are being made about life-sustaining treatments, the person making the decision should not be motivated to bring about the individual's death
- consideration should be given to the individual's past and present wishes, feelings, beliefs and values
- other relevant people, such as family members, partners and carers should be consulted.[11]

Double effect

The principle of double effect states that:

A single act having two possible foreseen effects, one good and one harmful, is not always morally prohibited if the good effect is intended and the means to that good effect is not through the bad effect. There must be no other safer way of achieving the same result.[1]

The principle is generally ascribed to Thomas Aquinas, a Thirteenth Century theologian and philosopher. It was originally enunciated in relation to self-defence: if an assailant is severely injured or killed, the victim of the attack can invoke this principle in defence against a charge of grievous bodily harm or murder.

The principle of double effect is thus a universal principle which is invoked to exculpate someone when a good action results in unintended harm. The practice of medicine would be impossible without such a principle. It is essential because all treatment has an inherent risk and, inevitably, things sometimes go wrong. However, it is *not* an excuse for harm resulting from incompetence.

Discussion of the principle of double effect often focuses on the use of morphine or other opioids to relieve pain in terminally ill patients. This gives the false impression that the use of morphine in this circumstance is a high-risk strategy.[12] When correctly used, morphine and other strong opioids are very safe drugs with little chance of causing significant harm.[13] Indeed, non-steroidal anti-inflammatory drugs (NSAIDs) may well cause more serious undesirable effects, sometimes fatal, particularly in certain groups of patients.

The use of both classes of analgesic is justified on the basis that the benefits of pain relief far outweigh the risk of serious undesirable effects, particularly in someone who is terminally ill. However, the balance between benefit and potential harm could change for both classes of analgesic, for example, in a patient with renal impairment.

The situation in the UK is encapsulated in a classic legal judgement:

> 'A doctor who is aiding the sick and the dying does not have to calculate in minutes or even in hours, and perhaps not in days or weeks, the effect upon a patient's life of the medicines which he administers or else be in peril of a charge of murder. If the first purpose of medicine, the restoration of health, can no longer be achieved, there is still much for a doctor to do, and he is entitled to do all that is proper and necessary to relieve pain and suffering, even if the measures he takes may incidentally shorten life.'[14]

Similar sentiments have been expressed in other countries, and reflect a broad international consensus.

Nonetheless, even in palliative care, the intended aim of treatment must be the relief of suffering and not the patient's death. Although a greater risk is acceptable in more extreme circumstances, measures which carry less risk to life should normally be used in the first place.

Thus, although in an extreme situation it may be acceptable to render a patient unconscious (because less extreme measures have failed to bring adequate relief; see p.27), it is still unacceptable intentionally to cause death. Indeed, because of a fundamental difference in the approach to patients (see p.22), the European Association for Palliative Care (EAPC) states that euthanasia should not be regarded as part of palliative care.[15]

Societal views on life are important in judging the intentions of actions. In the UK and most countries, respect for life underpins all actions and professional codes of conduct. However, some countries and some sections of society take a different view: when someone is terminally ill, death may be anticipated and desired, and so regarded as a good outcome.[16] The interpretation of the intention and outcome must take into account societal views as enshrined in law.

Ethical tensions

Alongside the four cardinal principles (p.13), when considering the ethics of actions (normative ethics), three major approaches are recognized:
- *Deontology*: decisions should be based around one's duties and other people's rights
- *Consequentialism*: the morality of an action is judged by its outcome
- *Virtue ethics*: focus on the character of the person carrying out an action, rather than the action itself.

The emphasis of these approaches is quite different and leads to situations where people may disagree vociferously on a particular action. For example, the principle of double effect depends on people regarding the *intention* of an action as being important. Whereas, for Consequentialists, their interest is in the *outcome* of the action. The tension between the two positions becomes apparent in considering specific ethical situations.

APPROPRIATE TREATMENT: WITHHOLDING AND WITHDRAWING

'Treatment that does not provide net benefit to the patient may, ethically and legally, be withheld or withdrawn and the goal of medicine should shift to the palliation of symptoms.'[17]

Some of the biggest challenges in end-of-life decision-making are about withholding or withdrawing a treatment which might prolong life, e.g. antibiotics, clinically-assisted nutrition and hydration, and ventilation.

Doctors must keep in mind the self-evident fact that all patients must die eventually. Thus, part of the skill of medicine is to weigh up the benefits, burdens and risks of a treatment; and decide when to intervene, and when to allow death to occur without prolonging dying or causing distress by using burdensome treatments.

A doctor is not obliged legally or ethically to preserve life 'at all costs'.[2] Priorities change when a patient is clearly dying. There is no obligation to employ treatments if their use can best be described as prolonging the process of dying.[18,19] A doctor has neither a duty nor the right to prescribe a lingering death. In palliative care, the primary aim of treatment is *not* always to prolong life but to make the life which remains as comfortable and as meaningful as possible.

Medical care is a continuum, ranging from complete cure at one end to symptom relief at the other. It is important to keep the therapeutic aim clearly in mind when employing any form of treatment. In deciding what is appropriate, the key points to bear in mind are:
- the goals and hopes of the individual patient
- the biological ability to benefit from a treatment
- the therapeutic aim and benefits of each treatment
- the burdens and risks of each treatment
- balancing the needs of those involved and using health resources wisely.

The benefits of a treatment may include:
- slowing disease progression
- sustaining life
- reducing disability or improving health
- relieving discomfort.

If a treatment does not have a realistic chance of achieving one of these aims, it is likely to be futile.

The burdens of a treatment may include:
- prolonging the dying phase
- treatment that is painful, exhausting, destructive, or intrusive.

Sometimes the correct course of action is a time-limited trial of a particular treatment: 'We will try this, but if there's no obvious benefit after 2–3 days, then we'll stop it'.

Health professionals generally find it harder to withdraw a treatment than to withhold it. However, there is no ethical difference; but not understanding this can lead to not starting treatment which may be of some benefit to the patient, or to continuing treatment which is of no overall benefit.[2]

There may be disagreements about the right course of action. Good communication with the patient, family and between team members, coupled with empathy and humility generally resolves most difficulties. It is important to allow time for adjustment and reflection. When there is persistent disagreement, a second opinion should be obtained. Occasionally, consultation with a clinical ethics committee, legal department, and/or defence organization may be necessary.

Clinically-assisted nutrition and hydration

Food and fluids can be emotive issues for patients and their families because they are seen as essential for maintaining life. Food and fluids are also considered part of basic care, and thus should always be offered to patients who can swallow without serious risk of choking or aspirating, providing additional help if necessary.[2]

Dysphagia is part of the disease process in some conditions, e.g. head and neck cancer and MND/ALS, and can have a major impact while the patient is still fairly active. To prevent starvation and dehydration when oral intake becomes inadequate, such patients should be considered for:
- clinically-assisted nutrition: IV feeding or feeding via a tube into the stomach or small bowel, e.g. nasogastric tube, percutaneous endoscopic gastrostomy (PEG)
- clinically-assisted hydration: IV or SC administration of fluids.

However, clincially-assisted nutrition and hydration are 'medical treatments'[20] and require a thorough ethical reflection before a decision is made. The literature is mixed on the outcomes, particularly in terms of prolonging life.[21] Individual decisions need to be considered in relation to the life expectancy, quality of life and impact with and without the intervention.

When deciding on clinically-assisted nutrition, potential goals of care include:
- increase in weight if the patient is underweight
- improvement of healing of pressure ulcers/wounds
- increased capacity for rehabilitation
- prolonging life.[22]

The burdens to consider include:
- risks of placement and reflux: PEG tube insertion carries a 30-day mortality of 6% with 10% morbidity; this rises significantly for certain conditions, e.g. MND/ALS
- being attached to a pump for up to 20h/day or needing bolus administrations every 1–2h
- socially becoming less involved in mealtimes, and losing the pleasure of eating
- alteration in body image.

Clinically-assisted hydration can also be considered in terms of the potential benefits (e.g. preventing thirst and dehydration) weighed up against the inconvenience, discomfort and undesirable effects (e.g. increased secretions, peripheral and pulmonary oedema, abdominal distension; see p.276).

In the last days of life, loss of interest in food and drink and a global deterioration in function is part of the dying process. Thus, generally, the benefits of clinically-assisted fluids and nutrition are likely to be small, and outweighed by the burdens. There is need for individual evaluation, clear explanation, and careful monitoring (see p.276).

However, it is essential to continue to offer drinks (or sips of fluid), and to provide good mouth care.

DO NOT ATTEMPT CARDIOPULMONARY RESUSCITATION (DNACPR) DECISIONS

Cardiopulmonary resuscitation (CPR) is the process of trying to restart a person's heart or breathing after a cardiac or respiratory arrest. DNACPR decisions are made to avoid patients having to suffer a futile resuscitation attempt.

In the UK there are national guidelines about making DNACPR decisions.[23] If a patient is at risk of a cardiac or respiratory arrest, clinicians need to weigh up the benefits, burdens and risks of attempting CPR. It is more likely to work in specific circumstances, to do with the type of arrest and the environment in which it occurs. *In dying patients CPR will not succeed.*

Futile treatments are not generally offered or discussed with patients unless they express a wish to do so. However, in 2014 in a ruling about communication in relation to DNACPR decisions, the courts ruled that *not* discussing a DNACPR order with a patient is a breach of the European Convention on Human Rights unless the doctor thinks that 'the patient will be distressed by being consulted and that that distress might cause the patient harm'.

Importantly, the ruling was not about the decision-making itself, and it affirmed the rights of patients to choose not to engage in CPR discussions.[10] The implication of this decision needs to be fully worked through. DNACPR decisions may be unique because they are emotive for the general public, and CPR is one of few treatments which require specific documentation to rule it out.

CPR decisions can be problematic because it is sometimes assumed that a DNACPR decision means that all active treatment will stop. National guidance is clear that CPR may well be futile even in those patients who are being actively treated in other respects, and that all patients in hospital should have their resuscitation status decided.[24]

Unfortunately, discussions are often carried out as an isolated discussion about CPR rather than in the context of an overall treatment strategy. Alternative approaches, e.g. the Universal Form of Treatment Options,[25] Treatment Escalation Plans,[26] or Emergency Care and Treatment Plans,[27] start by clarifying the goals of treatment for the patient and include a range of decision-making. These are more acceptable to patients and families.

In cases where CPR might work, the benefits and risks/burdens should be sensitively discussed with patients so that they can make an informed decision. Some patients may choose not to discuss this, often because it involves engaging with the prospect of dying. For patients lacking capacity, a decision will be taken on the basis of best interests. When disagreements occur, although it is a clinical decision, allowing time and sensitive communication should resolve most issues, offering a second opinion if necessary.

MEDICALLY-ASSISTED DYING: EUTHANASIA AND ASSISTED SUICIDE

'Assisted dying' (AD) refers to a medical intervention with the explicit intent to hasten death *at a person's voluntary and competent request*:

- *assisted suicide (AS) or physician-assisted suicide (PAS)*: a doctor intentionally helps a person commit suicide by providing drugs for self-administration
- *euthanasia (active euthanasia)*: a doctor intentionally kills a person by the administration of drugs.[28]

AS can also be defined more broadly as a health professional providing the means or knowledge to allow a person to take their own life, in the form of information, advice, prescription or supply. An alternative definition of euthanasia includes reference to the use of the most gentle and painless means possible, motivated solely by the best interests of the person who dies.[29]

'Non-voluntary euthanasia' relates to patients who no longer have capacity and thus cannot give valid consent, e.g. because of dementia or other brain damage, and the decision is taken on their behalf as a 'best interests' decision. In contrast, 'involuntary euthanasia' relates to patients who still have capacity but have made no request to die (this is essentially murder).

'Indirect euthanasia' has been used in the past to describe the administration of opioid analgesics to terminally ill patients. However, giving a *proportionate dose* of a drug to lessen pain cannot be equated with giving a *lethal overdose* deliberately to hasten death.

Thus, the following are *not* medically-assisted dying:

- 'allowing nature to take its course' in someone imminently dying
- stopping biologically futile treatment
- stopping treatment when the burdens outweigh the benefits
- using morphine and/or other drugs to relieve pain following best practice guidelines.

Requests for euthanasia and assisted suicide

Although patients may express a desire to hasten death, *persistent* requests for AD are uncommon:[30]

'Patients requesting a physician's assistance [to hasten death] are usually telling us that they desperately need relief from their mental and physical distress and that without such relief they would rather die. When they are treated by a physician who can hear their desperation, understand the ambivalence most feel about their request, treat their depression, and relieve their suffering, their wish to die usually disappears.'[31]

In other words, most of those who demand help to die are asking for help to live.

The common denominator in patients who desire to hasten death is despair, described as a sense of hopelessness, helplessness, lack of control, isolation, or endlessness. This may relate to actual or anticipated:
- severe pain or other physical distress, e.g. breathlessness, choking, vomiting
- increasing dependence
- slow deterioration over many months
- being a burden on family and friends
- being kept alive with machines and tubes when quality of life is unacceptably low or when in coma.

Despair also stems from:
- a short-term *adjustment disorder* on discovering one has a fatal disease with limited life expectancy
- *demoralization* ('no point in struggling on')
- *depression* (meaning a depressive illness, not just sadness or demoralization).

Depression or other significant psychiatric disorder is the underlying cause of the despair in about half of those desiring to hasten death.[32] Further, it seems that, without despair, there is no perception of unbearable suffering; and, unless associated with depression, feelings of unbearable suffering are not generally persistent.[33]

A persistent feeling of despair (and thus persistent unbearable suffering) may also relate to a philosophy of life in which self-worth depends on being robustly healthy and 'in control'.[34]

Listening to the patient non-judgementally should allow the clinician to determine the cause(s) underlying the desire to hasten death. For patients with a clinical depression, treatment is indicated (see p.189). For most other patients, the desire for death wanes when they experience the benefits of palliative care:
- unconditional positive regard (respect)
- good communication
- goal-setting
- holistic support
- sense of urgency
- high-quality pain and symptom management
- ongoing commitment (non-abandonment).

Current status

In the UK, no form of AD is legal and helping someone to commit suicide is punishable with a prison sentence. Attempts to legalize AS were defeated in both Scotland and England and Wales in 2015.

Partly because the law has not changed, around 30 UK residents per annum go to the Dignitas Clinic in Switzerland for AS, a country where assisting suicide has never been illegal. The Director of Public Prosecutions in London has issued guidance about when *not* to prosecute someone for helping a terminally ill person travel to Switzerland.[35] Thus, for several years, no family member or friend has been prosecuted for aiding and abetting suicide in these circumstances.

In several countries and jurisdictions, euthanasia and/or assisted suicide is permitted in adults ± 'emancipated minors' (16+) provided certain criteria are met. In the Netherlands, AD is permitted from the age of 12 and, in Belgium, there is no lower age limit but the child requesting euthanasia must have 'capacity for discernment'.[36,37] This excludes the very young, those with intellectual disability, or impaired consciousness. In the Netherlands, non-voluntary euthanasia of severely ill newborns is permitted under the Groningen Protocol.[38,39]

Ongoing debate

The debate about AD is generally conducted along pragmatic, utilitarian and consequentialist lines. To argue from mutually exclusive philosophical positions can never lead to the consensus which every society must strive for.

Since the time of Hippocrates the medical profession has opposed AD, although there have been historical examples of AD from ancient Greece onwards, and attitudes have changed in countries or jurisdictions where AD is now permitted.

In the UK, surveys indicate that 60–80% of the general public support a change in the law but that 60–70% doctors are opposed.[40-42] The highest opposition is in palliative care, where only around 10% of doctors favour a change.[40,42]

It is important to try and understand this paradox. In many cases, popular support for AD is associated with fear of future suffering generated by the unknown or past bad experience of a relative dying in great distress, coupled with a lack of understanding about what palliative care services can provide. In some cases, it is associated with an intolerable sense of indignity should progressive illness lead to increasing weakness and dependence, a viewpoint commonly expressed in terms of a right to self-determination or individual autonomy (Box A).

However, for many clinicians, the approach enshrined in palliative care provides a powerful contrasting set of positives (see p.1).

These can renew and maintain hope which, in turn, allows people to 'live until they die', complete unfinished (psychosocial) business, and to die peacefully ('with dignity') with no need for AD.[15]

Further, in a society governed by the Rule of Law, restrictions on individual autonomy are legitimate if other people are considered to be endangered. This requires us to balance all four cardinal principles, in particular justice (p.13). Ultimately, society should act in such a way that the common good is upheld.

Thus, the central question in the debate about AD is: can a law be devised which would allow those with progressive incurable illnesses or progressive general debility in old age to end their lives should they wish to without endangering others? Advocates for AD claim that it should be possible, whereas those against claim that a change to permit AD would lead to more harm than good.

However, unlike individual autonomy in relation to AD, there is probably no single 'trump card' which can be played by those against a change in the law. On the other hand, the reasons listed in Box B collectively make strong case against any change.

> **Box A** Arguments in support of Assisted dying (AD)
>
> People have a right to self-determination (individual autonomy) and should have the right to choose the time and mode of their death.
>
> People now live much longer than their forebears, and often have to suffer many years of physical debility ± progressive undignified dementia.
>
> It is compassionate to assist someone to die who is suffering unbearably; it is cruel to force them to continue to suffer.
>
> Palliative care cannot always relieve distressing symptoms adequately; AD is necessary as a 'long-stop' option.
>
> AD is necessary to avoid being subject to overzealous treatment ('therapeutic obstinacy').
>
> AD enables people to die with dignity rather than linger on for months or years, increasingly dependent on other people for even the most basic physical needs.
>
> Covert forms of AD are widespread; a clear legal framework would ensure proper safeguards and prevent abuse.
>
> There is no evidence of harmful outcomes or 'mission creep' in jurisdictions where AD is legal.

Regrettably, comments such as, 'We treat animals better than we do humans' and 'If he was an animal, he'd be put down' are heard too often for comfort. Although on one level such comments can be easily countered, these statements reflect a depth of compassion and anguish which can easily be lost or ignored in a detached discussion of philosophical and ethical principles.[44]

Those in favour of AD also stress that there is a level of existence where most people would wish not to be kept alive. If conscious, they might ask for AD, emphasizing that life no longer has meaning or purpose for them. Patients in irreversible coma would be one category and persistent vegetative state another.

In countries considering AD, it is imperative to ensure there is comprehensive palliative care provision to meet the needs of dying patients. However, palliative care cannot 'sanitize' all forms of dying. For example, when cancer erodes the face and replaces familiar features with a malodorous ulcerating fungating mass or when a similar process affects the perineum and results in distressing and humiliating double incontinence. These are powerful images and must be acknowledged by those who oppose AD. Indeed, a doctor who:

- has never been tempted to kill a patient probably has had limited clinical experience or is not able to empathize with those who suffer
- abandons a patient to suffer intolerably is morally more reprehensible than the doctor who (in ignorance of any alternative) opts for AD.

Box B Arguments against Assisted dying (AD)

Prognosis is based more on probability than certainty; some patients live much longer than anticipated.

Doctors will more often be feared as potential killers if AD is legalized, and more people will refuse to be referred for palliative care – and will suffer unnecessarily in consequence.

AD will alter the dynamics of the doctor-patient relationship.

Overworked doctors may encourage AD in order to reduce their work-load.

Implicit coercion, e.g. as one Dutch doctor commented, 'In the past, if I suggested euthanasia, nine times out of 10, the patient would choose euthanasia; now when I suggest palliative care, they choose palliative care.'[43]

An expressed wish by a terminally ill person to hasten death does *not* mean they want AD; *they want to be heard*, to express their frustrations and fears, to be understood.

Patients change their minds, particularly when receiving high quality palliative care.

A wish to hasten death is generally not persistent unless the patient has a depressive illness – which normally will respond to treatment.

A wish to hasten death is almost always associated with despair (a sense of hopelessness and helplessness); palliative care generally restores hope and overcomes despair by setting new goals with the patient.

Societal attitudes to disability and infirmity will become less tolerant if AD is available.

Pressure to opt for AD could increase as health budgets are further squeezed.

'Mission creep' is inevitable: the experience in the Netherlands (euthanasia and AS) and Belgium (euthanasia) provides irrefutable evidence of this, and the situation in Oregon is far from satisfactory (see below).

Oregon's Death with Dignity Act

Oregon is of particular interest because the proposals for AD currently being discussed in the UK are based on Oregon's Death with Dignity Act 1994. Annual statistics have been published annually since the Act came into force in 1997. Over 70% of those dying by AS in Oregon are college-educated people who are not suffering physically but whose major concerns are losing autonomy, being less able to do enjoyable activities, and loss of dignity.

It is concerning that:
- 67% of prescriptions for AS are issued by a small number of doctors; 29 out of about 10,000 doctors in the State[45]

- almost all those dying by AS are clients of Compassion and Choices (the AD advocacy organization in Oregon),[45] and discussion of alternatives may well have been cursory
- a review by two medically qualified doctors of five cases whose details were in the public domain revealed inadequate exploration of patients' concerns and a bias in favour of AS[31]
- although the incidence of depression in those who have a genuine desire to hasten death is possibly as high as 40%,[32] only 3% of patients in Oregon seeking AS are currently referred for psychiatric assessment (down from 30–40% in 1998–99)
- a study by a professor of psychiatry of 18 patients who requested AS found three of them had undiagnosed (and thus untreated) depression (17%); all three died by AS within two months[46]
- although the criteria for receiving a prescription for AS include a prognosis of less than six months, 10% or more live longer, some for 1–3 years (*estimates derived from Oregon Public Health Division's DWDA annual reports*).

'Mission creep'

Once the barrier of legislation is passed, AD tends to take on a dynamic of its own, and extends beyond the agreed restrictions, despite earlier explicit assurances that this would not happen.[47] This is predictable and inevitable because, to achieve popular support, activists tend to dilute their demands. However, once the law is changed, they work to evolve the legislation so as to achieve more fully their broader aim.

In the Netherlands, the intent of the 2002 Statute was to allow those with incurable progressive disease to opt for AD if there was no prospect of improvement. A Dutch ethicist who was an initial supporter of AD and a member of a Regional Euthanasia Review Committee for 12 years writes:

> 'Euthanasia is on the way to becoming a "default" mode of dying for cancer patients. Whereas the Law sees euthanasia as an exception, public opinion is shifting towards considering them rights, with corresponding duties on doctors to act.'[48]

The Netherlands Right to Die Society has founded a network of travelling doctors ('End of Life Clinic') to facilitate euthanasia and is campaigning for a lethal pill to be made available to anyone over 70 years who wishes to die.

Considerable mission creep has also occurred in Belgium,[49] and extends to psychiatric patients. Of 100 consecutive requests for euthanasia over four years at one outpatient psychiatric clinic, nearly 1/2 were accepted.[50] Diagnoses included depression, bipolar disorder, personality disorder, schizophrenia, post-traumatic stress disorder, chronic fatigue syndrome, and complicated grief.

Further, families in Belgium tend much more to consider the dying process as undignified, useless, and meaningless, even when peaceful. Requests from family members for fast and active interventions for their elderly parents are now often coercive, resulting in the doctor feeling obliged to hasten death deliberately.[47]

At present the Law in the UK prohibits AD. This is a clear 'bright line'; it may occasionally be crossed by doctors (and others) but it remains unambiguous.[51] It is perfectly consistent to argue that, ethically speaking, AD is permissible in some extreme cases but that it would be unwise to change the law. Law is a blunt instrument for dealing with ethical complexities. As at present, it could be better to allow hard cases to be taken care of by various expedients than to introduce new legislation which most likely would become too permissive.

Finally, it should be noted that, if the law is changed, there is no absolute reason why doctors and nurses should be involved. A suicide service comprising non-clinically registered individuals able to prescribe or administer a single lethal overdose for a patient who fulfilled the legal criteria could be set up and closely monitored.[52]

PALLIATIVE SEDATION

Palliative sedation is a term commonly used in relation to dying patients to describe the monitored use of drugs intended to induce a state of decreased or absent awareness (unconsciousness) in order to relieve intolerable suffering from refractory (intractable) symptoms (see p.253).[53,54]

Intolerable suffering is defined by the patient as a symptom or state which they do not wish to endure. Refractory symptoms are those for which treatment has failed, or it is considered that there is no treatment which would work within an acceptable time-frame, or with acceptable risks.

However, palliative sedation is often used more loosely as an umbrella term for all levels and patterns of sedation in the dying,[55] making it difficult to interpret and compare much of the literature. There is much to be said for abandoning the term, and using more precise terminology (Table 1).

In certain specified circumstances, all these forms of sedation can be justified on the grounds of necessity (the need to relieve suffering, while minimizing risk to consciousness or life as far as possible). However, because continuous deep sedation (CDS) has *an inevitable life-shortening effect*, it should never be regarded as 'routine' (see below).

In practice, most instances of the use of sedation in the last days of life are secondary, e.g. a patient with an agitated delirium is given an antipsychotic drug (e.g. haloperidol, levomepromazine) as a specific treatment for the delirium with sedation as a secondary effect. A benzodiazepine (e.g. midazolam) is often also given as a specific treatment of the anxiety; this too will have a sedative effect.

Initial doses are small and increased according to requirements, i.e. *the sedation is proportionate*. It is only when severe distress persists despite all usual non-drug and drug measures that increasing doses of sedatives would be used with the intention of achieving primary continuous deep sedation until death (see p.253).

Table 1 Contrasting varieties of sedative use in the dying

Primary		Secondary	
Primary	Sedative drugs used with the specific intent of easing anxiety ± inducing drowsiness/coma	Secondary	Unintended consequence of drugs with sedative properties used appropriately for symptom management
Light	Consciousness unaffected or easily rousable	Deep	Patient rendered unconscious
Intermittent (respite)	Repeated episodes each limited to a few hours or days at most	Continuous	Maintained until death
Progressive (proportionate)	Aim to limit impact on awareness by starting with a low dose, then if necessary titrating slowly upwards to achieve a relaxed patient	Sudden (emergency)	Deliberate large dose to rapidly induce coma
For physical distress	In response to intolerable refractory symptoms	For existential distress	In response to intolerable refractory mental distress

CONTINUOUS DEEP SEDATION (CDS) UNTIL DEATH

Various aspects of continuous deep sedation (CDS) until death are highly contentious (Box C).[56]

Box C Continuous deep sedation (CDS) until death: contentious issues

'Normal' treatment or 'last resort' measure?

Do guidelines help or hinder?

Does CDS shorten survival?

Is existential distress a legitimate indication for CDS?

At what point does CDS become 'slow euthanasia'?

Is it ethical to withhold clinically-assisted nutrition and hydration?

Does the practice of CDS lead to 'mission creep'?

'Normal' treatment or 'last resort' measure?

CDS is a 'normal' treatment in that it is considered acceptable medical practice *in certain circumstances*; it is how it is sometimes applied which is contentious.

Because it means the end of a person's 'biographical' or social life, it should always be regarded as an *exceptional 'last resort' measure*, and *never as routine* or, worse, the default option.[57]

Thus, it is of concern that, in the generalist setting in some countries, CDS is increasing, e.g. in Netherlands and Flanders (Belgium), it features in 12% of all non-sudden deaths.[58,59]

Although there is concern in these countries to differentiate CDS from euthanasia, rapid inducement of deep unconsciousness is typical.[60] This is perceived to be a proportionate response to unbearable suffering in a context where there is often considerable pressure from relatives and others to hasten dying. Indeed, CDS is sometimes organized like euthanasia, with a family farewell before the patient is rendered permanently unconscious.[60]

In contrast, at a palliative care centre in Belgium, the incidence of CDS fell from 7% to 3% over a six year period.[61] The decrease was attributed to an improved standard of palliative care and a team approach to decision-making. This raises the question: should CDS be permitted only if the patient has been seen by, and cared for, by a specialist palliative care team?

In the UK, clinical practice tends to reflect the guidelines produced by the EAPC for palliative sedation,[54] with an emphasis on titrating doses proportionately against symptoms, maintaining consciousness if at all possible (see p.253).[60]

Do guidelines help or hinder?

Guidelines are created to instruct clinicians, and as such will help to improve practice by ensuring that appropriate drugs and doses are used. However, guidelines for CDS differ considerably, and there is a clear need for convergence.[62]

Whereas some stress that death should be expected within hours or a few days,[53] the Royal Dutch Medical Association guidelines[63] (among others) state that death should be expected within two weeks. Unsurprisingly, this allows for widely differing practices between countries.

Most guidelines suggest midazolam as the sedative of first choice. This has limitations because the two most common reasons given for CDS are delirium and extreme breathlessness.[64] Delirium may be exacerbated by midazolam or other benzodiazepines (see p.278) precipitating a downward spiral: more distress → more midazolam → more agitation → more midazolam until deeply sedated, possibly unnecessarily.

In relation to extreme breathlessness, although midazolam may settle the associated fear and agitation, morphine and midazolam are best used in combination to achieve maximum benefit (see p.277).

Further, guidelines can lead to an uncritical 'one-size-fits-all' solution to difficult-to-manage symptoms, lowering rather than raising the standard of analytical symptom-specific management.[65]

Does CDS shorten survival?

Despite claims to the contrary, CDS predictably shortens life.[66] Thus, CDS (when justified) is an example of the principle of double effect (see p.15).

The doses of drugs necessary for CDS (good effect) simultaneously and inevitably suppress vital centres located in the brainstem which control respiration, blood pressure, heart rate, and pharyngeal muscles for swallowing and cough (bad effect). Thus, there will be a definite and increasing life-shortening impact if the patient's prognosis is more than a few hours.

Is existential distress a legitimate indication for CDS?

'Existential' refers to issues surrounding meaning and purpose in life. Existential is more profound than psychological and, by convention, does not include agitated delirium.

Most palliative care specialists accept that there are rare occasions when CDS for existential suffering is justifiable. Accordingly, it is essential that clear criteria are established for this. These should include:

- the designation of the distress as refractory should be made only after repeated (skilled) psychological evaluation has excluded concurrent depression and failed to help the patient move to a more positive outlook
- initially, deep sedation should be on a respite (intermittent) basis, and *not* continuous
- the decision to proceed to CDS must be a team decision; individual feelings or burn-out inevitably bias decision-making
- if the patient is *not* imminently dying, clinically-assisted hydration should be given unless refused by the patient.[67]

In a Japanese nationwide survey of some 9,000 patients in specialist palliative care units, only 90 (1%) were treated by CDS because of refractory existential distress. Of these, about 60% received specialist psychological/psychiatric or religious support, and 94% had at least one episode of intermittent (respite) sedation before progressing to CDS.[68]

Survival after starting CDS varied. About two thirds died in <1 week, suggesting that these patients could be classed as 'imminently dying' when CDS was started. Only rarely did a patient survive >1 month.[68] Although not explicitly stated, most patients probably received clinically-assisted hydration during CDS.

The low incidence of CDS for existential distress in palliative care units suggests that existential distress is significantly reduced when patients have access to high quality palliative care. Indeed, palliative care doctors are generally reluctant to offer CDS for existential suffering alone, particularly if the prognosis is months rather than days, and because it is almost impossible to be sure that the suffering is refractory.[69]

If the patient is *not* imminently dying, even with clinically-assisted hydration, CDS for existential distress alone will tend to become 'slow euthanasia'.

At what point does CDS become 'slow euthanasia'?

Provided the patient is imminently dying, it is possible to distinguish between CDS until death and euthanasia (Table 2). On the other hand, if *not* imminently dying, CDS is indistinguishable from 'slow euthanasia' *unless time-limited and clinically-assisted hydration is provided.*

Table 2 Comparison of continuous deep sedation and euthanasia

	CDS	Euthanasia
Intention	Relief by reducing awareness	Relief by killing the patient
Method	Dose titration	Standard doses
Drugs	Sedative	Lethal cocktail
Proportionate	Yes, at least in theory	Definitely not
Criterion of success	Relief of distress	Immediate death

It should be noted that in the Netherlands some doctors actively encourage patients to opt for CDS rather than euthanasia, simply because it is associated with less bureaucracy (Table 3).[60,70,71]

Table 3 Selected regulatory requirements for continuous deep sedation vs. euthanasia in the Netherlands

	CDS	Euthanasia
Prognosis	<2 weeks	No time limit[a]
Competence	Not essential	Yes
'Cooling off' period	No	Yes
Second opinion	No	Yes
Paperwork	No	Yes

a. the patient must be suffering unbearably without any prospect of improvement.

Is it ethical to withhold clinically-assisted nutrition and hydration in CDS?

If death is imminent (within hours), clinically-assisted hydration is irrelevant, and may cause harm (see p.18). However, as a general rule in patients receiving CDS for existential distress, clinically-assisted hydration should be maintained. Although it cannot be totally ignored, nutrition is less of an issue.

Does the practice of CDS lead to 'mission creep'?

The answer to this question is almost certainly yes:
- CDS is sometimes substituted for euthanasia in the Netherlands[71]
- there are reports of CDS which can be described only as non-voluntary (unrequested) euthanasia[72]
- the Norwegian Medical Association recently widened its guidelines from 'palliative sedation for the dying' (prognosis of <2 weeks) to 'palliative sedation at the end of life' (prognosis unstated)[73]

- in the USA, it has been proposed that the 'last resort' criterion should be dropped, and CDS allowed for any patient with a prognosis of <6 months[74]
- the French Government plans to legalize CDS as a specific substitute for euthanasia.

Proportionate sedation

The appropriate use of sedation for overwhelming distress is discussed elsewhere (see p.253). Meanwhile, the testimony of a doctor working in palliative care is noteworthy:

'I haven't given anyone continuous sedation: there have been lots of patients who have become agitated at the end of their lives and in those cases it's appropriate to give [drugs] to relieve that agitation and that restlessness. So we are giving drugs that do have sedative effects but the aim is not necessarily to sedate, the aim is to relieve that agitation and restlessness and make them more comfortable.' (UK doctor)[70]

Key points:

- involve palliative care specialists before proceeding to CDS
- good palliative care reduces the need for CDS
- CDS is only rarely necessary.

Final thought

'Patients tend to be sedated when the carers have reached the limit of their resources and are no longer able to stand the patient's problems without anxiety, impatience, guilt, anger or despair. Perhaps many of the desperate treatments in medicine can be justified by expediency, but history has the awkward habit of judging some as fashions, more helpful to the therapist than to the patient.'[75]

REFERENCES

1 Beauchamp T and Childress J (2013) *Principles of Biomedical Ethics. 7th edition.* Oxford University Press, New York.
2 General Medical Council (2010) *Treatment and care towards the end of life: good practice in decision making.* www.gmc-uk.org/guidance
3 Gillon R (1994) Medical ethics: four principles plus attention to scope. *British Medical Journal.* **309**: 184–188.
4 National Health and Medical Research Council (2011) *An ethical framework for integrating palliative care principles into the management of advanced chronic or terminal conditions.* National Health and Medical Research Council, Commonwealth of Australia.
5 Roy DJ (1990) Need they sleep before they die? *Journal of Palliative Care.* **6**: 3–4.
6 Stirrat GM and Gill R (2005) Autonomy in medical ethics after O'Neill. *Journal of Medical Ethics.* **31**: 127–130.
7 Re T (1992) Adult: refusal of treatment. *All England Reports.* **4**: 649–670.
8 Re MB (1997) An adult: medical treatment. *Family Court Reports.* **2**: 541.
9 Fleming JG (1998) *Law of Torts (9e).* LBC Information Services, p. 29.
10 Royal Courts of Justice (2014) *Tracey versus Cambridge University Hospitals NHS Foundation Trust and others.* Royal Courts of Justice, London. www.judiciary.gov.uk/wp-content/uploads/2014/2006/tracey-approved.pdf

11 Department for Constitutional Affairs (2007) *Mental Capacity Act Code of Practice*. TSO, London.

12 Gilbert J and Kirkham S (1999) Double effect, double bind or double speak? *Palliative Medicine*. **13**: 365–366.

13 George R and Regnard C (2007) Lethal opioids or dangerous prescribers? *Palliative Medicine*. **21**: 77–80.

14 Devlin P (1985) *Easing the Passing. The trial of Dr John Bodkin Adams*. The Bodley Head, London.

15 Radbruch L et al. (2015) Euthanasia and physician-assisted suicide: A white paper from the European Association for Palliative Care. *Palliative Medicine*. **30**: 104–116.

16 Allmark P et al. (2010) Is the doctrine of double effect irrelevant in end-of-life decision making? *Nursing Philosophy*. **11**: 170–177.

17 BMA (1999) *Withholding or withdrawing life-prolonging medical treatment. Guidance for decision making.* BMA, London.

18 Gillon R (1999) End-of-life decisions. *Journal of Medical Ethics*. **25**: 435–436.

19 London D (2000) Withdrawing and withholding life-prolonging medical treatment from adult patients. *Journal of the Royal College of Physicians of London*. **34**: 122–124.

20 Airedale NHS Trust v Bland (1993) 1 All ER 821.

21 Department of Health (2007) *Improving Nutritional Care*. A Joint action plan from the Department of Health and Nutrition Summit stakeholders. DOH, Leeds.

22 Royal College of Physicians and British Society of Gastroenterology (2010) *Oral feeding difficulties and dilemmas: A guide to practical care, particularly towards the end of life*. Royal College of Physicians, London.

23 BMA, the Resuscitation Council (UK) and the RCN (2014) *Decisions relating to cardiopulmonary resuscitation. 3rd edition.* www.resus.org.uk/dnacpr/decisions-relating-to-cpr/

24 NCEPOD (2012) *Time to intervene.* www.ncepod.org.uk/2012cap.htm

25 Fritz Z et al. (2013) The Universal Form of Treatment Options (UFTO) as an alternative to Do Not Attempt Cardiopulmonary Resuscitation (DNACPR) orders: a mixed methods evaluation of the effects on clinical practice and patient care. *PLoS One*. **8**: e70977.

26 Obolensky L et al. (2010) A patient and relative centred evaluation of treatment escalation plans: a replacement for the do-not-resuscitate process. *Journal of Medical Ethics*. **36**: 518–520.

27 National Emergency Care and Treatment Plan. www.resus.org.uk/consultations/emergency-care-and-treatment-plan/

28 Materstvedt LJ et al. (2003) Euthanasia and physician-assisted suicide: a view from an EAPC Ethics Task Force. *Palliative Medicine*. **17**: 97–101.

29 Draper H (1998) Euthanasia. In: R Chadwick (ed) *Encylopaedia of Applied Ethics, 2* . Academic Press p 176.

30 Zylicz Z and Janssens M (1998) Options in palliative care: dealing with those who want to die. *Bailliere's Clinical Anaesthesiology*. **12**: 121–131.

31 Hendin H and Foley K (2008) Physician-assisted suicide in Oregon: a medical perspective. *Michigan Law Review*. **106**: 1613–1639.

32 Wilson KG et al. (2014) Mental disorders and the desire for death in patients receiving palliative care for cancer. *British Medical Journal Supportive Palliative Care*. www.spcare.bmj.com/content/early/2014/03/04/bmjspcare-2013-000604.short

33 Dees MK et al. (2011) Unbearable suffering: a qualitative study on the perspectives of patients who request assistance in dying. *Journal of Medical Ethics*. **37**: 727–734.

34 Krag E (2014) Rich, white, and vulnerable: rethinking oppressive socialization in the euthanasia debate. *Journal of Medical Philosophy*. **39**: 406–429.

35 Director of Public Prosecutions (2014) *Policy for prosecutors in respect of cases of encouraging or assisting suicide.* CPS, London.

36 Dan B et al. (2014) Self-requested euthanasia for children in Belgium. *Lancet*. **383**: 671–672.

37 Siegel AM et al. (2014) Pediatric euthanasia in Belgium: disturbing developments. Journal of the American Medical Association. **311**: 1963–1964.

38 Verhagen E and Sauer PJ (2005) The Groningen protocol-euthanasia in severely ill newborns. New England Journal of Medicine. **352**: 959–962.

39 Jotkowitz A et al. (2008) A case against justified non-voluntary active euthanasia (the Groningen Protocol) American Journal of Bioethics. **8**: 23–26.

40 Seale C (2009) Legalisation of euthanasia or physician-assisted suicide: survey of doctors' attitudes. Palliative Medicine. **23**: 205–212.

41 Royal College of Physicians (2014) RCP position on assisted dying. www.rcplondon.ac.uk/ press-releases/rcp-reaffirms-position-against-assisted-dying

42 Association for Palliative Medicine (2014) Survey on physician assisted suicide. www. apmonline.org/documents/142134248840564.pdf

43 Oostveen M (2001) Spijt. Voorvechters van euthanasie bezinnen zich. NRC Handelsblad. November 10.

44 Hurst SA and Mauron A (2006) The ethics of palliative care and euthanasia: exploring common values. Palliative Medicine. **20**: 107–112.

45 Stevens KR (2011) Concentration of Oregon's AS prescriptions and deaths from a small number of prescribing physicians. Analysis and critique of Hedberg et al. 2009. Journal of Clinical Ethics. **20**: 124–132.

46 Ganzini L et al. (2008) Prevalence of depression and anxiety in patients requesting physicians' aid in dying: cross sectional survey. British Medical Journal. **337**: a1682.

47 Vandenberghe P (2013) Assisted dying: the current situation in Flanders. European Journal of Palliative Care. **20**: 266–272.

48 Boer T (2014) Assisted dying: don't go there. Daily Mail on-line July 2014.

49 de Diesbach et al. (2012) Dossier of European Institute of Bioethics: Euthanasia in Belgium 10 years on.

50 Thienpont L et al. (2015) Euthanasia requests, procedures and outcomes for 100 Belgian patients suffering from psychiatric disorders: a retrospective, descriptive study. BMJ Open. **5**: e007454.

51 Finlay I (2006) Crossing the 'bright line'–difficult decisions at the end of life. Clinical Medicine. **6**: 398–402.

52 Finlay IG et al. (2005) The House of Lords Select Committee on the Assisted Dying for the Terminally Ill Bill: implications for specialist palliative care. Palliative Medicine. **19**: 444–453.

53 de Graeff A and Dean M (2007) Palliative sedation therapy in the last weeks of life: a literature review and recommendations for standards. Journal of Palliative Medicine. **10**: 67–85.

54 Cherny NI and Radbruch L (2009) European Association for Palliative Care (EAPC) recommended framework for the use of sedation in palliative care. Palliative Medicine. **23**: 581–593.

55 Papavasiliou ES et al. (2013) From sedation to continuous sedation until death: how has the conceptual basis of sedation in end-of-life care changed over time? Journal of Pain and Symptom Management. **46**: 691–706.

56 Schildmann E and Schildmann J (2014) Palliative sedation therapy: a systematic literature review and critical appraisal of available guidance on indication and decision making. Journal of Palliative Medicine. **17**: 601–611.

57 Van Delden JJM (2013) The ethical evaluation of continuous sedation at the end of life. Stercks S, Raus K, Mortier F (eds). Cambridge University Press, Cambridge, pp 218–227.

58 Onwuteaka-Philipsen BD et al. (2012) Trends in end-of-life practices before and after the enactment of the euthanasia law in the Netherlands from 1990 to 2010: a repeated cross-sectional survey. Lancet. **380**: 908–915.

59 Chambaere K et al. (2015) Recent trends in euthanasia and other end-of-life practices in Belgium. New England Journal of Medicine. 372: 1179–1181.

60 Seale C et al. (2015) The language of sedation in end-of-life care: The ethical reasoning of care providers in three countries. Health 19: 339–354.

61 Claessens P et al. (2007) Palliative sedation and nursing: The place of palliative sedation within palliative nursing care. Journal of Hospice and Palliative Nursing. 9: 100–106.

62 Gurschick L et al. (2015) Palliative Sedation: An Analysis of International Guidelines and Position Statements. American Journal of Hospice and Palliative Care. 32: 660–671.

63 KNMG (2009) Guideline for palliative sedation. www.knmg.artsennet.nl/Publicaties/ KNMGpublicatie/Guideline-for-palliative-sedation-2009.htm

64 Maltoni M et al. (2012) Palliative sedation in end-of-life care and survival: a systematic review. Journal of Clinical Oncology. 30: 1378–1383.

65 Scott JF (2015) The case against clinical guidelines for palliative sedation. In: Taboada P (ed.). Sedation at the end-of-life: an interdisciplinary approach. Spinrger, Heidelberg, pp 143–159.

66 Rady MY and Verheijde JL (2010) Continuous deep sedation until death: palliation or physician-assisted death? American Journal of Hospice and Palliative Care. 27: 205–214.

67 Cherny NI (1998) Commentary: sedation in response to refractory existential distress: walking the fine line. Journal of Pain and Symptom Management. 16: 404–406.

68 Morita T (2004) Palliative sedation to relieve psycho-existential suffering of terminally ill cancer patients. Journal of Pain and Symptom Management. 28: 445–450.

69 Weddington WW, Jr. (1981) Euthanasia. Clinical issues behind the request. Journal of the American Medical Association. 246: 1949–1950.

70 Seymour J et al. (2015) Using continuous sedation until death for cancer patients: a qualitative interview study of physicians' and nurses' practice in three European countries. Palliative Medicine. 29: 48–59.

71 Anquinet L et al. (2013) Similarities and differences between continuous sedation until death and euthanasia - professional caregivers' attitudes and experiences: a focus group study. Palliative Medicine. 27: 553–561.

72 Harrison PJ (2008) Continuous deep sedation: Please, don't forget ethical responsibilities. British Medical Journal. 336: 1085.

73 Forde R et al. (2015) Palliative sedation at the end of life - revised guidelines. Tidsskrift for Den Norske Laegeforen. 135: 220–221.

74 LiPuma SH and DeMarco JP (2015) Expanding the use of continuous sedation until death: moving beyond the last resort for the terminally ill. Journal of Clinical Ethics. 26: 121–131.

75 Main T (1957) The ailment. British Journal of Medical Psychology. 30: 129–145.

3. COMMUNICATION

GOOD COMMUNICATION IS ESSENTIAL

'Communication skills are not an optional add-on extra; without appropriate communication skills, our knowledge and intellectual efforts are easily wasted.'[1]

'Communications, like tumours, may be benign or malignant. They may also be invasive, and the effects of bad communication with a patient may metastasise to the family. Truth is one of the most powerful therapeutic agents available to us, but we still need to develop a proper understanding of its clinical pharmacology and to recognise optimum timing and dosage in its use. Similarly, we need to understand the closely related metabolisms of hope and denial.'[2]

Good communication is an essential component of palliative care. Most complaints made by patients and families centre on poor communication. Particularly in those with a life-limiting condition, poor communication can have a significant negative impact on the quality of care, the patient's and family's well-being, and how the family copes in bereavement.[3,4]

The aims of communication are to:
- share information
- reduce uncertainty
- facilitate choice and joint decision-making
- create, develop and maintain relationships[5].

The basic message a patient wants to hear at a time of increasing uncertainty is:
'No matter what happens, we won't desert you.' (*non-abandonment*)
'You are important to us.' (*acceptance and affirmation*)

Only part of this can be said in words:
'We can relieve your pain, and can ease most other symptoms.'
'I will see you regularly.'
'One of us will always be available.'
'Let's work out how best we can help you and your family.'

A large part of the message is conveyed to the patient non-verbally:
- facial expression
- eye contact
- posture, including whether sitting or standing
- pitch of voice and pace of speech
- touch.

Eye contact indicates that you are focused on the patient and are listening to them. It also emphasizes that what they are saying is important to you and that you are keen to be involved in their care. This does not mean that you need to stare fixedly; it is a matter of finding a happy medium.

Posture or positioning can influence the dynamics of any consultation. Standing when the patient is sitting or lying in bed, changes the perceived balance of power or control, and is generally intimidating for the patient. Being at the same eye level as the patient makes the conversation more of a shared experience.

Touch is an important means of establishing a sense of connectedness with other people and with the world in general. A hand, perhaps only briefly, on the patient's hand or arm may be all that is needed to reduce the sense of isolation, although cultural norms should be borne in mind.

Getting started

To facilitate effective communication:

- prepare for the consultation, e.g. read through the clinical notes, talk with the nurses beforehand
- make time for unhurried conversation without interruption; no pagers or mobile phones; place a 'do not disturb' sign on the door
- privacy in a comfortable setting is important
- introduce yourself by name and shake hands if culturally appropriate
- explain who you are and why you are there
- check how the patient wishes to be addressed
- sit down to indicate you have time to listen; avoid looking at a clock or watch
- make eye contact; let the patient talk without interruption
- avoid medical jargon; check the patient understands what you have said.

Identifying concerns

One of the main aims of a consultation is to elicit the patient's feelings and concerns. Allowing the patient to set the agenda is particularly important when they have a number of symptoms or concerns, which is generally the case.

Starting with a formal systematic enquiry may frustrate or upset the patient, as the issues most important to them may not be acknowledged. Once a doctor focuses on physical symptoms, it can be difficult to move onto psychosocial or spiritual issues.

It may be helpful for a new patient to tell their story from the start of illness, even if this was some time ago. For example, 'We've not met before; it would help me if you could start from the beginning'. This often throws up unresolved concerns or resentments from the past which may be crucial to present management and support. It is important to let the patient tell their story with minimal interruption.

Useful ways of starting subsequent conversations include:

'How can I help you today?'

'Is there anything in particular you'd like to talk about first?'

'Is there anything you think we should be doing which we've ignored so far?'

The way in which questions are asked can either restrict or facilitate the amount of information shared by the patient:

* *leading* questions tend to produce the answer the questioner wants to hear, e.g. 'Are you feeling better today?'
* *closed* questions tend to produce the answer yes or no, e.g. 'Have you any pain?', but are necessary in any systematic enquiry.

In contrast:

* *open (how)* questions allow the patient to express their feelings or concerns, e.g. 'How are you feeling today?' or 'How have you been coping since we last spoke?'
* *open (what)* questions elicit more specific information, e.g. 'What worries you most about your situation?' or 'What causes you the most distress?'

Only with open questions is it possible to discover how the patient is really feeling, and to find out what their main concerns are.

Active listening

Listening is much more than just hearing what the patient is saying. Facilitation of effective communication involves letting the patient know that what they are telling you is important to you. This includes:

* nodding from time to time to show that you are still paying attention
* if the patient stops in the middle of a sentence, repeat their last few words; this often helps them to continue, and shows you have been listening to them
* pick up on cues, e.g. 'It's like Granny's illness': 'What do you mean "It's like Granny's illness"?'
* reflect questions back, e.g. 'What do you think the operation was for?'
* ask about feelings, e.g. 'How did/does that make you feel?'
* validate feelings, e.g. 'It's understandable that you should feel like that'
* watch body language and pick up on non-verbal cues
* summarize to check the accuracy of your understanding of the patient's problems
* if there is a long list of problems, ask the patient if they can prioritize them.

Barriers

It is also important to recognize the common barriers to effective communication. These relate to the patient, the professional, the illness, and the health system.

Patient factors:

* current physical condition and co-morbidities, e.g. drowsiness, fatigue, hearing difficulties, poor eyesight, dementia
* coping mechanisms, e.g. denial
* psychosocial state, e.g. anxiety, depression
* language, e.g. patient's first language not being English.

Professional factors:
- language, e.g. jargon, using complex sentences, professional's first language
- ability, e.g. feelings of failure or impotence where cure isn't possible
- assumptions, e.g. patient's ability to cope with information
- emotion, e.g. a reminder of one's own vulnerability, personal experience
- fear, e.g. of blame, of the patient's reaction, of not knowing what to say.

Illness factors:
- symptoms, e.g. fatigue, pain, breathlessness, confusion
- prognosis, e.g. when to discuss the implications of uncertainty.

Health system factors:
- co-ordination, e.g. multiple hospital/clinic appointments
- continuity, e.g. different professionals at each appointment/admission
- communication, e.g. poor transfer of information between professionals
- planning, e.g. absence of integrated planned care
- support, e.g. lack of specialist support in the community
- time, e.g. short appointments.

Although some barriers are difficult to eliminate or overcome, it is important that they are recognized and minimized as far as possible.

Behaviours

In our dealings with patients and families, it is important to move from paternalism to partnership (see p.14). Certain behaviours are *not* acceptable:
- dominance, e.g. issuing orders, moralizing, lecturing, criticizing
- categorizing, e.g. 'She's a breast cancer', 'The pancreas in bed 10', 'That difficult patient'
- being dismissive, e.g. 'Don't worry', 'It could be worse'
- distancing (blocking, deflecting), thereby not facilitating the expression of concerns, anxieties and fears.

Doctors and other health professionals are generally unaware when they are distancing. Common ways by which doctors and others distance themselves include:
- negative non-verbal messages:
    too busy
    facial expression/too important
    tone of voice/exasperated
- paying selective attention to 'safe' physical aspects
    Patient 'I'm very worried about myself. I'm losing weight and the pain in my back has come back again'
    Doctor 'Tell me about the pain'
- never enquiring beyond the physical, i.e. *not* asking
    'How are you feeling today?'
    'How have you been coping?'

- using only closed questions
- premature normalization, e.g. when a patient starts to cry, saying
    'Don't worry, everyone in your position feels upset' instead of,
    'Can you tell me exactly what's upsetting you?'
- premature or false re-assurance, e.g.
    'Don't worry. You leave it to me. Everything will be all right'
- using euphemisms to mislead (a 'conspiracy of words'), e.g.
    'There's a small shadow on your lung/polyp in your stomach; but leave it to us, we'll fix it'
- 'jollying along'/expecting the patient to keep up a brave face, e.g.
    'Come on, the sun's shining; there's no need to look so glum!'
- concentrating on physical tasks
- inappropriate humour
- disappearing from the stressful situation.

Note: people's ability to express thoughts and feelings, particularly negative ones, varies greatly. For some people, deep verbal communication is virtually impossible. However, they may obtain considerable benefit from non-verbal means of expression, e.g. through music or art therapy.

Summary
- patients, families, professionals and health services all benefit from good communication
- effective communication is more than what is said
- use of a structured approach can help when discussing important issues (see SPIKES below)
- elicit information by allowing the patient to talk, and by asking open questions
- active listening lets the patient know that what they are saying is important to you
- recognition of the potential barriers to effective communication can help you avoid them.

BREAKING BAD NEWS

'Bad news' is any information that drastically alters a person's view of their future for the worse. How we break bad news can profoundly affect our patients. It is easy to shy away from breaking bad news but, in practice, it is seldom a question of 'to tell or not to tell', but more a matter of 'when and how to tell'.

There can be a significant difference between how much information professionals *think* patients and their families want and how much they *actually* want, with patients often wishing for more.

Breaking bad news is generally upsetting for both patient and the news giver. It is necessary to be prepared for a strong emotional reaction, e.g. tears, anger, denial.

Anger can be both understandable and healthy, but it is difficult if it is directed at you. Denial is a coping mechanism which initially may be necessary. However, imparting significant news to the patient and family together can avoid later difficulties and mistrust. It also gives the opportunity for open discussion and mutual support.

Gradual communication of the truth within the context of continued support and encouragement almost always leads to enhanced hope (see p.43). Remember: the doctor–patient relationship is based on trust; it is nurtured by honesty, but damaged by deceit.

Patients and their relatives will retain only a small proportion of the information shared with them, and maybe not accurately. This can be the result of the news itself, which may be overwhelming or because of other factors, e.g. the environment, anxiety, use of language the patient doesn't understand, feelings of loss of control. It is important to avoid jargon and be prepared to repeat information given.

An approach to breaking bad news

Preparation is important before breaking bad news. Following a structured approach is generally helpful (Box A).

Box A The SPIKES protocol for breaking bad news (adapted)[5]

Setting (the physical environment, the news giver's body language)

Perception (what does the patient/relative already know?)

Invitation or information (how much does the patient/relative want to know?)

Knowledge (give a warning shot, communicate the information)

Empathy (demonstrate understanding; show support)

Summarize and strategize (iterate key points, make plans)

The *setting* is important. A quiet comfortable environment free from interruptions (e.g. pagers, mobile phones) and which provides privacy is optimal. However, in hospital, the patient may wish to remain in or at their bed.

The patient and family's *perception* of their illness 'journey' and knowledge of the current situation should be explored. This prevents discussing issues which the patient already feels they know enough about and identifies gaps in knowledge or understanding. This enables the news giver to plan how to deliver news at a pace and in quantities which the patient and their family can cope with.

   'Can you tell me what has been happening so that I know what you have been told and understand so far?' *(perception)*

The patient and family should then be offered an *invitation* to receive further information. Do they want to know more about their illness at the moment? How much information would they prefer, and in what way? Some patients want to know everything at once, some may want to hear a simple explanation and arrange to meet later to explore in more depth, and others may not want any information at all. It is important to remember that it is their choice on whether, or how they want to discuss their illness.

'Are you the sort of person who likes to know what's happening, or do you prefer to leave it all to the doctors?' (*invitation*)

'I've got the results of your tests. Would you like me to talk to you about them?' (*invitation*)

If the patient and their family do want to know more, imparting this *knowledge* should be done in stages. It is often useful to provide a 'warning shot', and then communicate the information in small amounts.

'The results of your tests tell us that we may be dealing with something serious.' (*warning shot*)

The 'chunk and check' approach is also useful: give a chunk of information, and then check the patient's understanding before giving more information and whether they want to know more.

'We've talked about a lot today. I want to be sure I explained everything clearly. Can you please explain it back to me so I can be sure that I did?' (*understanding*)

Try to avoid using technical language, and also euphemisms (e.g. 'growth' or 'mass' when you are talking about a cancer) in order to prevent misunderstanding.

The news giver needs to demonstrate *empathy* with the patient and family. Anger is a normal response to bad news and may be directed at the news giver. It is important not to become defensive. Instead, listen carefully to what is being expressed, clarify the causes and acknowledge that you recognize they are angry. Judgements about the appropriateness of the focus of the anger are not helpful. Silence can be a useful tool.

'Given what you're having to cope with, you've every right to feel angry.' (*empathy*)

'I know that I've just told you some very upsetting news and that this must be a lot to take in at the moment.' (*empathy*)

Finally, it can be useful for patients and their families if the news giver briefly *summarizes* what has been discussed, and also outlines a *strategy* for what happens next. This emphasizes that there are things which can be done to support the patient and their family, and will help to maintain appropriate hope.

'We've talked about your test results – that they tell us you have cancer and it may not be curable. However, we've talked about some of the ways we can manage problems which may arise, and how we help you to maintain the best possible quality of life, and support you and your family.' (*summarize*)

'You may have lots of questions once you've had time to think about what we've discussed. I, and other members of the team, are available to talk again with you when you want to.' (*strategy*)

'We're going to make sure you know who will be your main contact in the team and how you can get in touch with them whenever you need to between regular appointments.' (*strategy*)

Breaking bad news is never easy. However, not talking to the patient and their family will not change their situation or future. You may think you are protecting them, but not being honest is generally an attempt to protect yourself.

Summary

- preparation is important before breaking bad news
- a structured approach is helpful (Box A)
- have a relative or friend present to support the patient
- ensure privacy and avoid interruptions
- know the facts about the patient's illness
- allow the expression of strong emotions, e.g. tears, anger
- allow denial, but do not collude with it
- never make assumptions
- demonstrate empathy
- acknowledge how hard it is to live with uncertainty, and explore the problems it creates (see below)
- arrange to meet again to deal with any 'matters arising'.

COPING WITH UNCERTAINTY

In relation to life-limiting illness, questions about prognosis are common. Although mean and median figures for survival may be available, these relate to 'Mr/Ms Average' and *not* to the patient sitting with you. Prognosis depends on many factors, both physical and psychological. Thus, a prognosis can never be more than an informed 'guesstimate'. In advanced cancer doctors tend to be overoptimistic.[6] However, gross underestimation by years is not uncommon.

Talking about prognosis is important because the information provides patients and their families with the opportunity to make plans and to re-order their priorities. Thus, when a patient asks about prognosis, often there is a specific reason for them asking. Clarification ensures that the question is addressed in the most helpful way:

Patient 'How long have I got, doctor?'

Doctor 'Before I try and answer that question, can I check exactly why you are asking it now? Understanding this will help me to provide the information you need.'

Patient 'Well, my daughter is getting married next year and I am worried that I might not make it...she has talked of bringing it forward and I don't know what to do.'

Having established what made them ask about prognosis, it is important to convey that nobody can really know an individual patient's prognosis, particularly with life-limiting illnesses other than cancer, because of the unpredictable nature of the illness, and a patient's ability to pull back from yet another acute-on-chronic exacerbation or superadded infection. Nonetheless, a 'rolling diary' approach may be useful:

Patient 'How long have I got, doctor?'

Doctor 'Unfortunately, that's something no one can tell you with any certainty. Anything we say is a 'best guess' and we are generally bad at guessing. However, as a rough guide, one way to look forward is to look back and consider how things have been changing for you. If things have been getting worse month by month, perhaps we are talking about planning ahead a few months at a time. If things have been changing week by week, maybe we're talking about planning a few weeks at a time. If day by day, maybe take things a few days at a time.'

Try and avoid giving a specific time, as some patients take this very literally. A 'definite' prognosis may drive some people to seemingly rash behaviour or, conversely, may make them a prisoner to their illness, becoming increasingly fearful as the doctor's 'deadline' approaches. Further, patients' and doctors' interpretations of the uncertainty can differ greatly:

Doctor 'It could be 2–3 months or it could be 2–3 years.'

Patient later to family 'The doctor said I had only 2 months to live' or 'The doctor said I had at least 3 years'.

Acknowledge that living with uncertainty is very hard, and discuss strategies to help them cope in a way that preserves hope if at all possible (see next section):

- *this sort of illness can feel a bit like being on a rollercoaster*
  'The illness can be unpredictable in some ways. You will have good times but probably also some bad times. It's hard when this happens, but it's important to enjoy the good times when you are feeling well.'
- *sometimes we have to hope for the best, but also plan for the worst*
  'It's important to maintain hope, while also being aware that you may want to do some things that we all usually put off.'
- *aim for specific events or anniversaries*
  'It's wonderful that you're going to be a grandparent in a few months. That's a great thing for you to focus on.'
- *as hard as it may be, take each day one at a time*
  'Planning ahead is important, but sometimes we may need to accept that we need to take each day as it comes, doing what we want or what we can.'

HOPE

'Hope is an expectation greater than zero of achieving a goal.'

Hope is important in providing direction and purpose in life, enabling people to be resilient, and to cope with adversity. Hope is crucial to maintaining a psychological equilibrium, and is particularly important when coping with life-limiting illness. Key elements underlying hope include:

- experience: accepting that events (triumphs or setbacks) are part of being human; satisfaction comes from being rather than achieving

- rationalization and acknowledgement of your past, present and future life
- relationships: being connected with other people.[7]

These elements may derive from external sources such as family, or internal sources such as personality traits. For hope to be nurtured, it needs an object. Setting realistic goals jointly with a patient is one way of restoring and maintaining hope. Sometimes, it is necessary to break down an ultimate (probably unrealistic) goal into a series of (more realistic) 'mini-goals'. Thus, if a patient says, 'I want to be cured' or a paraplegic says, 'I want to walk again', an initial reply could be:

> 'I hear what you're saying ... that is your ultimate goal. But I think it will be helpful if we can agree on a series of short-term goals. Reaching these would give everyone a sense of achievement. How does that seem to you?'

Setting goals is an integral part of caring for patients with life-limiting disease, and is an essential component of palliative care. In one study, doctors and nurses in two palliative care units set significantly more goals than did their counterparts in a general hospital.[8]

Communication of painful truth does *not* equal destruction of hope. However, when people lose control of their situation, life may lose meaning and lead to a sense of hopelessness. Honesty, acknowledgement of the patient's predicament, and specifically enabling a greater sense of control by setting small achievable goals often increases hope. Thus, it is possible for hope to increase when a person is close to death, provided care and comfort are adequate (Table 1).[9] When little else is left to hope for, it should still be realistic to hope for a peaceful death.

Table 1 Factors that influence hope in the terminally ill[9]

Decrease	Increase
Feeling devalued	Feeling valued

Abandonment and isolation
  'conspiracy of silence'
  'conspiracy of words'
  'there's nothing more I can do for you'
	Meaningful relationship(s)
	  reminiscence
	  humour

Lack of direction/goals	Realistic goals
Unrelieved pain and discomfort	Pain and symptom relief

FAMILY MATTERS

Supporting a patient's relatives and close friends is an integral part of palliative care. A supported and involved family increases the likelihood of a patient who feels supported and cared for. Family-doctor communication generally needs to be initiated and maintained by the doctor. It is easy to neglect the family as the patient is the main focus of clinical encounters. However, the family is your strongest ally in providing excellent care and need to be involved to enable them to cope through what is a very emotional and challenging time.

Family dynamics

Cancer always changes family psychodynamics, either for better or worse. Dysfunctional family psychodynamics may pre-date the life-limiting diagnosis. Health professionals need to recognize both the scope (and limit) of their remit and abilities, as well as the priorities for care for the patient and support for their relatives.

Within families, conflict can arise between a wish to confide and to receive emotional and practical support on the one hand, and a wish to protect loved ones from distress on the other, particularly children or frail parents. A conspiracy of silence (collusion) is not uncommon, and can be a source of tension by impeding the discussion of feelings, fears, the future and preparation for dying. How collusion is managed can be complex.

Sharing information

Ultimately, a patient with capacity has a right both to know about their diagnosis and to decide with whom such information is shared. It can be difficult to explain this to relatives, who may feel they are protecting the patient by keeping potentially upsetting news from them. Such situations need to be handled sensitively and diplomatically, but health professionals should always be mindful of their responsibilities and the legal framework within which they operate.

Thus, health professionals must ensure that they know from the patient with whom information can be shared, as well as how much. For the patient and family to be too far out of step in relation to knowledge about the diagnosis, management plans, and prognosis can create a barrier between them.

Common initial reactions include:

'You won't tell him, will you, doctor?'

'We'd prefer you not to tell him, doctor.'

These should be seen as an initial shock reaction, stemming from the relative's own instinctive desire to protect a loved one from hurt. It should not be used as an excuse for saying nothing to the patient. If family and patient are to be mutually supportive, it is necessary to help the family move forward from this initial reaction to a position of greater openness and trust.

The family cannot forbid the doctor from discussing diagnosis and prognosis with the patient. Indeed, given the ethic of medical confidentiality, it is clear that relatives can be told only with the implicit or explicit permission of the patient, and not the other way round. It can be useful to say:

'We would never force information on your relative. However, this is their information and, if they ask specifically, we would have to discuss this with them. Obviously, we'd really prefer you to be involved if this situation arose.'

In practice, there is much to be said for joint discussions at the time of communicating the diagnosis and later, i.e. patient, relative, doctor and nurse. This prevents collusion and a 'conspiracy of silence' by which the patient is excluded from the process of information sharing. In addition, the presence of a nurse can help facilitate subsequent clarification of what has been discussed.

The doctor may also make an opportunity to see both the patient and the family apart from each other. As with the patient, and as mentioned earlier, discussing the diagnosis with the family should be done sensitively, as they also need time to adjust to the implications of hearing such news.

Involvement in in-patient care

The family may see admission to hospital or a palliative care unit as a defeat. They may feel that they should have been able to manage all of the patient's care at home, particularly if this is what the patient wanted. It helps to emphasize how well they have been caring for the patient, and that specific circumstances have meant that admission is necessary. It should also be emphasized that the presence of family while the patient is in the unit is regarded as important. If practical, unrestricted visits should be encouraged.

The family's separation anxiety may be reduced by encouraging them to continue to help in the care of the patient, e.g. by adjusting pillows, refilling a water jug, assisting at meals, performing mouth care. Some relatives need to be taught how to visit, e.g. to behave as if they were at home and to sit and read a book or newspaper, knit, or watch the television together. They need to know that they don't have to keep up a tiring patter of conversation.

Overnight accommodation should be arranged when necessary and where possible, particularly if the patient cannot return home at the end of their life.

Planning for discharge

A proportion of patients with life-limiting illness become well enough to go home, or reach the end of their lives but want to die at home. Understandably, many families have fears about what will happen when the patient is discharged. When possible, a supervised daytime visit or a weekend at home can do much to allay fears, or confirm that discharge is impractical.

Discharge plans should be fully discussed with the family before the patient goes home. They need to know who the patient's key worker is, and who to call for routine queries and in an emergency.

Families sometimes overprotect the patient at home by doing too much. This can be tiring for them and frustrating for the patient. The clinical team should support the patient by explaining to the family what the patient can and cannot do, and the importance of allowing as much independence as possible.

Explanation of treatment

All aspects of the patient's care should be explained at each stage of the in-patient stay so that the family feels involved. When the patient is close to death, possible approaches to their care should be explained. For example, if swallowing becomes difficult, it may be necessary to give medication by injection to prevent pain or other symptoms from recurring.

When the patient dies

Palliative care does not end when the patient dies. Health professionals have a duty of care to the family of the deceased patient.[10] It is important to allow relatives to be involved in the care of their loved one immediately after the death, should they wish to be.

Time should be made to talk with them, and ensure they know that further conversations can be arranged if they have questions or concerns. Families often have false feelings of guilt:

'If only I'd done this!'

'If he'd gone to the hospital sooner, maybe he wouldn't have died.'

Opportunity should be given for such feelings to be aired. This can easily be overlooked when other patients are urgently needing our attention.

REFERENCES

1 Silverman J et al. (2005) *Skills for communicating with patients* (2nd ed). Radcliffe Publishing Ltd, Abingdon.
2 Simpson M (1979) *The Facts of Death.* Prentice-Hall, Englewood Cliffs, New Jersey.
3 Fallowfield LJ et al. (2002) Truth may hurt but deceit hurts more: communication in palliative care. *Palliative Medicine.* **16:** 297–303.
4 Edmonds P and Rogers A (2003) 'If only someone had told me' - a review of the care of patients dying in hospital. *Clinical Medicine.* **3:** 149–152.
5 Buckman RA (2005) Breaking bad news: the S-P-I-K-E-S strategy. *Community Oncology.* **2:** 138–142.
6 Glare P et al. (2003) A systematic review of physicians' survival predictions in terminally ill cancer patients. *British Medical Journal.* **327:** 195–198.
7 Macleod R (1999) Health professionals' perception of hope: Understanding its significance in the care of people who are dying. *Mortality.* **4:** 309–317.
8 Lunt B and Neale C (1987) A comparison of hospice and hospital: care goals set by staff. *Palliative Medicine.* **1:** 136–148.
9 Herth K (1990) Fostering hope in terminally ill people. *Journal of Advanced Nursing.* **15:** 1250–1259.
10 General Medical Council (2010) Treatment and care towards the end of life: good practice in decision making. www.gmc-uk.org/guidance/ethical_guidance/end_of_life_care.asp

FURTHER READING

Dunphy J (2011) *Communication in palliative care: clear practical advice, based on a series of real case studies.* Radcliffe Publishing Ltd. Abingdon.
Kissane D et al. (eds) (2010) *Handbook of communication in oncology and palliative care.* Oxford University Press, Oxford.

4. PSYCHOLOGICAL ASPECTS

IMPACT OF LIFE-LIMITING ILLNESS

Learning that you have a life-limiting illness is devastating, and is associated with a range of strong emotions and serious implications. It is vital for health professionals to recognize this if they are to be maximally supportive. With few exceptions, patients initially will be very upset and fearful of what the future may hold, and may feel lost and alone amidst all the uncertainty about what may happen as the disease progresses.

Health professionals who understand the psychology of loss are in a much better position to empathize with patients and their families, and thus to be truly supportive.

Remember: the impact on both patient and family is heavily influenced by how they learn about their diagnosis and prognosis, how health professionals communicate with them, and how supported they feel.

LOSS AND CHANGE OF ROLE

When diagnosed with a life-limiting illness, a patient may experience a range of losses, including:
- loss of independence and control
- loss of hopes for the future
- loss of employment
- loss of place in the family as 'breadwinner'.

Families can experience similar losses: loss of the head of the family, the organizer or the 'strong one', loss of the person they knew, loss of future plans and hopes.

Similar psychological responses occur with any kind of major loss, e.g. redundancy, amputation, divorce, bereavement (Table 1). These responses do not necessarily occur in any logical or predictable sequence. Several may occur together and some may not occur at all. A rollercoaster of emotions and reactions from patients and those close to them is common.

In patients with cancer, more marked responses can be seen at various points in the illness:
- at or shortly after the time of diagnosis
- at the time of the first recurrence
- as function declines
- as death approaches.

Table 1 Psychological responses to loss

Phase	Symptoms	Typical duration
Disruption	Disbelief	Days → weeks
	Denial	
	Shock/numbness	
	Despair	
Dysphoria	Anxiety	Weeks → months
	Insomnia	
	Poor concentration	
	Anger	
	Guilt	
	Activities disrupted	
	Sadness	
	Depression	
Adaptation (adjustment)	*(as dysphoria diminishes)*	Weeks → months
	Implications confronted	
	New goals established	
	Hope refocused and restored	
	Activities resumed	

Adjustment is a complex psychosocial transition, and can be either helped or hindered by those close to the patient (Figure 1); also see p.44.[1]

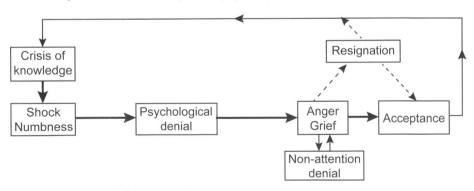

Figure 1 Adjustment: the route from the crisis of knowledge to acceptance. Reproduced from Stedeford 1984 with permission.[2]

The route to acceptance can be tortuous and prolonged (Figure 2); and some may never achieve a renewed psychological equilibrium.[3]

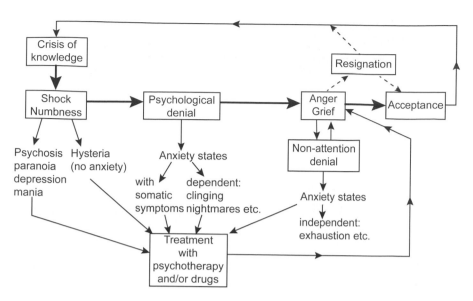

Figure 2 Detours on the route to acceptance. Reproduced from Stedeford 1984 with permission[2]

Typical coping strategies include:
- denial/avoidance (see below)
- fighting spirit
- fatalism
- helplessness/hopelessness
- anxious pre-occupation.[4]

Denial and fighting spirit are often associated with less psychological distress, and the last three strategies with anhedonia (unhappiness, loss of pleasure in life).[5]

Unlike some major losses in life where there may be an end-point to adjustment, with an incurable progressive life-threatening condition, adjustment is likely to be an ongoing or recurrent psychosocial process as the initial loss is compounded by further losses.

For each individual, this process can include both negative and positive consequences (see p.3).

DENIAL

'A psychological anaesthetic to an otherwise unbearable reality'

'The psychological shock-absorber that allows us to suppress mentally what we cannot accept emotionally'

Denial is a common coping strategy (defence mechanism) used by people when in receipt of news which significantly affects them in either the short- or longer-term.

The threat is effectively obliterated or minimized by ignoring it, thereby offering a 'temporary solution'.

Denial can happen subconsciously or consciously, although this can be difficult to determine and does not necessarily alter how the patient can be supported. It may also be constant or intermittent. Denial may be associated with physiological and other non-verbal manifestations of anxiety (see p.185).

The ongoing fluctuating use of denial by most patients and relatives reflects the conflict between a wish to know the truth and a wish to avoid upsetting news and the associated anxiety.

Specific support and intervention may be needed if denial persists and interferes with:
- the ability to make decisions about treatment
- planning for the future (although patients have the right not to be forced to do this)
- interpersonal relationships.

ANGER

Anger is common among both patients and their relatives, and may be an appropriate short-term reaction to the implications of the diagnosis or the way it was disclosed. Patients may focus their anger on:
- themselves, e.g. 'Why didn't I notice something was wrong?'
- their carers, e.g. 'Why didn't the doctor do something sooner?'
- life's unfairness, e.g. 'Why is this happening to me?'.

Persistent anger is difficult for relatives and health professionals to cope with if it is directed at them. It is all too easy to react with like for like. However, this is almost always counterproductive, and is likely to lead to alienation.

Recognition and understanding of the cause(s) of a patient's (or relative's) anger, together with a calm response, generally helps to defuse the situation and enables the patient to move on.

Anger can also interfere with the acceptance of limitations, and may prevent a patient from making positive adjustments to physical disability and, as with denial, prevent planning for the future. Further, if anger is suppressed, the patient may become withdrawn, unco-operative, and/or depressed.

ANXIETY AND DEPRESSION

Anxiety and depression are common concomitants of incurable progressive life-limiting illness. Management is discussed in Chapter 11 (see p.185).

GENERAL SUPPORT

Supporting the patient through the psychological turmoil is enhanced by:
- excellent staff–patient and staff–staff communication and relationships to promote trust and continuity of care

- provision of information according to individual need, in a format and manner appropriate and acceptable to the recipient, i.e. not the information the professionals may think they need, but the information the patient and family actually want or ask for (see p.35)
- partnership between patient and staff, emphasising equality rather than hierarchy, showing mutual respect (see p.9).

Broadly speaking, the adage 'a trouble shared is a trouble halved' remains true; and 'a listening ear' is generally crucial. Patients often feel better for just having discussed their worries, fears or anxieties with someone outside their own family or social circle.

Patients and carers with greater levels of need may benefit from the support provided by specialist palliative care teams, a counsellor or clinical psychologist. Psychiatric interventions may be necessary for patients with the most complex needs, including those with a history of panic attacks, post-traumatic stress disorder, depressive or other psychiatric illness, war veterans, holocaust survivors, victims of abuse or torture.

Remember: there is no one 'right' way of responding and adjusting to a poor prognosis. The health professional's task is to help the patient adjust in the best way possible, given the individual patient's family, cultural and spiritual background. However, many people have a combination of inner resources and good support from their family and friends which enable them to cope without prolonged disabling distress.

OTHER PROBLEMS

Patients diagnosed with a life-limiting illness can experience numerous psychological problems:
- *illness-related,* e.g. an impact on sexual function (see p.180), difficulty in accepting living with paraplegia or the effects of cerebral metastases, fear of the process of dying, death itself or 'being' dead.
- *treatment-related,* e.g. hair loss, surgical scars/deformity, difficulty accepting a stoma
- *concurrent,* e.g. a bereavement (see p.67), relationship difficulties, pre-existing psychological or psychiatric illness.

THE WITHDRAWN PATIENT

Some patients appear withdrawn and seem to be psychologically inaccessible. Although this may not be detrimental to the patient, there are times when the patient's facial expression and behaviour suggest considerable underlying psychological distress. Withdrawal can make the acceptance of treatment very difficult, and can have a profound negative effect on the patient's family and those who care for them.

Causes

There are numerous causes of withdrawal, some of which may co-exist (Box A).

Box A Causes of withdrawal[6]

Personality

Pathological
Brain tumour(s)
Cerebrovascular disease
Secondary mental disorders, e.g. caused by drugs, organ failure
Concurrent illness, e.g. hypothyroidism

Pharmacological
Over-sedation
Tardive dyskinesia

Psychological

Anger	
Collusion	'no point in talking about my feelings'
Distrust	
Fear	'too painful'
Guilt	'too embarrassed'
Shame	

Psychiatric
Depression   'no point in talking about my feelings'
Paranoia   'dangerous'

Management

Management depends on the cause. If a psychological cause seems likely, try to find a 'window' in the patient's protective shell in order to help them acknowledge the problem and to begin to move forward to a healthier/more comfortable frame of mind. Good communication skills are essential to achieve this:

- acknowledge your difficulty, 'We seem to be finding it difficult to get into conversation'
- offer the patient an invitation which they can accept or reject, e.g. 'Are you able to tell me why you find it difficult to talk about things?'
- if the patient then gives a clue as to the reason for the reticence, this should be gently but firmly followed up, e.g. 'Can you tell me exactly what's troubling you?'
- it is important to establish the frequency and intensity of any mood disturbance in case the patient is psychiatrically ill rather than just psychologically disturbed
- ask for specialist help if you feel you are getting nowhere.

PATIENTS WHO ARE DIFFICULT TO CARE FOR

It is not possible to be equally positive towards all patients. However, it is important to remember that the problem is primarily *ours* and not the patient's, although it could be a joint problem. Thus, it is better to say, 'I find Mrs Brown difficult to look after' and not, 'Mrs Brown is difficult'.

Causes

There are many reasons why a patient may be difficult to care for (Box B). The difficulties elicit feelings of impotence and inadequacy in us; we feel we have failed and that we have come to the end of our therapeutic resources.

Box B Reasons why patients can be difficult to care for

Patients or relatives perceived as	**Patient's behaviour**
Unpleasant	Withdrawn
Seductive	Psychologically volatile, angry
Ungrateful	Depressed
Critical	
Antagonistic	**Patient's symptoms**
Demanding	Gross disfigurement
Manipulative	Malodour
Over-dependent	Poor response to symptom management
	Somatization

Negative transference and countertransference reactions

Negative transference and countertransference reactions are negative feelings evoked by behaviour or personality traits in the patient reflecting your past experiences (transference), or by your personality evoking negative feelings in the patient (countertransference). Both parties sense the 'vibes' and react negatively to them.

Management
- acknowledge your difficulty with the rest of the team
- explore possible reasons why the patient is difficult to look after.

Agree on a management plan with the rest of the team and record it in the notes, including short-term goals and time to be spent with the patient and family. Accept that some problems cannot be solved.

REFERENCES

1 Brennan J (2001) Adjustment to cancer - coping or personal transition? *Psychooncology.* **10:** 1–18.
2 Stedeford A (1984) *Facing death: patients, families and professionals.* Heinemann Medical Books, Oxford.
3 Jaiswal R *et al.* (2014) A comprehensive review of palliative care in patients with cancer. *International Reviews of Psychiatry.* **26:** 87–101.
4 Watson M *et al.* (1984) Reaction to a diagnosis of breast cancer. Relationship between denial, delay and rates of psychological morbidity. *Cancer.* **53:** 2008–2012.
5 Watson M *et al.* (1991) Relationships between emotional control, adjustment to cancer and depression and anxiety in breast cancer patients. *Psychological Medicine.* **21:** 51–57.
6 Maguire P and Faulkner A (1993) Handling the withdrawn patient - a flow diagram. *Palliative Medicine.* **7:** 333–338.

FURTHER READING

Holland JC *et al.* (eds). (2014) *Psycho-Oncology: A Quick Reference on the Psychosocial Dimensions of Cancer Symptom Management (2nd edn).* Oxford University Press, Oxford.
Kellehear A (2014) *The inner life of the dying person.* Columbia University Press, New York.
Lloyd-Williams M (ed) (2008) *Psychosocial issues in palliative care (2nd edn).* Oxford University Press, Oxford.
Robinson S *et al.* (2015) A systematic review of the demoralization syndrome in individuals with progressive disease and cancer: a decade of research. *Journal of Pain and Symptom Management.* **49:** 595–610.

5. SPIRITUAL ASPECTS

INTRODUCTION

Spirituality is a broad concept which encompasses the search for meaning, personal values and development, a sense of connection to something bigger than ourselves, and extends to the transcendent, i.e. beyond intellectual knowledge or normal sensory experience (Box A).

Box A Aspects of spirituality[1]

Finding meaning ('Why are we here?')

'What is the purpose of life?'

'Do things happen for a reason?'

Becoming ('Who am I?)

Motivation

Values and beliefs

Creativity and achievements

Self-esteem

Connecting ('Who are we?')

Relationships

Community

Culture

Transcending ('Beyond the senses')

Awe and wonder

Mystery

God or higher power

Spirituality is a universal aspect of human nature, and throughout life people attribute meanings to their experiences. Changes in one's circumstances, such as the diagnosis of a life-limiting disorder or an increasing awareness of one's mortality, often brings spiritual concerns into sharp focus and may move a person towards assigning 'final meanings'.[2]

Indeed, spiritual development can be seen as a movement towards greater integration and 'wholeness'. This generally includes the need for *inner healing*, i.e. achieving and maintaining a right relationship with one's self, others, the environment, and God or a higher power. As one patient said, 'You can't die cured, but you can die healed'.

The aim of inner healing is not to be cured, or to survive, but to become 'whole'. This includes being able to say (or convey non-verbally) to one's family and friends: 'I love you', 'Forgive me', 'I forgive you', 'Thank you', 'Good-bye'.

The basis of spiritual care in practice is *acceptance* and *affirmation*, i.e. treating patients with deep genuine respect, demonstrating that you regard them as fellow humans of worth, with intrinsic dignity no matter who, what, and how they are.

Many practices recommended for enhancing spiritual wellbeing are similar to those recommended for improving emotional wellbeing. This is because spiritual and emotional wellbeing overlap and influence one another. Because spirituality often includes seeking a meaningful connection with something bigger than one's self, this can result in positive emotions such as *awe, contentment, gratitude, peace, acceptance*. It is clearly difficult to find meaning and connection in life if you are ensnared by negative emotions.

Likewise, it is difficult to cultivate positive emotions such as *gratitude* and *compassion* if you don't have a sense of connectedness with the world. Thus, emotions and spirituality are deeply integrated with one another. Indeed, the spiritual dimension of 'human being' is best viewed as the all-embracing integrating dimension (Figure 1).

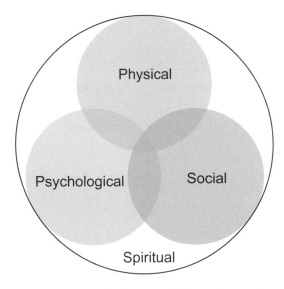

Figure 1 A model of 'human being'; the spiritual dimension embraces and integrates the physical, psychological and social dimensions.

Although spirituality and religion are *not* synonymous, nor are they entirely distinct. Religion can be defined as a shared framework of beliefs and rituals which gives a social context within which spirituality is expressed and nurtured, and the meaning of life explored.

In the 2011 Census for England and Wales, two thirds of the population recorded a religious affiliation.[3] However, many religious people are not wholly orthodox in their beliefs; they may not accept all the traditional dogmas of their religion. In other words, a specific religious label does not necessarily mean a specific set of personal beliefs.

CAUSES OF SPIRITUAL DISTRESS

In practice, the impact of a person's spirituality (or religion) is either positive or negative. When positive, it is generally supportive in the face of illness and death; whereas, when negative, it may exacerbate fear and distress.

People approaching the end of their lives commonly have deep existential questions (Table 1). There is commonly an increased need for affirmation and acceptance, and a corresponding need for forgiveness and reconciliation ('completion').

Table 1 Common spiritual concerns at the end of life

Area of concern	Possible comments by patients or family
Personal identity	'Who am I?' 'Will I be remembered?'
Meaning of suffering and pain	'Why does God allow me to suffer like this?'
	'Why is this happening to me? It is so unfair.'
	'There's absolutely no point in carrying on… I want out now.'
Meaning of life	'What's the meaning of life now that I am dying?'
	'What's the point of it all?'
Value systems	'This is making me rethink what's important in life.'
	'At the end of the day, it's love and people that matter….'
Quest after God	'What do I really believe?'
	'Is there a God?'
	'How can God allow suffering like this?'
Guilt feelings	'Looking back, I've got real regrets.'
	'I've done many wrong things; how can they be put right?'
	'Can I be forgiven?'
Life after death	'Is there life after death?' 'What's it like?'
	'How can I believe in life after death?'

Suffering is experienced by whole persons, not bodies. Thus, suffering does not correlate with physical status. The patient may have much pain or other symptoms but no anguish. Conversely, the patient may be free of physical symptoms, yet suffer greatly.[4] 'Demoralization syndrome' is a term sometimes used to describe spiritual distress marked by hopelessness and despair (see p.189).

Existential suffering commonly perpetuates and magnifies existing physical symptoms, rendering them intractable (Box B).

Box B Case history of spiritual distress and pain

Joan was in her mid-30s with two children aged 3 and 6. Her ovarian cancer caused severe pelvic and sciatic pain which was difficult to control. Her supportive partner was finding it very difficult to discuss with her plans for the care of the children after her death. She frequently woke in the night in severe pain.

Night after night, the hospice staff gave her 'permission' to express her thoughts and feelings (see p.52), listening a lot and saying little. She was very distressed because she would not live to see her children grow up, and had a sense of failure for not seeing her GP much earlier about her abdominal pain. She felt it was grossly unfair to be losing everything which she and her partner had struggled so hard to achieve.

She had been brought up in a church-going family, and obtained some help from visits by a Catholic priest. She continued to express anger at God for allowing all this to happen. The hospice staff helped her to produce memory boxes for the children. Over time, her pain eased considerably, although she remained intermittently tearful and distressed.

EVALUATING SPIRITUAL CONCERNS

Sensitive communication skills are needed when evaluating spiritual concerns. Spirituality is intensely personal and, although some patients may be comfortable discussing such matters, others may never before have disclosed their hopes, fears and beliefs.

Asking about a patient's 'inner life' may help avoid ambiguity and incomprehension surrounding 'existential' and 'spiritual'. Useful open questions include:

'What gives you strength during hard times, like now?'

'What do you find is most supportive when life is difficult?'

'How are you making sense of all that's happening to you?'

'In all this, what causes you the most distress?'

'What place does religion or God have in your life, if any?'

'Are you part of a religious/faith community?'

Following through on a patient's initial response may well elicit clear evidence of spiritual need (Box C).

Note: patients are unlikely to raise existential questions with health professionals unless given the opportunity to do so – and even then may choose not to do so.[6] Further, patients can be very perceptive, and are unlikely to embarrass their carers if they sense that communication at this level will cause discomfort.

However, if a patient does raise such issues with a carer who prefers not to get involved at this level, the carer should find out if the patient knows a priest or other religious leader. If so, the carer can offer to let them know about the patient's concerns.

Box C Possible indicators of spiritual need, pain, or disease[5]

Sense of hopelessness, helplessness, meaninglessness (patients may become withdrawn and suicidal): 'I'd be better off dead than living like this', 'What's the point of going on like this?'

Intense suffering (includes loneliness, isolation, vulnerability): 'I can't endure this anymore.' 'If this is the best you can do, I'd rather be dead'

Remoteness of God, break with religious ties: 'I don't believe in God any more', 'I can't ask him for help'

Anger towards God, religion, clergy: 'Why? Why me?', 'What have I done to deserve this?'

Undue stoicism and desire to show others how to do it: 'I must not let God/my church/my family down'

Sense of guilt or shame, being punished, bitterness, unforgiving of self or others: 'I deserve to be ill.' 'I don't deserve to get better'

Bitter and unforgiving of others: 'I'll hate him for ever for what he did to me/the family.' 'No way! He's not welcome here. Tell him I don't want to see him – ever!'

Vivid dreams/nightmares: e.g. about being trapped in a box or falling into a bottomless pit.

MANAGING SPIRITUAL CONCERNS

A listening ear is what patients are primarily looking for; they are generally *not* asking the doctor for spiritual guidance. They want to be treated holistically and have a relationship in which they can share their fears.[7]

The very process of asking a patient about their spirituality and giving them space to talk around it can play a significant role in addressing and resolving existential concerns. This can be particularly helpful for patients who have not previously acknowledged a possible spiritual cause for their distress. Allowing a patient to realize the true source of their discomfort is a big step on the way to spiritual healing.

Some patient's spiritual needs may have clear practical solutions. For example, if someone feels the need to ask for forgiveness from or reconciliation with a relative or friend, help can be offered to arrange a meeting, and to support the patient through it if necessary.

Further, obtaining permission from a patient to share information with other team members enables better suited colleagues to address the concerns raised. Nurses typically spend longer with patients than doctors, and those working in palliative care often become skilled in communicating about spirituality.

Hospitals and palliative care teams generally have access to multi-faith chaplaincy services. These can help patients of any faith or none explore spiritual concerns within a safe and non-judgemental environment.

Those with particularly complex spiritual distress may benefit from more formal therapies. There are various evidence-based interventions,[8] such as meaning-centered psychotherapy based on the work of Viktor Frankl.[9]

RELIGIOUS NEEDS

For religious people, their spiritual needs are likely to be facilitated by maintaining the relationship with their faith community, where this applies, and continued access to and involvement in religious activities.

The healthcare team should ask the patient and family about their religious practices, in order to facilitate these. Generally, when in hospital or hospice, visits from a chaplain or spiritual care counsellor will be welcomed.

In the UK, most hospitals and hospices have a multi-faith chapel or quiet room. Many patients value its peace and quiet, sometimes commenting that 'I feel a lot better after sitting there'.

As already noted, religious people are not always wholly orthodox in their beliefs: a specific religious label does *not* necessarily mean a specific set of personal beliefs. It is thus important not to make assumptions but, as always, to listen to the patient.

Some religious practices have implications for carers (Table 2). Although the care of the body after the patient has died ('Last offices') is normally undertaken by nurses, in some religions, washing and preparing the body for the funeral must be undertaken by family members or religious leader.[10]

Note: even in a broadly secular post-Christian culture, many families welcome the presence of a chaplain 'to say a few words' or a prayer after their loved one has died as they collectively stand at the threshold between life and death.

Table 2 Summary of religious needs and end-of-life care

Religion	Dietary restrictions	Attitude to healthcare	Religious practices approaching death	Funeral	Mourning	Belief in after-life
Buddhism	May be vegetarian	Some may decline analgesics or sedatives; clarity of thought is important. 'Helping people' is a fundamental ideal; consult family about specific needs and wishes	May like to contact a Buddhist monk	Cremation or burial. Anyone may wash the body	Black or white is the colour of mourning	Rebirth
Christianity	No restrictions; personal choice	Generally very positive; but some sects discourage reliance on doctors and drugs	Priest or minister may visit regularly and share responsibility with chaplain. Some will want sacraments, e.g. reconciliation, anointing, communion	Cremation or burial. Anyone may wash the body. Priest/minister officiates at the funeral	Black is the traditional colour of mourning	Resurrection in heaven
Hinduism	Often vegetarian. No beef. Some want food prepared by a member of same caste	Some may decline analgesics or sedatives. Autopsies are distasteful	Some may prefer to die on the floor 'near mother earth'. When death imminent, family member may place Ganges water on the patient's lips or in their mouth	Normally cremation. The relatives may prefer to wash the body	Official mourning lasts 7–41 days and involves the extended family and friends	Re-incarnation

continued

Table 2 Contd.

Religion	Dietary restrictions	Attitude to healthcare	Religious practices approaching death	Funeral	Mourning	Belief in after-life
Islam	No alcohol Halal diet No pork or shellfish	Modesty is important: may dislike being bathed or nursed by someone of the opposite sex, or undressing for physical examination Autopsy only if legally required	Friends may read from the Qur'an and whisper the Muslim articles of faith in order to bring peace to the soul The whole family visit as often as possible	Burial in <24h Bed moved so that the deceased faces Mecca Staff should use disposable gloves for last offices The staff should *not* wash the body; this is done by a Muslim undertaker or a family member of the same sex as the deceased	Practices vary	Resurrection in heaven
Judaism	Kosher diet No pork or shellfish	Sometimes restrictions on organ donation Autopsy only if legally required	Local Jewish community may organize a group of people to care for patient in hospital	Burial in <24h Staff should use disposable gloves for last offices The staff should *not* wash the body; this is done by members of the Jewish community, who may also wish to stay in hospital with the body	Relatives are encouraged to express their grief openly: 3 days of intense grief, then grieving periods of 7 and 30 days for re-adjustment	Beliefs vary considerably; there is often an over-riding ethical concern for preserving this life

continued

Table 2 Contd.

Religion	Dietary restrictions	Attitude to healthcare	Religious practices approaching death	Funeral	Mourning	Belief in after-life
Sikhism	No alcohol No halal food Normally no beef Often vegetarian	Most Sikhs have a positive attitude towards healthcare and are willing to seek medical help and advice when unwell	When death is close, relevant parts of Sikh scriptures are read There is need to respect the symbols of the Sikh religion	Normally cremation Sikh hymns are read over the dead body Staff may handle the body, but normally the family will wash the body	White is the colour of mourning Official mourning lasts about 10 days and concludes with a special ceremony	Re-incarnation

THE IMPACT OF THE DOCTOR'S OWN BELIEFS

When delivering holistic patient care, it is important to be aware of the impact of your own spirituality.[11] Just as spirituality forms a lens through which a patient interprets their own world and needs, a clinician's spirituality will profoundly affect their motives and methods of providing care.

It is important *not* to think that you can understand the spiritual pain a patient is suffering. Spirituality is deeply personal, and providing neat answers to a patient's questions is essentially a distancing tactic (see p.38). Instead, active listening and being present with them in their confusion and distress is more likely to provide support and comfort.

Respect for patients as individuals does not allow the imposition on them of one's own faith (or lack of faith). However, many patients are comforted by the discovery that their doctor (or other carer) has a religious faith. Although there may be occasions when mentioning this is appropriate, care is needed *not* to impose your own beliefs on a patient or family.

REFERENCES

1 Wright M (2004) Hospice care and models of spirituality. *European Journal of Palliative Care.* 11: 75–78.
2 MacKinlay EB and Trevitt C (2007) Spiritual care and ageing in a secular society. *Medical Journal of Australia.* 186: S74–S76.
3 Census for England and Wales (2011) www.ons.gov.uk
4 Mount BM et al. (2007) Healing connections: on moving from suffering to a sense of well-being. *Journal of Pain and Symptom Management.* 33: 372–388.
5 Speck P (1984) *Being there: pastoral care in time of illness.* Society for Promoting Cristian Knowledge, London.
6 Best M et al. (2015) Doctors discussing religion and spirituality: a systematic literature review. *Palliative Medicine.* 30: 327–337.
7 Best M and Olver P (2014) Spiritual support of cancer patients and the role of the doctor. *Support Care Cancer.* 22: 1333–1339.
8 Best M et al. (2015) Treatment of holistic suffering in cancer: a systematic literature review. *Palliative Medicine.* 29: 885–898.
9 Breitbart W et al. (2015) Meaning-centered group psychotherapy: an effective intervention for improving psychological well-being in patients with advanced cancer. *Journal of Clinical Oncology.* 33: 749–754.
10 Neuberger J (2004) *Caring for dying people of different faiths* (3rd edition). Radcliffe Medical Press, Oxford.
11 Best M et al. (2015) Creating a safe space: a qualitative inquiry into the way doctors discuss spirituality. *Palliative and Supportive Care.* 1–13.

FURTHER READING

Frankl VF (1988) The will to meaning: foundations and applications of logotherapy. Expanded edition. Penguin Books, New York.
Nolan S (2012) Spiritual Care at the End of Life. Jessica Kingsley, London.

6. BEREAVEMENT

INTRODUCTION

Bereavement is one of the greatest personal crises of life which, for a substantial number of people, has serious health consequences.[1] Bereavement care is a core element of palliative care. It encompasses both care for the patient after death and care for their family and friends. With patients whose death is expected there may be 'anticipatory grief' and bereavement care may start before the patient has died.

'Bereavement' refers to the experience of the death of a loved one, whereas 'grief' refers to the response of sorrow or distress following a death. Grief is a transitional process through which people assimilate the reality of their loss and find a way of living without the deceased.[2] Grief is not just an emotional experience; it has behavioural, cognitive, physical, social, and spiritual dimensions.[3] Thus, it needs an holistic approach (Box A).

Box A Common reactions to bereavement

Emotions
Agitation
Anger
Anxiety
Depression
Guilt
Loneliness
Relief

Attitudes
Hopelessness
Low self-esteem
Self-reproach
Sense of unreality
Social withdrawal
Suspicion
Yearning/pining for the deceased

Behaviours
Alcohol abuse
Fatigue
Tearfulness

Physiological changes
Dry mouth
Hair loss
Headaches
Indigestion
Insomnia
Loss of appetite, weight loss
Muscular pains
Palpitations
Shortness of breath
Stress-related illness, infection
Substance use
Visual complaints

Bereavement is associated with increased mortality, particularly from cardiovascular disease in the months after the death.[4] There is increased morbidity from physical and mental illness, infection and alcohol abuse,[5] and increased use of health services and psychotropic drugs.[5,6]

MODELS OF GRIEF

Grief is an intensely personal experience and varies significantly between individuals. Even so, it is possible to identify a number of typical phases, which has resulted in several models of grief.

Although these can be helpful when supporting bereaved people, models are always simplifications, and must be applied with care. Linear progression through the phases is *not* the norm. People generally oscillate in a way which can perplex both themselves and those around them:

> 'In grief nothing "stays put". One keeps emerging from a phase, but it always recurs. Round and round. Everything repeats. Am I going in circles, or dare I hope I am on a spiral?'[7]

Thus, it is important to avoid hasty judgements about where bereaved people are, or ought to be, in their grief.

Personality has a major influence.[3] People who are primarily in touch with their feelings tend to experience grief more as described in the traditional models, whereas people who are primarily thinkers tend to experience grief more as a cognitive process, and may cope more by seeking information, thinking through problems, taking action, and seeking diversion – a pattern which is not necessarily problematic.[3]

There is also significant variation in the way grief is experienced and expressed across cultures.[8] In the UK and the USA, greater emphasis is placed on self-reliance and independence, which exert a social pressure on bereaved people to suppress emotions and hide distress, particularly men.

Traditional model

The traditional model depicts the process in defined stages but, in reality, there will be overlap and unexpected variation.[9]

Numbness

The initial reaction is shock and disbelief, accompanied by feelings of unreality and the feeling of being on 'auto-pilot'. Somatic symptoms may or may not be evident.

Separation and pain

Numbness gradually gives way to episodes of intense pining, anxiety, tension, anger and self-reproach. There is a deep desire to recover the deceased. This may manifest through dreams, auditory and sensory awareness of the deceased and a pre-occupation with memories. There may also be an obsession with reviewing events surrounding the death. Somatic symptoms are common.

Despair

This occurs as the realization develops that the lost person will not return. Common features include poor concentration, apathy, social withdrawal, lack of purpose and extreme sadness.

Acceptance

Despair gradually gives way to an acceptance of the loss. Acceptance of its finality first comes intellectually, and later emotionally. Sadness and emotional swings may continue for more than a year.

Resolution and reorganisation

Eventually the bereaved person begins to adapt to life without the deceased: they rebuild their identity and purpose, acquiring new skills and taking on new roles. Gradually, more positive feelings emerge, energy returns, and new interests and relationships develop. The dead person can be remembered without being overwhelmed by emotion, although anniversaries and special days often continue to trigger episodes of grief.

Denver Grief Wheel

This model diagrammatically represents concepts which are similar to the traditional model (Figure 1).

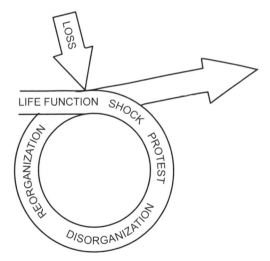

Figure 1 Denver Grief Wheel[10]

Normal *life function* is interrupted by *loss*, leading initially to *shock* with numbness and denial. This is followed by *protest*, with anger and guilt, which gives way to *disorganization*, with sadness, loneliness and emptiness. Ultimately, *re-organization* generally allows a person to return to their previous level of functioning, often with a changed attitude to life and values.

Dual process model

This model emphasizes that bereaved people oscillate between loss-oriented activity which confronts grief (e.g. thinking about the deceased, pining, holding onto memories, expressing feelings) and restoration-oriented activity which seeks distraction in order to manage everyday life (e.g. suppressing memories, regulating emotions, keeping busy) (Figure 2).[11]

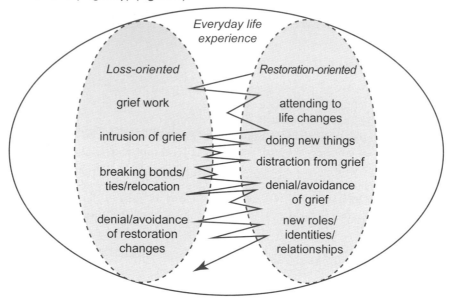

Figure 2 Dual process model of coping with loss. Reproduced with permission from Stroebe and Schut 1999.[11]

Restoration-orientation enables people to make adjustments and build a new identity, but as daily living is full of reminders of what has been lost, people oscillate between the two behaviours. The dominant behaviour and degree of oscillation for any one individual will depend on personality factors, gender, and cultural background. Over time there is generally a shift from predominantly loss-oriented behaviour to predominantly restoration-oriented behaviour.

This model helps to explain why someone may appear to be coping well one day and full of grief the next. Difficulties may emerge if the balance of behaviour is oriented exclusively on loss (chronic grief) or on restoration (absent grief).

Bereaved parents may grieve very differently: one parent predominantly loss-orientated grief and the other largely restoration orientated, leading to strain between them as each fails to understand the way the other is grieving.

BEREAVEMENT CARE

Bereavement care is based on excellent general care before the death, good communication, and the rapport built up with the family. Prompt verification and certification of death, removal of drugs and equipment from the home, and being available to answer questions goes a long way to reducing ongoing distress.

Health professionals who offer bereavement support include GPs, district nurses, community specialist palliative care nurses, along with various bereavement organizations, e.g. Cruse Bereavement Care. Specific groups are available to support those bereaved by trauma or suicide, stillbirth or the death of a child (Compassionate Friends), and for bereaved children (see p.307).

After the death of a patient under the care of a hospice, formal bereavement support is generally offered to families with risk factors for complicated grief (see below).

For most bereaved people, a simple 'supportive-expressive' approach will suffice: inviting the individual to talk about their feelings and listening attentively. This has great therapeutic value, and is something which all health professionals should be able to offer. Indeed, the most positive factor in favour of a good bereavement outcome is a supportive family and friends who allow the bereaved person to express grief and to talk unconditionally about feelings for as long as needed.[12] It may be helpful to offer written information about grief and details of bereavement organizations.

The goal is to enable people to build on their strengths and to develop their own coping strategies. Because individuals may be reluctant to seek help, it is important to ask how they are coping. Often they are seeking assurance that their experience of grief is normal.

Reactions to bereavement range from immediate to delayed, brief to prolonged, and mild to severe. Most bereaved people work through their grief with support from family and friends, and the listening ear of an empathic health professional. About 10% need volunteer bereavement counselling or a support group, and about 5% develop complicated (pathological) grief for whom specialist psychological or psychiatric input is required.

Apart from the family, it is also important to consider the needs of the professional carers who looked after the patient, particularly if the death was traumatic (see p.282). For most, a 'supportive-expressive' approach will suffice.

COMPLICATED GRIEF

Complicated grief refers to grief associated with prolonged impairment of physical and/or psychological health. Risk factors include:
- untimely or unexpected death
- unduly disturbing death
- over-dependent, ambivalent or difficult relationship with the deceased
- poor social support networks
- lack of opportunity for open conversations and planning before the death

- anger, if it results in the deflection of support and in social isolation
- concurrent life events reducing time and space to grieve, e.g. financial concerns, unemployment, dependent children/elderly relatives
- previous bereavement
- pre-existing physical or psychological illness
- history of alcoholism, drug abuse or suicidal behaviour.

The manifestations of complicated grief are generally the extremes of those of normal grief. The formal diagnosis of complicated grief remains controversial. DSM5 does not include complicated grief as a psychiatric diagnosis, but it no longer includes bereavement as an exclusion criterion for major depression.[13]

Those suffering from complicated grief require expert psychological or psychiatric help. Interventions include guided mourning, interpersonal psychotherapy, cognitive behavioural therapy, and family focused grief therapy.

Short-term drug treatment with benzodiazepines/hypnotics is sometimes helpful, but it is important to monitor closely to prevent dependence.

For those who develop a recognizable psychiatric disorder (e.g. depression, anxiety disorder, substance abuse, post-traumatic stress disorder, psychosis), management will follow standard psychiatric practice.

CARE AFTER DEATH

There are many practical issues to be dealt with immediately after a person dies.[14] It is part of bereavement care to advise families about these, or at least to direct them to sources of further support and information (Table 1). In hospitals, bereavement offices co-ordinate care after death. In the community, funeral directors are a valuable source of advice.

Table 1 Commonly asked questions after the death of a loved one

Question	Comment
My relative has just died: can I stay with him?	A junior doctor will have been called to verify the death. Nurses (or family in certain cultures) will then wash and dress the body of the deceased. Although likely to be transferred to the hospital mortuary within a few hours, the family can generally spend as much time as they like with the deceased.
Can I come and view her tomorrow?	Generally it is possible to view the deceased in the 'chapel of rest' of the hospital or in the funeral director's parlour. An appointment needs to be made; appointment slots are typically for one hour.

continued

Table 1 Contd.

Question	Comment
What paperwork needs to be completed?	Once the death has been verified and recorded in the patient's case-notes, a Medical Certificate of Cause of Death (MCCD) is issued. This must be completed by a doctor who had been involved in the patient's care within two weeks, generally a junior hospital doctor or GP.
	GMC guidelines emphasize the importance of completing the MCCD as soon as possible after the death because funeral arrangements cannot be made until this has been done.
	The relatives take the MCCD to the Registrar of Births, Deaths and Marriages to register the death ($\leq$5 days in England/Wales; $\leq$8 days in Scotland) and obtain the formal Death Certificate. This is sufficient to allow a burial.
	If cremation is planned, further medical forms need to be completed, one by the junior doctor or GP who issued the MCCD and a second by an independent second doctor who has been on the medical register for at least five years (in hospital, generally a Consultant Pathologist; in the community, a senior GP in another practice).
	These doctors need to examine the body, ensure pacemakers and other implants have been removed and give additional information regarding the final illness. The medical referee at the crematorium will then authorize cremation (also see Appendix 2).
When does the Coroner/ Procurator Fiscal need to be involved?	The back of the MCCD form lists those deaths that should be Coroner in England and Wales or the Procurator Fiscal in Scotland. These are predominantly those for whom the cause of death is uncertain, or deaths from unnatural causes.
	Coroner's officers are happy to give advice about completing MCCDs and referrals to the Coroner. They may obtain the Coroner's permission for you to issue the MCCD or arrange for further investigation, which may include a Coroner's post-mortem examination and/or an inquest. Out of hours, Coroner's officers are not available, and the police serve as locum Coroner's officers, contacted via the local police station.

continued

Table I Contd.

Question	Comment
My relative has just died at home. What happens now?	If someone dies at home, the GP should be called as soon as possible. If the death is expected and the GP had seen them in the previous two weeks, they should be able to issue the MCCD. The family then need to choose a funeral director who will take the deceased to the firm's refrigerated storage facility.
	If the death was not expected, the cause of death is uncertain, or there is a reason for compulsory referral to the Coroner such as a suicide, an MCCD cannot be issued: the deceased will be taken to a hospital mortuary and a post-mortem performed.[14]
What does a post-mortem involve?	It is helpful to attend a post-mortem while a medical student so you can respond appropriately to this question. A technician removes all of the major organs via a large midline incision from the clavicle to the pubis, with a scalp incision to remove the brain. Any pathology is noted, and the organs then replaced. The incisions are stitched up, and it is not obvious that a post-mortem has taken place when the body is dressed and laid out for viewing.
I don't want a post-mortem to be done. Can I stop it?	When requested by a Coroner, a post-mortem examination is a legal requirement and the family cannot refuse even if cultural traditions regard autopsies as unacceptable or burial before sunset is important. In hospital, if an autopsy is requested for research or educational purposes, a senior doctor will request this of the family who are entitled to refuse.
Can I speak to someone senior about the care my relative received?	Sometimes relatives may have questions about the care the patient received beyond those you feel able to answer as a junior doctor. In this case, a meeting should be arranged with minimal delay with a senior doctor or nurse.
How do I arrange the funeral?	Most people choose a local funeral director. They are normally on call '24/7' to collect the deceased from home. They will collect them from the hospital mortuary when the official death certificate has been issued. Then, as requested by the family, they liaise with a religious leader and the cemetery or crematorium.
	Some people visit a funeral director to arrange and pay for their funeral before their death in order to make it easier for their families after they die.

continued

Table 1 Contd.

Question	Comment
My faith requires burial before sunset on the day of death: is this possible?	This is common request in some cultures and religious traditions, e.g. Islam and Judaism. Provided death occurs in the morning and it is possible to issue an MCCD promptly, this may well be feasible. You will need to liaise with the hospital chaplaincy and mortuary team or community funeral director who will know who to contact and how to make the necessary arrangements.
What about the Will?	Unless the wishes of the deceased are known, the Will should be checked in case there are specific requests about funeral arrangements (e.g. burial or cremation).
	The Registrar of Births, Deaths and Marriages can advise about obtaining probate (permission to deal with the deceased's estate in accordance with the terms of the Will). If complicated, the solicitor who prepared the Will may need to be involved.
What about their pension and life insurance?	The family or the executors of the Will need to inform governmental organizations of the death (e.g. local Council, HM Revenue and Customs). In England and Wales, the *Tell Us Once* system can be used in some areas.
	Insurance companies require an official copy of the Death Certificate before a claim is settled.

REFERENCES

1 Stroebe W and Stroebe M (1987) *Bereavement and Health*. Cambridge University Press, Cambridge.
2 Parkes C (1993) Bereavement as a psychosocial transition: processes of adaptation to change. In: M Stroebe *et al.* (eds) *Handbook of Bereavement*. Cambridge University Press, Cambridge, pp. 91–101.
3 Martin T and Doka K (2000) *Men Don't Cry...Women Do*. Taylor and Francis, Philadelphia.
4 Kaprio J et al. (1987) Mortality after bereavement: a prospective study of 95,647 widowed persons. *American Journal of Public Health*. **77**: 283–287.
5 Guldin MB et al. (2013) Healthcare utilization of bereaved relatives of patients who died from cancer. A national population-based study. *Psychooncology*. **22**: 1152–1158.
6 Osterweiss M et al. (1984) *Bereavement Reactions: Consequences and Care*. National Academy Press, Washington.
7 Lewis C (1961) *A Grief Observed*. Faber and Faber, London.
8 Parkes C et al. (1997) *Death and Bereavement Across Cultures*. Routledge, London.
9 Parkes C (1986) *Bereavement: Studies of Grief in Adult Life*. Pelican, London.
10 Grief Education Institute Denver (1986) *Bereavement Support: Leadership Manual*.

11 Stroebe M and Schut H (1999) The dual process model of coping with bereavement; rationale and description. *Death Studies*. **23:** 197–224.

12 Raphael B (1977) Preventive intervention with the recently bereaved. *Archives of General Psychiatry*. **34:** 1450–1454.

13 American Psychiatric Association (2013) *Diagnostic and Statistical Manual of Mental Disorders 5th Edition*. American Psychiatric Publishing, Arlington, USA.

14 UK Government. *What to do when someone dies*. www.gov.uk/after-a-death/overview

7. SYMPTOM MANAGEMENT: PRINCIPLES AND PAIN

SYMPTOMS AT THE END OF LIFE

Symptoms are common in end-stage disease, both cancer and non-cancer. Prevalence varies between studies, but the over-arching message is clear: most dying patients need relief from a range of symptoms, notably pain, fatigue and breathlessness.[1] Other common symptoms include anorexia, nausea/vomiting, constipation, anxiety, low mood/depression, delirium. Certain symptoms are associated with certain conditions, e.g. breathlessness in COPD (90–95%) and diarrhoea in AIDS (30–90%), but also occur to a lesser extent in other end-stage diseases.[1]

GENERAL PRINCIPLES

The scientific approach to symptom management can be encapsulated in the acronym **'EEMMA'**:

- **E**valuation: diagnosis of the cause of each symptom before treatment
- **E**xplanation: explanation to the patient before treatment
- **M**anagement: individualized treatment plan
- **M**onitoring: ongoing review of the impact of treatment
- **A**ttention to detail: no unwarranted assumptions.

Evaluation

Evaluation must always precede treatment and is based on *probability* and *pattern recognition*.

Patients may be reluctant to bother their doctor about symptoms such as dry mouth, altered taste, anorexia, pruritus and insomnia. Enquiries should be made rather than relying entirely on spontaneous reports.

What is the cause of the symptom?

The primary disorder is not always the cause of a symptom. Causal factors also include:

- treatment
- debility
- concurrent disorders.

Some symptoms are caused by several factors. All symptoms are made worse by insomnia, exhaustion, anxiety, fear, helplessness, hopelessness and depression.

What is the underlying pathological mechanism?

Particularly in cancer, a symptom may be caused by different mechanisms, e.g. vomiting from hypercalcaemia and from raised intracranial pressure. Treatment varies accordingly.

What has been tried and failed?

This helps by excluding certain treatment options, provided they were used optimally. If not, a further trial of a given drug may be indicated.

What is the impact of the symptom on the patient's life?

The following questions help to determine how big an impact a symptom is having on the patient's life:

'How much does [the symptom] affect your life?'

'What makes it worse and what makes it better?'

'Is it worse at any particular time of the day or night?'

'Does it disturb your sleep at all?'

Explanation

Explain the underlying mechanism(s) in simple terms

Treatment begins with an explanation by the doctor of the reason(s) for the symptom, e.g. 'The shortness of breath is caused partly by the cancer itself and partly by fluid at the bottom of the right lung. In addition, you are anaemic'. Such information often does much to reduce the negative psychological impact of the symptom, and thereby reduces the severity of the symptom itself.

If explanation is omitted, patients continue to think that their condition is shrouded in mystery. This is frightening because 'Even the doctors don't know what's going on'. Explanation generally enables a patient to understand the rationale behind the recommended treatment, thereby improving adherence.

Discuss treatment options with the patient

As far as possible, the doctor and the patient should decide together on the course of action. Few things are more damaging to a person's self-esteem than to be excluded from discussions about one's self.

Management

Correct the correctable

Palliative care includes disorder-specific treatment when it is practical and not disproportionately burdensome. For example, patients with breathlessness and bronchospasm benefit from bronchodilator therapy. Likewise, an emollient cream applied topically will moisturize dry skin, and thereby relieve the associated pruritus.

Use non-drug as well as drug treatments

Examples of non-drug treatment are contained in the sections dealing with individual symptoms. Relaxation therapy is a non-drug treatment with wide applicability.

Prescribe drugs prophylactically for persistent symptoms

When treating a persistent symptom with a drug, it should be administered regularly on a prophylactic basis, and also prescribed 'as needed' (p.r.n.). Giving drugs just 'as needed' instead of regularly 'by the clock' is the cause of much unrelieved distress.

Keep the treatment as straightforward as possible

When an additional drug is considered, ask yourself the following questions:

'What is the treatment goal?'

'How can it be monitored?'

'What is the risk of undesirable effects?'

'What is the risk of drug interactions?'

'Is it possible to stop any of the current medications?'

'Will the patient actually take it?'

Written advice is essential

Precise guidelines are necessary to achieve maximum patient co-operation. 'Take as much as you like, as often as you like' is a recipe for anxiety, poor symptom relief and increased undesirable effects.

The drug regimen should be written out in full for the patient and his family to work from (see p.321 and p.322). Times to be taken, names of drugs, reason for use (for pain, for bowels, etc.) and dose (x ml, y tablets) should all be stated.

Also patients should be advised how to obtain further supplies. Generally this will be from their general practitioner.

Seek a colleague's advice in seemingly intractable situations

No one is an expert in all aspects of patient care. For example, the management of an unusual genito-urinary problem is likely to be improved by advice from a urologist or gynaecologist.

Never say 'I have tried everything' or 'There's nothing more I can do'

It is generally possible to develop a repertoire of measures. Without promising too much, assure the patient that you are going to do all you can to help, e.g. 'No promises but we'll do our best'.

Often it is a case of chipping away at symptoms, a little at a time, and not expecting immediate, complete relief. When tackled in this way, it is surprising how much can be achieved with determination and persistence.

Monitoring

Review! Review! Review!

Patients vary and it is not always possible to predict the optimum dose of opioids, laxatives and psychotropic drugs. Undesirable effects put adherence in jeopardy. Arrangements must be made for monitoring and adjusting medication. Further, with any progressive disease, new symptoms may develop. These must be dealt with urgently.

Sometimes it is necessary to compromise on complete relief in order to avoid unacceptable undesirable effects. For example, antimuscarinic effects such as dry mouth or visual disturbance may limit dose escalation and, with inoperable bowel obstruction, it may be better to reduce vomiting to once or twice a day rather than seeking complete relief.

Attention to detail

Attention to detail makes all the difference to palliative care; without it success may be forfeited and patients suffer needlessly. Attention to detail requires an inquisitive mind, one which repeatedly asks 'Why?'

'Why is this patient with breast cancer vomiting? She's not taking morphine; she's not hypercalcaemic. Why is she vomiting?'

'This patient with cancer of the pancreas has pain in the neck. It does not fit with the typical pattern of metastatic spread. Why does he have pain there?'

It is important not to make unwarranted assumptions. Remember: to ass-u-me means to make an ass of u and me.

Attention to detail is important at every stage: in evaluation, explanation (avoid jargon, use simple language), when deciding management (e.g. drug regimens which are easy to follow, providing written advice) and when monitoring treatment

Attention to detail is equally important in relation to the non-physical aspects of care. All symptoms are exaggerated by negative emotions, e.g. anxiety and fear.

'GOOD ENOUGH' RELIEF

It is important to remember that:
- response to treatment varies; relief may be incomplete
- some symptoms continue to be exacerbated by activity
- relief is often *not* 'once and for ever'; e.g. old pains may recur as the disease progresses and/or new pains develop.

In these circumstances, the primary goal of symptom management needs to be redefined as *helping patients move from being overwhelmed by a particular symptom to exercising mastery over it.* For example, when a patient is overwhelmed by pain, the pain becomes all-embracing. When sufficiently improved, a patient may say:

'I still have the pain, but it doesn't worry me anymore.'
'It's still there, but it's not what you'd call pain.'
'I can get on with things and forget it now.'

Of course, the ultimate goal remains complete relief and it is important to follow the principles of holistic symptom control, and to seek the help of specialist teams when symptoms are challenging. But, having done so, partial relief may be acceptable provided the patient is much more comfortable, mentally rested, and both patient and family are demonstrating 'mastery' of the situation. In these circumstances there is little need to pursue relentlessly the ultimate goal using more invasive techniques which would not guarantee success but might well cause distressing complications, or prevent the patient achieving other goals, e.g. being at home.

PAIN

Although the focus here is on cancer, the general principles are equally applicable to non-cancer pain. However, with increasing use of opioids for chronic non-cancer pain, there have been corresponding increases in rates of addiction and fatal overdose.

Because benefits are generally lower and risks higher with opioids in non-cancer pain,[2] specialist advice should be followed (e.g. British Pain Society guidelines)[3] and/or sought from chronic pain teams.

However, in patients with a short prognosis (weeks–months), pain relief is paramount, and benefit from opioids is likely to far outweigh any risk, and should be used if necessary regardless of the primary disorder.

'Pain is what the patient says hurts.'

Pain is an unpleasant *sensory* and *emotional* experience associated with actual or potential tissue damage or described in terms of such damage.[4] In other words, pain is a somatopsychic phenomenon modulated by:
- the patient's *mood* and *morale*
- the *meaning* of the pain for the patient.

The meaning of persistent pain in advanced cancer is 'I am incurable; I am going to die'. Common factors affecting pain threshold are shown in Table 1. Because pain is multidimensional, it is helpful to think in terms of *total pain*, encompassing the physical, psychological, social and spiritual aspects of suffering (Figure 1).

Table 1 Factors affecting pain sensation

Pain increased	Pain decreased
Anger	Acceptance
Anxiety	Reduction in anxiety, relaxation
Boredom	Creative activity
Depression	Elevation of mood
Discomfort	Relief of other symptoms
Grieving	Vent feelings, empathic support
Insomnia → fatigue	Sleep
Lack of understanding about condition	Explanation
Mental isolation, social abandonment	Companionship

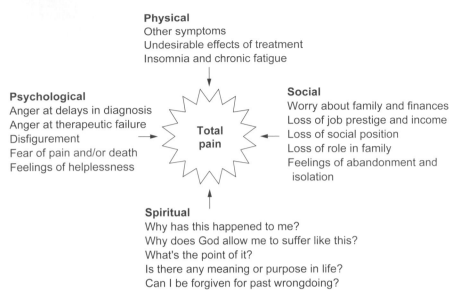

Physical
Other symptoms
Undesirable effects of treatment
Insomnia and chronic fatigue

Psychological
Anger at delays in diagnosis
Anger at therapeutic failure
Disfigurement
Fear of pain and/or death
Feelings of helplessness

Total pain

Social
Worry about family and finances
Loss of job prestige and income
Loss of social position
Loss of role in family
Feelings of abandonment and
  isolation

Spiritual
Why has this happened to me?
Why does God allow me to suffer like this?
What's the point of it?
Is there any meaning or purpose in life?
Can I be forgiven for past wrongdoing?

Figure 1 The four dimensions of pain.

People with chronic pain generally do not look in pain because of the absence of autonomic concomitants (Table 2). In cancer, acute pain concomitants may be evident particularly if the pain is severe and of recent onset, or is paroxysmal.

Table 2 Temporal classification of pain

	Acute	Chronic	
Time course	Transient	Persistent	

Meaning to patient	Positive
	  draws to injury or
	  illness
		Negative
		  serves no useful
		  purpose
			Positive
			  patient obtains
			  secondary gain

Concomitants	Fight or flight
	  pupillary dilation
	  increased sweating
	  tachypnoea
	  tachycardia
	  shunting of blood
	    from viscera to
	    muscles
		Vegetative
		  sleep disturbance
		  anorexia
		  decreased libido
		  no pleasure in life
		  constipation
		  somatic pre-occupation
		  personality change
		  lethargy	

PAIN MANAGEMENT

Evaluation

About half of those receiving anticancer treatment report pain.[5] Even with advanced cancer, pain is not universal. Overall, about:
- 3/4 experience pain
- 1/4 do not.[5]

In those who have pain, multiple concurrent pains are common. Approximately:
- 1/3 have a single pain
- 1/3 have two pains
- 1/3 have three or more pains.[6]

Evaluation is a multidimensional process. It is partly sequential and partly synchronous. It begins by asking the patient to identify the location of the pain ('Where exactly is your pain?') and its duration ('When did it start?'). Then while the patient describes the pain (Box A), the practitioner reflects on:
- the cause of the pain (cancer vs. non-cancer)
- the underlying mechanism (functional vs. pathological; nociceptive vs. neuropathic)
- the contribution of non-physical factors.

Causes of pain

Pain in advanced cancer can be grouped into four causal categories:
- *cancer*, e.g. soft tissue, visceral, bone, neuropathic
- *treatment*, e.g. chemotherapy-related mucositis
- *debility*, e.g. constipation, muscle tension/spasm
- *concurrent disorder*, e.g. spondylosis, osteo-arthritis.

Even in advanced cancer, sometimes none of the patient's pains are caused by the cancer itself.

Box A Evaluating pain: SOCRATES	
Site	'Where is it? '
Onset	'When did the pain start?'
Characteristics	'What does it feel like?'
Radiation	'Does it spread anywhere?'
Associated symptoms	'Any other symptoms associated with the pain?'
Timing	'Is it there all the time or does it come and go?' 'Is it worse at any particular time of the day or night?'
Exacerbating/alleviating factors	'What makes it worse?' 'What makes it better?'
Severity	'How severe is it?' 'How much does it affect your life?'

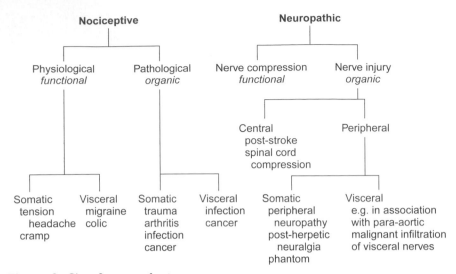

Figure 2 Classification of pain.

Mechanisms of pain

It is important to distinguish between functional and pathological pains (Figure 2). Functional muscle pains are part of everybody's life experience:
- somatic muscle-tension pains, e.g. tension headache, cramp, myofascial
- visceral muscle-tension pains, e.g. distension and colic.

Myofascial pain is a specific form of cramp related to myofascial trigger points. These occur most commonly in the muscles of the pectoral girdle and neck, and are likely to be more troublesome in physically debilitated and anxious people.[7] Functional muscle pains are common in patients with advanced cancer, and may become persistent.

Pathological pains can be divided into:
- nociceptive:
  ▷ associated with tissue distortion or injury activating nociceptors
  ▷ sensory nerves (somatic or visceral) functioning *normally*
- neuropathic:
  ▷ associated with nerve compression or injury
  ▷ sensory nerves (somatic or visceral) functioning *abnormally*.

Pain in an area of abnormal or absent sensation is always neuropathic.

There are many potential causes of neuropathic pain in cancer (Box B). Note:
- when directly caused by the cancer, nerve compression generally precedes nerve injury
- pain associated with compression of a single peripheral nerve or plexus is typically a deep ache of variable intensity, neurodermatomal in distribution
- pain associated with peripheral nerve injury is often superficial and burning ± a spontaneous stabbing/lancinating component (± a deep aching component as well), but with a similar neurodermatomal distribution
- the distribution (and associated pain) of paraneoplastic, diabetic, and drug-induced peripheral polyneuropathy is typically 'glove and stocking'(Box C).

Box B Causes and distribution of neuropathic pain in advanced cancer

Cancer
Mononeuropathy (neurodermatomal)
Plexopathy (neurodermatomal)
Polyneuropathy ('glove and stocking')[a]
Spinal cord compression
Thalamic tumour (variable distribution)

Anticancer or other treatment
Chronic surgical incision pain
Drugs → polyneuropathy ('glove and stocking')
    chemotherapy
    thalidomide
Phantom limb pain
Radiation fibrosis → plexopathy

Debility
Postherpetic neuralgia (neurodermatomal)

Concurrent disorders
Diabetic polyneuropathy ('glove and stocking')

Post-stroke pain (variable distribution within an area of altered sensation)

a. paraneoplastic.

Box C Clinical features of nerve injury pain

Quality
One or more of the following:
- superficial burning/stinging pain, particularly if a peripheral lesion
- spontaneous stabbing/lancinating pain
- a deep ache.

Concomitants
Often there is:
- allodynia (light touch exacerbates pain), e.g. unable to bear clothing on the affected area
- a sensory deficit, generally numbness.

Occasionally there is a sympathetic component manifesting as:
- cutaneous vasodilation → increased skin temperature
- sweating.

Patients also become exhausted and demoralized, particularly if there is insomnia.

Relief from analgesics
About 50% of nerve injury pains caused by cancer respond to the combined use of a NSAID and a strong opioid; the rest need adjuvant analgesics.[11]

The characteristics of nerve injury pain stem from pathological changes in the nervous system:

- neuronal hyperexcitability and spontaneous activity at the site of injury
- a cascade of neurochemical and physiological changes in the CNS, particularly in the dorsal horn of the spinal cord ('central sensitization').[8]

These changes result in:[9]

- a variable response to opioids
- spontaneous pain, hyperalgesia (i.e. mild noxious stimuli become more intensely noxious) and allodynia (i.e. non-noxious stimuli become noxious) in the areas adjacent to the nerve damage
- ongoing generation, amplification, and maintenance of pain.

The prolonged and amplified pain signals are relayed to higher cortical and midbrain centres important in sensation (e.g. thalamus, cortex), emotion (e.g. limbic system) and level of arousal.

The relative importance of the various mechanisms differs between patients, and probably contributes towards the variation seen in the clinical presentation and responses to drug treatment.[10]

Non-physical factors

Because non-physical factors influence pain intensity, psychosocial evaluation is essential. Most patients benefit if they are enabled to express their fears and anxieties. Sometimes there is need for specific intervention, e.g. treatment of depression.

The help of a clinical psychologist or psycho-oncologist may be necessary if the patient seems to be using pain to express otherwise inexpressible negative emotions ('somatization'). The aim is to encourage the patient to discover and utilize coping strategies which help them:

- control pain or continue to function despite the pain
- accept and adapt to their situation, e.g. switching their focus to activities and goals less affected by pain
- to pursue a meaningful and valued life.[12]

Explanation

Given that many patients have pain which is not caused by the cancer, the positive value of an explanation of the causes and mechanisms of their pains is self-evident. In relation to neuropathic pain which is not responding to standard analgesics, it is important to tell the patient that:

- nerve compression pain 'often needs a corticosteroid as well as painkillers'
- nerve injury pain 'does not always respond to painkillers like morphine... Because of this we need to use a different type of painkiller... And an important step is to get you a good night's sleep'.

Management

In cancer pain, multiple mechanisms may co-exist, and optimal relief may require a combination of therapies.

Different types of pain may well need different types of treatment (Table 3). A broad-spectrum multimodal approach is often necessary (Box D). For pain caused by the cancer itself, drugs may well give adequate relief (provided the right drugs are administered in the right doses at the right time intervals) but, with bone metastases in particular, palliative radiotherapy is often crucially important.

If anticancer treatment is recommended, analgesics should be given until the treatment ameliorates the pain; this may take several weeks.

It is often best to aim at incremental pain relief:
• relief at night
• relief at rest during the day
• relief on movement (not always completely possible).

Relief should be evaluated in relation to each pain. If there is severe anxiety and/or depression, it may take 3–4 weeks to achieve maximum benefit. Re-evaluation is a continuing necessity; old pains may get worse and new ones develop.

Correct the correctable

When possible and appropriate, modification of the pathological process can improve and sometimes eliminate the pain. Treatments include radiotherapy, hormone therapy (e.g. in breast, endometrial and prostate cancers), chemotherapy and surgery.

Non-drug treatment

The perception of pain requires both consciousness and attention. Pain is worse when it occupies a person's whole attention. Activity, particularly when creative, does much more than pass the time; it aids coping and diminishes pain. Further, professional time spent exploring a patient's worries and fears is time well spent, and relates directly to pain management.

In addition to the use of analgesic drugs and the non-drug measures detailed above, pain on movement may be helped by suggesting modifications to the patient's way of life and environment. This is where the help of a physiotherapist and an occupational therapist is often invaluable.

Table 3 Mechanisms of pain in cancer and implications for treatment

Type of pain	Mechanism	Example	Response to opioid	Typical first-line treatment
Nociceptive	Stimulation of nerve endings			
Muscle spasm		Cramp	–	Skeletal muscle relaxant
Somatic		Soft tissue, bone pain	±	NSAID ± opioid
Visceral		Liver pain	±	NSAID ± opioid
Neuropathic				
Compression				
Peripheral nerve	Stimulation of nervi nervorum	Brachial plexus compression by apical lung cancer	±	Corticosteroid + opioid
CNS (central)	Neural ischaemia (→ irreversible injury if prolonged)	Spinal cord compression	±	Corticosteroid + opioid
Injury				
Peripheral nerve	Neural injury	Neuroma or nerve infiltration, e.g. brachial or lumbosacral plexus	±	NSAID + opioid and/or TCA ± anti-epileptic
CNS (central)	Neural injury	Thalamic metastasis	±	TCA ± anti-epileptic

Box D Examples of treatment modalities for cancer pain management

Explanation
Tends to reduce the negative psychological impact of unexplained pain

Modification of the pathological process
Radiotherapy
Hormone therapy
Chemotherapy
Percutaneous interventions
   vertebroplasty
   kyphoplasty
Surgery
   orthopaedic
   other

Analgesics
Non-opioid
Opioid
Adjuvant
   corticosteroids
   antidepressants
   anti-epileptics
   NMDA-receptor-channel blockers
   muscle relaxants
   bisphosphonates

Non-drug methods
Physical
   massage
   heat pads
   transcutaneous electrical nerve
     stimulation

Psychological
Identify and address psychological issues
Relaxation
CBT

Neural blockade and neurosurgery
Local anaesthesia
   lidocaine
   bupivacaine
Neurolysis
   chemical, e.g. alcohol, phenol
   cryotherapy
   thermocoagulation
Neurosurgery, e.g.
   cervical cordotomy

Modification of way of life and environment
Avoid pain-precipitating activities
Immobilization of the painful part
   cervical collar
   surgical corset
   slings
   orthopaedic surgery
Walking aid
Wheelchair
Hoist

USE OF ANALGESICS

Also see respective sections in The Essential Palliative Care Formulary, p.317.

For convenience, analgesics can be divided into three classes (Figure 3):
- non-opioid (p.323)
- opioid (p.326 and p.327)
- adjuvant (p.93).

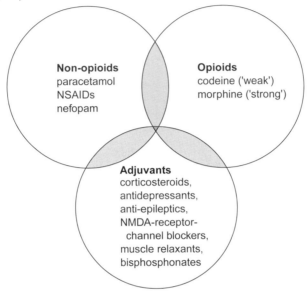

Figure 3 Broad-spectrum analgesia; drugs from different categories are used alone or in combination according to the type of pain and response to treatment.

The principles governing their use for persistent pain are summarized in the WHO Method for Relief of Cancer Pain:[13]
- 'By the mouth', the oral route is the standard route for analgesics, including opioids
- 'By the clock', persistent pain requires preventive therapy; analgesics should be given regularly and as needed (p.r.n.)
- 'By the ladder', use the analgesic ladder (Figure 4); after optimizing the dose, if a drug fails to relieve, move up the ladder
- 'Individual dose titration', titrate the dose upwards until the pain is relieved or undesirable effects prevent further escalation
- 'Use adjuvant drugs' (see p.93)
- 'Attention to detail' (see p.77).

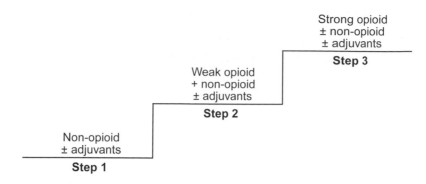

Figure 4 The World Health Organization 3-step analgesic ladder.[13]

The original reason for Step 2 was because, 30 years ago, morphine was effectively unavailable in many countries. Step 2 was to encourage doctors to use what was already available, while at the same time negotiating for morphine to be made available. There is *no* pharmacological rationale for using a weak opioid before progressing to a strong opioid.[14]

Generally, pain management in children is comparable with adults. However, because codeine is no longer recommended in children, the WHO analgesic ladder for children has been reduced to two steps (see p.304).

In adults, compared with a weak opioid, benefit from low-dose morphine (30mg/24h) is greater and more rapid.[15] Thus, in countries where morphine is readily available, by-passing Step 2 is likely to become standard practice in adults as well as in children.

Because cancer pain typically has an inflammatory component, it is generally appropriate to optimize treatment with an NSAID and an opioid before introducing adjuvant analgesics.

However, with treatment-related pains (e.g. chemotherapy-induced neuropathic pain, chronic postoperative scar pain) and pains unrelated to cancer (e.g. post-herpetic neuralgia, muscle spasm pain), an adjuvant may be an appropriate first-line treatment, e.g. an antidepressant or an anti-epileptic for neuropathic pain.

Episodic pain

Some pains in cancer are transient and intermittent rather than persistent:
- predictable (incident) pain caused or exacerbated by weight-bearing and/or activity (including swallowing, defaecation, coughing, nursing/medical procedures)
- unpredictable (spontaneous) pain unrelated to movement or activity, e.g. colic, stabbing pain associated with nerve injury.

In patients receiving analgesics regularly 'by the clock', such episodes are often referred to as 'episodic pain'. It is common in both cancer patients (up to 90%) and non-cancer patients (up to 75%) receiving regular opioid medication.[16,17]

Patients with poorly relieved persistent pain are not included in the definition; they need upward adjustment of the regular dose of their analgesic medication. Similarly, pain recurring shortly before the next dose of a regular analgesic is due ('end-of-dose-interval pain') is not regarded as true episodic pain.

Patients may experience more than one episodic pain, and they may have different causes. Episodic pain may not be at the same location as the background controlled (persistent) pain.[18,19] Various strategies reduce the impact of such pain (Figure 5).[20]

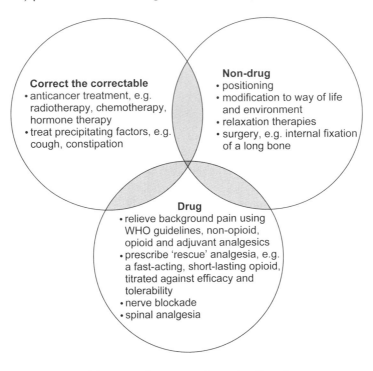

Figure 5 A multimodal approach to managing episodic pain.

Before modified-release (m/r) opioid products were available, it was traditional to give an extra dose of the regular q4h dose of oral morphine (i.e. one sixth of the total daily dose). However, many episodic pains are short-lived and this approach effectively doubles the patient's opioid intake for the next 4h. Many centres now recommend that the patient initially takes, as an immediate-release formulation, 10% of the total daily regular dose as the p.r.n. dose.[21,22]

A standard fixed-dose is unlikely to suit all patients and all pains, particularly because the intensity and the impact of the pain vary considerably. For patients who have been encouraged to optimize their rescue dose, the dose varies from 5–20% of the total daily dose.[23,24]

Generally, episodic pain has a relatively rapid onset and short duration (e.g. 20–30min, ranging from <1min to >3h), whereas oral morphine has a relatively slow onset of action (30min) and long duration of effect (3–6h).[25] This helps to explain why many patients choose not to take a rescue dose of PO opioid with every episode of pain, particularly when predictable, mild–moderate in intensity, and of relatively short duration.[16,26]

Strategies to circumvent the mismatch between episodic pain duration and drug effect latency include:

• timing a predictable painful activity or procedure to coincide with the peak plasma concentration after a regular or rescue PO dose of morphine (1–2h) or other strong opioid

• using routes of administration, e.g. buccal, intranasal, SL, which permit more rapid absorption of some (lipophilic) opioids, e.g. fentanyl.[27]

Transmucosal fentanyl products cost substantially more than PO opioids. Experience with them indicates:

• there is little or no correlation between the dose of the regularly administered strong opioid and the satisfactory rescue dose

• that the rescue dose needs to be individually titrated

• that different products are not bio-equivalent and cannot be substituted for one another

• serious adverse events and deaths can occur with inappropriate:
  ▷ patient selection, e.g. opioid non-tolerant, transient acute pain
  ▷ product use, e.g. exceeding recommended frequency of administration, dose for-dose substitution of one product with another.

Thus, their use should be limited to those with the necessary expertise (see Chapter 18, p.334).

ADJUVANT ANALGESICS

Adjuvant analgesics are drugs whose effect on pain is *circumstance-specific*. Some reduce the painful stimulus directly:

• cancer-related bone pain (bisphosphonates)

• skeletal muscle spasm (skeletal muscle relaxants)

• smooth muscle spasm (antispasmodics)
  ▷ cancer-related oedema (corticosteroids).

Others correct changes in pain transmission caused by persistent severe pain and/or damage to the nervous system:

• peripheral sensitization (NSAIDs, corticosteroids)

• ectopic foci caused by nerve damage (some anti-epileptics)

• central sensitization (NMDA-receptor-channel blockers, some anti-epileptics)

• altered descending pain modulation (some antidepressants).

Many act in more than one way (Figure 6). Most are marketed for indications other than pain.

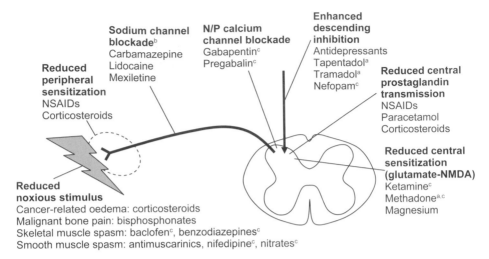

Figure 6 Overview of the peripheral and spinal non-opioid sites of action of analgesics

a. also act as μ-opioid receptor agonists
b. reduces ectopic nerve signal transmission by damaged neurones; the higher concentrations of lidocaine used in local/regional anaesthesia completely inhibit nerve signal transmission
c. also have additional actions.

Some adjuvant analgesics take longer to act than standard analgesics, and complete pain relief is not always possible. Undesirable effects are often a limiting factor, particularly in frail patients.[28] As with any analgesic, it is important to discuss with the patient desired outcomes, potential problems and the likely timing of benefits.

Generally, with neuropathic pain the crucial first step is to help the patient obtain a good night's sleep. The second is to reduce pain intensity and allodynia to a bearable level during the day. Initially there may be marked diurnal variation in relief, with more prolonged periods with less or no pain rather than a decrease in worst pain intensity around the clock.

Low-dose combined treatment may be preferable if a single drug (appropriately titrated) does not provide adequate relief. For example, used together for neuropathic pain, nortriptyline and gabapentin are more effective than either drug alone.[29]

Use relative to other measures

Because cancer pain typically has an inflammatory component, it is generally appropriate to optimize treatment with an NSAID (p.324) and an opioid (p.327) before introducing adjuvant analgesics. Subsequently, adjuvant analgesics are added to:

• relieve those pains which fail to respond *and/or*
• reduce undesirable effects, e.g. by reducing opioid dose requirements.

However, with treatment-related pains (e.g. chemotherapy-induced neuropathic pain, chronic postoperative scar pain) and pains unrelated to cancer (e.g. post-herpetic neuralgia, muscle spasm pain), an adjuvant may be an appropriate first-line treatment.

Antidepressants and anti-epileptics

First-line choices for neuropathic pain include amitriptyline (p.337) and gabapentin (p.345). Their efficacy and tolerability are comparable with alternatives: pregabalin, duloxetine and nortriptyline. Choice is thus influenced by cost and individual circumstances, e.g. concurrent co-morbidity, low mood, poor sleep.

Drugs which act via different mechanisms can be combined if patients do not respond to a single drug (Figure 7).

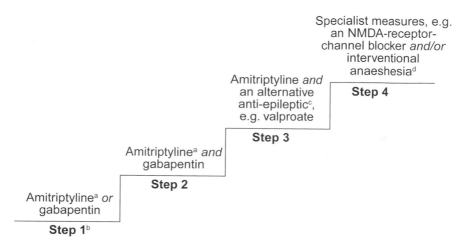

Figure 7 Suggested adjuvant analgesics for neuropathic pain.

a. consider nortriptyline or duloxetine if amitriptyline is poorly tolerated, but *not* if it is ineffective because their mechanism of action are similar
b. systemic corticosteroids are an alternative for *cancer-related* neuropathic pain, particularly if pain is associated with limb weakness or awaiting benefit from another treatment, e.g. radiotherapy
c. it is unknown if patients with an inadequate response to gabapentin are best switched to pregabalin or to an anti-epileptic which differs in its mechanism of action, e.g. valproate. Gabapentin can be switched directly to pregabalin; for all others, generally, the gabapentin is withdrawn once the new anti-epileptic has been titrated to an effective dose
d. e.g. spinal analgesia, nerve block.

Bisphosphonates

Bisphosphonates (see p.359) are osteoclast inhibitors and are used to relieve metastatic bone pain which persists despite analgesics and radiation therapy ± orthopaedic surgery. Although published data relate mainly to breast cancer and myeloma, benefit is also seen with other cancers. About 50% of patients benefit, typically in 1–2 weeks, and this may last for 2–3 months. Benefit may be seen only after a second treatment but, if there is no response after two treatments, nothing is gained by further use.[30,31] In those who respond, continue to treat p.r.n. for as long as there is benefit.

Corticosteroids

Systemic corticosteroids are used for various types of pain (see Chapter 18, Box K, p.365) particularly for those associated with:
- nerve root/nerve trunk compression
- spinal cord compression
- raised intracranial pressure.

Systemic corticosteroids do not help in pure non-cancer nerve injury pain, e.g. chronic postoperative scar pain, post-herpetic neuralgia. However, in cancer-related nerve injury pain, a 5–7 day trial of dexamethasone may be beneficial.

Epidural depot corticosteroids are sometimes used to relieve radicular pain associated with a spinal metastasis.

NMDA-receptor-channel blockers

NMDA-receptor-channel blockers include:
- ketamine
- methadone
- magnesium.

They are most commonly used when neuropathic pain does not respond well to standard analgesics together with an antidepressant and an anti-epileptic. They have also been used in ischaemic pain, bone pain, and severe mucositis. Their use is limited to those with the necessary expertise.

Skeletal muscle relaxants

These include diazepam and baclofen. Although non-drug treatment is generally preferable for painful skeletal muscle spasm (cramp) and myofascial pain, e.g. physical therapy (local heat, massage), some patients also benefit from relaxation therapy ± diazepam (see p.356). Myofascial trigger points often benefit from acupuncture or direct injection of local anaesthetic.[7,32] *However severe, morphine is ineffective for the relief of cramp and trigger point pains.*

Smooth muscle relaxants (antispasmodics)

This is a mixed bag of drugs encompassing antimuscarinics, glyceryl trinitrate, and calcium-channel blockers (e.g. nifedipine).

Antimuscarinics are used to relieve visceral distension pain and colic. Hyoscine *butylbromide* and glycopyrronium are quaternary drugs which are widely regarded as the antispasmodics of choice because they do not cross the blood-brain barrier and are thus free from central effects (see p.349).

Glyceryl trinitrate and calcium-channel blockers can be used for the same range of indications, but tend to be reserved for painful spasm of the oesophagus, rectum and anus.

ALTERNATIVE ROUTES OF ADMINISTRATION

Not all patients are able to swallow tablets or capsules and those experiencing nausea and vomiting may not be able to retain them. A range of alternative routes is available. In practice, choice is largely determined by local availability (Figure 8).

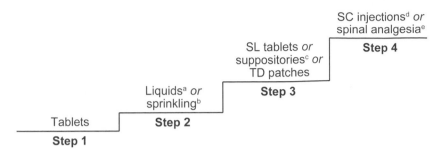

Figure 8 Alternative routes of administration.

a. solutions or suspensions
b. on semisolid food
c. can use m/r tablets in an emergency
d. in the UK, CSCI generally used in preference to intermittent SC injections
e. the use of spinal analgesia is generally decreasing in palliative care.

'Sprinkling' refers to the practice of emptying the contents of an m/r morphine capsule onto a teaspoon of semisolid food immediately before swallowing, e.g. apple sauce, puree, jam, yoghurt, ice-cream. Although sachets of m/r morphine granules are available for use as a suspension, they are much more expensive.

Available buccal and SL tablets include lansoprazole and buprenorphine. Orodispersible lansoprazole (FasTab®) is in fact a soluble oral preparation, i.e. the dissolved tablet still has to be swallowed. On the other hand, SL buprenorphine is absorbed locally, and swallowing it results in a major loss of efficacy because of first-pass hepatic metabolism.

Buprenorphine and fentanyl TD patches are an alternative in selected patients. For the relief of episodic pain, buccal, SL and intranasal formulations of fentanyl are available (see p.334).

Morphine administered SL is poorly absorbed through the buccal mucosa, with most absorption resulting from it being swallowed.[33] However, it has been successfully used by this route in moribund patients cared for at home. Morphine suppositories are available for PR administration, but are not always feasible.

Continuous SC infusions (CSCI)

Battery-driven portable syringe drivers are a convenient method for administering many drugs by CSCI to patients with severe nausea and vomiting, or who cannot swallow medication for various reasons. The advantages of CSCI infusion include:
- better control of nausea and vomiting (guarantees drug absorption)
- constant analgesia (no peaks or troughs)

- generally reloaded once in 24h (saves nurses' time)
- comfort and confidence (minimal number of injections)
- does not limit mobility (lightweight and compact).

Detailed information about CSCI is available in *PCF* and at www.palliativedrugs.com. In patients with venous access, e.g. a Hickman line, the IV route is an obvious alternative but CSCI is generally preferable.

Topical morphine

Nociceptive afferent nerve fibres contain peripheral opioid receptors which are silent except in the presence of local inflammation. Topical morphine, has been used successfully to relieve otherwise intractable pain associated with cutaneous ulceration, often decubitus ulcers.

Generally it is applied as a 0.1% (1mg/mL) gel, made by thoroughly mixing 1mL of morphine sulfate 10mg/mL injection with an 8g sachet of IntraSite® gel. Higher concentrations, namely 0.3–0.5%, have been used when managing pain associated with:
- vaginal inflammation associated with a fistula
- rectal ulceration.

The amount of gel applied varies according to the size and the site of the ulcer, but is typically 5–10mL applied b.d.–t.d.s. The topical morphine is kept in place with:
- a non-absorbable pad or dressing, e.g. Opsite
- gauze coated with petroleum jelly.

Other opioids, e.g. diamorphine, methadone, and other carriers, e.g. Stomahesive® paste, medronidazole gel have also been used.

Spinal morphine

In the UK, few cancer patients receive morphine spinally (epidural or intrathecal). The main indications are:
- intractable pain despite appropriate combined use of standard and adjuvant analgesics
- intolerable undesirable effects with systemic opioids.

This route of administration is normally undertaken by an anaesthetist. Particularly with neuropathic pain, morphine is generally combined with a local anaesthetic (e.g. bupivacaine) and sometimes with clonidine.

REALISTIC EXPECTATIONS

Many cancer patients with long-standing pain have a low expectation of relief. Thus, when first seen, all patients should be assured that the situation can be improved. With few exceptions, it is possible to achieve *at least* some improvement within 48h. However, particularly with pain exacerbated by activity, it is generally wise to aim at incremental relief, with the initial target a pain-free sleep-full night, and then comfort at rest during the day (see p.87).

However, the doctor and other carers must be determined to succeed, and be prepared to spend time evaluating and re-evaluating the patient's pain and other distressing symptoms. In addition, a balance is needed between 'marking time' therapeutically (capitalizing on the impact of improved sleep and morale) and pressing on decisively with further initiatives.

If this skill is not developed, the doctor and patient become trapped in the 'one step behind' syndrome. Most of the right things will be done, but always several days or weeks too late.[34] The 'one step behind' syndrome is graphically illustrated in the account of a 90 year-old man admitted to a University hospital with bone pain and who died still in pain three months later.[35]

REFERENCES

1   Solano J et al. (2006) A comparison of symptom prevalence in far advanced cancer, AIDS, heart disease, chronic obstructive pulmonary disease and renal disease. Journal of Pain and Symptom Management. 31: 58–69.

2   Manchikanti L et al. (2012) American Society of Interventional Pain Physicians (ASIPP) guidelines for responsible opioid prescribing in chronic non-cancer pain: Part I-evidence assessment. Pain Physician. 15: S1–S65.

3   British Pain Society (2010) Opioids for persistent pain: Good practice. London. www.britishpainsociety.org

4   IASP Task Force on Taxonomy (2011) www.iasp-pain.org/Education/Content.aspx?ItemNumber=1698&navItemNumber=576

5   Van den Beuken-van Everdingen MH et al. (2007) High prevalence of pain in patients with cancer in a large population-based study in The Netherlands. Pain. 132: 312–320.

6   Grond S et al. (1996) Assessment of cancer pain: a prospective evaluation in 2266 cancer patients referred to a pain service. Pain. 64: 107–114.

7   Lavelle ED et al. (2007) Myofascial trigger points. Anesthesiology Clinics. 25: 841–851.

8   Baron R (2000) Peripheral neuropathic pain: from mechanisms to symptoms. Clinical Journal of Pain. 16: S12–S20.

9   Romero-Sandoval EA et al. (2008) Neuroimmune interactions and pain: focus on glial-modulating targets. Current Opinion in Investigational Drugs. 9: 726–734.

10   Sindrup S and Jensen T (1999) Efficacy of pharmacological treatments of neuropathic pain: an update and effect related to mechanism of drug action. Pain. 83: 389–400.

11   Grond S et al. (1999) Assessment and treatment of neuropathic cancer pain following WHO guidelines. Pain. 79: 15–20.

12   Van Damme S et al. (2008) Coping with pain: a motivational perspective. Pain. 139: 1–4.

13   WHO (1986) Cancer Pain Relief. World Health Organization, Geneva.

14   Caraceni A et al. (2012) Use of opioid analgesics in the treatment of cancer pain: evidence-based recommendations from the EAPC. Lancet Oncology. 13: e58–e68.

15   Bandieri E et al. (2016) Randomized trial of low-dose morphine versus weak opioids in moderate cancer pain. Journal of Clinical Oncology. 34: 436–442.

16   Davies AN et al. (2009) The management of cancer-related breakthrough pain: recommendations of a task group of the Science Committee of the Association for Palliative Medicine of Great Britain and Ireland. European Journal of Pain. 13: 331–338.

17   Douglas I et al. (2000) Central issues in the management of temporal variation in cancer pain. In: R Hillier et al. (eds) The Effective Management of Cancer Pain. Aesculapius Medical Press, London, pp. 93–106.

18 Davies A (ed) (2006) *Cancer-related breakthrough pain*. Oxford University Press, Oxford. UK.

19 Portenoy RK *et al.* (2006) Prevalence and characteristics of breakthrough pain in opioid-treated patients with chronic noncancer pain. *Journal of Pain*. **7**: 583–591.

20 Zeppetella G and Ribeiro MD (2002) Episodic pain in patients with advanced cancer. *American Journal of Hospice and Palliative Care*. **19**: 267–276.

21 Davis MP *et al.* (2005) Controversies in pharmacotherapy of pain management. *Lancet Oncology*. **6**: 696–704.

22 Davis MP (2003) Guidelines for breakthrough pain dosing. *American Journal of Hospice and Palliative Care*. **20**: 334.

23 Portenoy K and Hagen N (1990) Breakthrough pain: definition, prevalence and characteristics. *Pain*. **41**: 273–281.

24 Mercadante S *et al.* (2002) Episodic (breakthrough) pain: consensus conference of an expert working group of the EAPC. *Cancer*. **94**: 832–839.

25 Zeppetella G (2008) Opioids for cancer breakthrough pain: a pilot study reporting patient assessment of time to meaningful pain relief. *Journal of Pain and Symptom Management*. **35**: 563–567.

26 Gomez-Batiste X *et al.* (2002) Breakthrough cancer pain: prevalence and characteristics in Catalonia. *Journal of Pain and Symptom Management*. **24**: 45–52.

27 Davies A *et al.* (2011) Multi-centre European study of breakthrough cancer pain: Pain characteristics and patient perceptions of current and potential management strategies. *European Journal of Pain*. **15**: 756–763.

28 Bennett MI (2010) Effectiveness of antiepileptic or antidepressant drugs when added to opioids for cancer pain: systematic review. *Palliative Medicine*. **25**: 553–559.

29 Gilron I *et al.* (2009) Nortriptyline and gabapentin, alone and in combination for neuropathic pain: a double-blind, randomised controlled crossover trial. *Lancet*. **374**: 1252–1261.

30 Mannix K *et al.* (2000) Using bisphosphonates to control the pain of bone metastases: evidence-based guidelines for palliative care. *Palliative Medicine*. **14**: 455–461.

31 Wong R and Wiffen PJ (2002) Bisphosphonates for the relief of pain secondary to bone metastases. *Cochrane Database Systematic Reviews*. **2**: CD002068. www.thecochranelibrary.com

32 Sola A and Bonica J (1990) Myofascial pain syndromes. In: J Bonica (ed) *The Management of Pain* (2e). Lea and Febiger, Philadelphia, pp. 352–367.

33 Coluzzi P (1998) Sublingual morphine: efficacy reviewed. *Journal of Pain and Symptom Management*. **16**: 184–192.

34 Fenton A. (1992) The ultimate failure. *British Medical Journal*. **305**:1027–1027.

35 Hunt JM *et al.* (1977) Patients with protracted pain. *Journal of Medical Ethics*. **3**: 61–73.

8. SYMPTOM MANAGEMENT: ALIMENTARY

DRY MOUTH (XEROSTOMIA)

There are many causes of dry mouth (Box A).

Box A Causes of dry mouth in advanced cancer

Cancer
Erosion of buccal mucosa
Hypercalcaemia ($\rightarrow$ dehydration)
Replacement of salivary glands by cancer

Treatment
Drugs, particularly
• antimuscarinics
• diuretics
• opioids
• oxygen
Local radical surgery ⎱ affecting salivary
Local radiotherapy ⎰ glands
Stomatitis associated with neutropenia

Debility
Anxiety
Dehydration
Depression
Infection
Mouth breathing
Zinc deficiency

Concurrent
Alcohol
Amyloid
Auto-immune disease
Diabetes mellitus
• autonomic neuropathy
• uncontrolled $\rightarrow$ dehydration
Hypothyroidism Caffeine
Sarcoid
Smoking

Management

Prevent the preventable

- ideally, patients should have a dental check and any necessary treatment before commencing radiotherapy to the head and neck
- maintain good oral hygiene and mouth care before, during and after radiotherapy.

Correct the correctable

- review drug regimen and stop or reduce the dose of antimuscarinic drugs if possible
- substitute a drug with less or no antimuscarinic effects, e.g. an SSRI instead of amitriptyline, and haloperidol instead of prochlorperazine or chlorpromazine
- treat oral candidosis (see p.103).

Non-drug treatment

Short-lived relief may be obtained by frequent sips of water, preferably ice-cold, or mineral water. Mix carbonated with plain in equal parts to maintain freshness but decrease excessive gas content, or according to personal preference.

Debride the tongue if furred with gentle brushing with a baby's soft toothbrush several times a day until the tongue is clean.

Artificial saliva is a poor substitute for natural saliva, and unless a main salivary duct is blocked, a saliva stimulant is preferable.

Chewing gum acts as a saliva stimulant and is as effective as, and preferred to, mucin-based artificial saliva. The gum should be sugar-free and, in patients with dentures, low-tack, e.g. Orbit®.

Drug treatment

Options include salivary stimulants (e.g. pilocarpine) and artificial saliva.

OROPHARYNGEAL CANDIDOSIS

Oropharyngeal candidosis is a common fungal infection with *Candida* in patients with advanced cancer.[1] Many patients will have concurrent oesophageal infection, and some develop systemic fungal infections. Oral candidosis is associated with:

- poor performance status
- dry mouth
- dentures
- topical antibacterials and/or corticosteroids
- a CD4 cell count <200cells/mm in AIDS.

Oral candidosis generally manifests as:

- white plaques on the buccal mucosa (thin and discrete) and/or tongue (thick and confluent) *or*
- a smooth red painful tongue and/or buccal mucosa or
- angular stomatitis.

Management

Correct the correctable

Correct underlying causal factors if possible, particularly dry mouth and poor denture hygiene.

Dentures must be thoroughly cleaned at least once daily, brushing the denture with a nailbrush or denture brush, and using soap and water or an appropriate commercial product. Dentures should also be soaked overnight in an appropriate antiseptic, e.g. chlorhexidine or dilute sodium hypochlorite. The latter should not be used for dentures with metal parts.

Failure to sterilize the denture will lead to failure of antifungal treatment. The dentures should be thoroughly rinsed before re-insertion to prevent drug inactivation.

Drug treatment

Nystatin is a good choice for mild oral candidosis in non-immunocompromised patients, whereas fluconazole is the preferred choice for moderate–severe infections, and in patients who cannot use nystatin (Table 1).[2] Alternatives include amphotericin lozenges, miconazole and itraconazole.

Cross-resistance and cross-infection do occur. If there is a high local prevalence of azole resistance, local guidelines should be followed.

Azole antifungals have an inhibitory effect on human cytochrome P450 enzymes and clinically relevant drug interactions can occur. These are generally less likely and less pronounced with fluconazole (a weaker CYP inhibitor).

Table 1 Typical antifungal treatment

Drug	Recommended regimen	Comments
Nystatin	Oral suspension 100,000 units/mL; 5mL q.d.s for 7 days (continue for 48h after lesions disappear); hold against lesions for at least 1min, and then swallow	Smaller volumes make it more difficult to hold against lesions
Fluconazole	Capsules 50mg, 150mg, 200mg Oral suspension 50mg/5mL and 200mg/5mL; 50–100mg once daily for 7 days	May need higher doses/longer courses in immunosuppressed patients, and patients with more severe infections

MOUTH DISCOMFORT

Mouth discomfort may be caused by dryness, infection (fungal, viral, bacterial), mucositis, various deficiency states (e.g. anaemia), trauma (e.g. ill-fitting dentures) and drugs (e.g. antibacterials, phenytoin).

Stomatitis is a general term applied to diffuse inflammatory, erosive and ulcerative conditions affecting the mucous membranes lining the mouth (synonym: sore mouth). The term 'mucositis' tends to be restricted to stomatitis caused by chemotherapy or local radiotherapy.

In contrast, aphthous ulcers are generally discrete small, round or ovoid ulcers with a definite margin, an erythematous halo and a yellow or grey floor. They are caused through a combination of auto-immunity and opportunistic infection with various precipitating factors, e.g. genetic tendency, stress, immunosuppression.

Management

It is important to determine the cause so that, if appropriate, specific as well as symptomatic treatment is given.

Correct the correctable

- review the drug regimen and, if possible, stop or reduce the dose of drugs which can cause stomatitis and/or a dry mouth
- mouth care before, during and after radiotherapy or chemotherapy treatment reduces the severity of mucositis
- check teeth and dentures; replace/reline ill-fitting dentures
- dry mouth (see p.101)
- candidosis (see p.102)
- aphthous ulcers.

Non-drug treatment

The following help to reduce pain when ulcers are present:
- avoid spicy foods, acidic fruit juices, and carbonated drinks
- drink through a straw to bypass the mouth
- avoid sharp foods, e.g. crisps.

Symptomatic drug treatment

Coating agents on the ulcerated areas can be difficult to apply, and do not relieve persistent oral inflammatory pain. However, by adhering to and coating the denuded surface, they may help to reduce contact pain, e.g. from eating or drinking. Available agents include:
- polyvinylpyrrolidine and sodium hyaluronate oral gel (Gelclair®) a.c.
- carmellose sodium (Orabase® paste, Orahesive® powder) p.c.

Topical analgesics include:
- NSAIDs, e.g. benzydamine 0.15% oral rinse
- local anaesthetics, e.g. lidocaine ointment 5% rubbed gently onto the affected area
- topical morphine, e.g. locally prepared solution or gel.

Systemic analgesics (non-opioids and opioids) may also be helpful.

ABNORMAL TASTE

Abnormalities of taste include:
- a reduction in taste (hypogeusia), 'Food does not taste the same'
- a loss of taste (ageusia), 'Everything tastes like cotton wool'
- an unpleasant taste (parageusia), 'I have a metallic taste in my mouth'
- altered taste (dysgeusia), 'I've given up eating meat, it tastes so bitter'.

Taste abnormalities may be caused by systemic inflammation, nutritional deficiencies (e.g. zinc), drugs (e.g. ACE inhibitors, antimicrobials, antipsychotics), chemotherapy and local radiotherapy.

Management
Correct the correctable
- review the drug regimen and, if possible, stop or reduce the dose of drugs which can affect taste or cause a dry mouth
- improve mouth care and dental hygiene
- treat oral candidosis.

Non-drug treatment
The advice of a dietician should be obtained, and an appropriate recipe book supplied. For those with reduced taste, the use of food enhancers may be useful.

General advice includes:
- encourage tart foods, e.g. pickles, lemon juice, vinegar
- recommend food which leaves its own taste like fresh fruit, hard candy
- add or reduce sugar as appropriate
- reduce the urea content of diet by eating white meats, eggs, dairy products
- mask the bitter taste of food containing urea, e.g.:
  ▷ add wine and beer to soups and sauces
  ▷ marinate chicken, fish, meat
  ▷ use more and stronger seasonings
  ▷ eat food cold or at room temperature
  ▷ drink more liquids.

ANOREXIA

Anorexia (poor appetite) is common in advanced disease.

Pathogenesis
The hypothalamus plays a key role in the regulation of food (energy) intake. In cancer, and many other chronic diseases, there is an increased expression of cytokines, e.g. IL-1 and TNF-α, in the hypothalamus which ultimately:
- inhibit the hypothalamic response to fasting signals
- inhibit orexigenic neurones
- stimulate anorexigenic neurones.

This results in anorexia, increased energy expenditure and weight loss.

Vagal afferent information arising from the GI tract, e.g. as a result of gastroduodenal distension, is processed by the brain stem and leads to satiety. Increased distension, caused by delayed gastric emptying, e.g. due to ageing, disease or drugs, will also lead to early satiety.

Early satiety can occur without concurrent anorexia ('I look forward to my meals but, then, after a few mouthfuls I feel full up and can't eat any more'); this is associated with various conditions, including:

- a small stomach (post-gastrectomy)
- hepatomegaly
- gross ascites.

One or more other factors may also contribute to anorexia (Table 2).

Table 2 Causes of poor appetite in advanced disease

Cause	Management possibilities
Unappetizing food	Choice of food by patient
Too much food provided	Small meals
Altered smell/taste	Adjust diet to counter smell/taste change
Dyspepsia	Antacid, antiflatulent, prokinetic (see p.115)
Nausea and vomiting	Anti-emetic
Early satiety	Prokinetic; 'small and often', snacks rather than meals
Gastric stasis	Prokinetic
Constipation	Laxatives
Sore mouth	Mouth care
Poor dentition, ill-fitting dentures	Dental review
Pain	Analgesics
Malodour	Treatment of malodour
Biochemical	
hypercalcaemia	Correction of hypercalcaemia (see p.245)
hyponatraemia	Demeclocycline if caused by inappropriate antidiuretic hormone secretion
Uraemia	Anti-emetic
Secondary to treatment	
drugs	
radiotherapy	Modify drug regimen; anti-emetics
chemotherapy	
Disease process	Appetite stimulant (see text)
Anxiety	Empathic support; anxiolytic (see p.185)
Depression	Empathic support; antidepressant (see p.189)
Social isolation, loneliness	Eat with others; attend a day centre

Management

Correct the correctable

When appropriate, identify and treat any causal factors. Early satiety is common yet poorly identified and managed.

Non-drug treatment

For general advice, see p.110.

Specific advice for those with a prognosis <2 months

Whose problem is it? The patient's or the family's?

Helping the patient and family accept and adjust to the reduced appetite is often the focus of management:
- listen to their fears; this can lead to discussion about the progressive impact of the illness
- explain that:
  - ▷ in the circumstances it is normal to be satisfied with less food
  - ▷ carer's can assist a fickle appetite by providing food when the patient is hungry (a microwave oven helps with this)
- a small helping looks better on a smaller plate
- offer specific dietary advice, particularly with early satiety
- discourage the 'he must eat or he will die' syndrome by emphasizing that a balanced diet is unnecessary at this stage in the illness:
  - ▷ 'Just give him a little of what he fancies'
  - ▷ 'I shall be happy even if he just takes fluids'
- recognize the 'food as love' and 'feeding him is my job' syndromes, encourage carer's to redirect their energies into other ways of caring and/or validate the importance of 'just being there'
- remember that eating is a social habit; people generally eat better at a table and when dressed.

Drug treatment

For patients with early satiety, consider a trial of a prokinetic (p.342).

Appetite stimulants can increase calorie intake and as such may be indicated in selected patients for anorexia. If used, they should be closely monitored and stopped if no benefit is perceived after 1–2 weeks:
- corticosteroid, e.g.:
  - ▷ prednisolone 15–40mg each morning or
  - ▷ dexamethasone 2–6mg each morning[3]
- progestogen, e.g. megestrol acetate
  - ▷ initially 80–160mg PO each morning
  - ▷ if response poor, consider doubling the dose after 2 weeks
  - ▷ maximum dose generally 800mg PO per 24h.[4]

Given the relatively poor benefit:risk ratio of progestogens, their use requires careful consideration, particularly in patients with conditions other than cancer or AIDS.[5]

Significant undesirable effects can also occur with corticosteroids. For both, starting doses should be low and titrated to the lowest effective dose.

Progestogens and corticosteroids are best *not* regarded as 'anticachexia' agents; any weight gain is likely to be because of an increase in fat and fluid retention, and the catabolism of skeletal muscle *increased*, particularly in inactive people.

CACHEXIA

Cachexia is common in cancer and other chronic diseases, impairing quality of life and increasing morbidity and mortality.[6,7] It is characterized by the loss of skeletal muscle ± body fat that cannot be fully reversed by conventional nutritional support.

Recommended diagnostic criteria for cancer cachexia are:
- involuntary weight loss >5% in the past 6 months *or*
- weight loss >2% in patients with either a BMI of <20kg/m^2 or skeletal muscle sarcopenia (absolute muscularity <5th centile of gender-specific norm).

Patients with lesser degrees of weight loss are considered to have pre-cachexia.

Causes

Cancer cachexia is a complex paraneoplastic phenomenon caused by multiple factors (Box B).

Box B Causal factors in cancer cachexia

Paraneoplastic
Cytokines and other substances produced by host cells and cancer, e.g. TNF-α, IL-1, IL-6, proteolysis-inducing factor, lead to:
- a pro-inflammatory state
- abnormal metabolism of:
  ▷ protein → increased acute phase proteins, decreased skeletal muscle (catabolism ↑, anabolism ↓)
  ▷ fat → increased lipolysis, fatty acid oxidation
  ▷ carbohydrate → increased glucose production and recycling, insulin resistance and glucose intolerance
- increased metabolic rate → increased energy expenditure

Concurrent
Anorexia → deficient food intake
Vomiting
Diarrhoea
Malabsorption
Bowel obstruction
Debilitating effect of treatment:
- surgery
- radiotherapy
- chemotherapy

Ulceration ⎫ excessive loss of
Haemorrhage ⎬ body protein

The two main mechanisms are a reduced food intake (anorexia) and abnormal host metabolism resulting from substances produced by the cancer, e.g. proteolysis-inducing factor, or by the host in response to the cancer, e.g. cytokines. One outcome of this is a chronic inflammatory state, as evidenced by a raised serum CRP, the level of which relates to the degree and rate of weight loss.

Cytokines such as IL-1 and TNF-α act on the hypothalamus and skeletal muscle leading to:
- anorexia
- inefficient energy expenditure
- loss of body fat
- wasting of skeletal muscle.

The management of cachexia needs to address both the reduced nutritional intake and the abnormal host metabolism; increasing nutritional intake alone is generally ineffective.[8]

Clinical features

The principal features of cancer cachexia are:
- weight loss
- anorexia
- weakness
- fatigue.

Associated physical features include:
- altered taste sensation
- loose dentures causing pain and difficulty with eating
- early satiety
- pallor (anaemia)
- oedema (hypo-albuminaemia)
- pressure ulcers.

Psychosocial ramifications extend to:
- ill-fitting clothes which increase the sense of loss and displacement
- altered appearance which engenders fear and isolation
- difficulties in social and family relationships.

Management

The optimal management of cachexia requires a multidisciplinary, multimodal approach which addresses both the reduced nutritional intake and the abnormal metabolism, and is offered *before* significant wasting has occurred.

A response to treatment is unlikely when cancer cachexia is advanced, e.g. the patient has severe muscle wasting, ECOG performance status 3–4, unresponsive metastatic disease, prognosis <3 months. In these circumstances the focus should be on symptom relief and psychosocial support.

For the management of concurrent anorexia, see p.107.

Prevent the preventable

Early detection and intervention is preferable and requires a pro-active approach to screening for malnutrition. A sedentary lifestyle will contribute to the loss of muscle mass through disuse atrophy. Thus, patients should be encouraged to be as physically active as possible.

Correct the correctable

When appropriate, identify and treat any causal factors limiting food intake. If oral intake is to be improved, particular attention must be paid to:
- the ability to obtain and prepare food
- oral problems, e.g. dry mouth, mucositis, oral candidosis (see p.101, p.104, p.102 respectively)
- uncontrolled nausea and vomiting (see p.119)
- dysphagia (see p.111).

Particularly in relation to neurogenic dysphagia, simple measures such as adding thickeners to liquids and to semi-solid foods may be enough. As a rule, patients with swallowing difficulties which put them at risk of aspiration should be assessed by a speech and language therapist.

Non-drug treatment

Because of abnormal metabolism, *aggressive nutritional supplementation (enteral or parenteral) alone is of minimal value in established cancer cachexia.*[9]

The aims of dietary advice vary according to the patient's prognosis:
- when <3 months, when cachexia is likely to be advanced, the focus should be on the psychosocial aspects of eating and drinking (see below)
- when ≥3months, the focus should be on the prevention or slowing of the rate of weight loss in patients by ensuring sufficient intake of energy, protein, electrolytes vitamins, minerals and trace elements.

Dietary advice might include:
- meal patterns, e.g. eat small amounts frequently
- milk-based drinks, e.g. hot chocolate, malted drinks, latte coffee, rather than water-based tea or coffee
- dietary fortification, e.g. use full-fat milk and cream, extra butter, margarine, oil and sugar (fats are the most concentrated source of energy)
- consider relaxing pre-imposed dietary restrictions, e.g. diabetic diet
- making use of microwave meals and convenience foods; quick and easy to prepare, often small portions, high in fat and salt. The latter may help patients with a reduced sense of taste.

Generally, weight gain is more likely with dietary advice and nutritional supplements than with dietary advice alone in patients with illness-related malnutrition.[10] Nonetheless, any increase in weight is likely to represent a gain in fat rather than muscle tissue.[11]

As cachexia progresses, the focus of treatment should shift from body weight to the amelioration of the psychosocial consequences for both the patient and the carer along with the physical complications (also see Anorexia, p.105):

- weight loss is generally seen as indicative of disease progression and shortened survival which may bring to the fore a wide range of concerns
- trying to eat 'to stay alive' when difficult to do so or unsuccessful (i.e. weight loss continues) can become a burdensome and distressing activity for both the patient and (often more so) the carer, causing feelings such as anxiety, incomprehension, loss of control, anger, frustration, helplessness, rejection and guilt
- health professionals can help the patient and carer to come to terms with the situation by exploring their understanding of the situation, allowing venting of emotions, providing explanation, and helping to set realistic goals
- reline dentures to improve chewing and facial appearance; as a temporary measure, this can be done at the bedside and lasts about 3 months
- if affordable, buy new clothes to enhance self-esteem
- supply equipment to help maintain personal independence, e.g. raised toilet seat, commode, walking frame, wheelchair
- educate the patient and carer about the risk of pressure ulcers and the importance of skin care.

Drug treatment

Currently, there are no established drug treatments for cancer cachexia. Several drugs, targeting either the inflammatory response and/or the abnormal metabolism, have shown some efficacy in clinical trials, including:

- thalidomide (inhibits TNF-α and other cytokines)
- indometacin, (inhibits inflammation)
- eicosapentaenoic acid, an omega-3 polyunsaturated fatty acid (inhibits inflammation); available as a high-dose constituent of some oral nutritional supplements
- ghrelin analogues (stimulates food intake and decreases fat metabolism).

DYSPHAGIA

Dysphagia (difficulty in swallowing) is generally caused by:
- mechanical obstruction and/or
- neuromuscular defects.

It is common in patients with cancer (Box C), MND/ALS, dementia and other neurodegenerative illnesses, and stroke. It is almost universal at the end of life due to extreme weakness.

Dysphagia can lead to dehydration, malnutrition, and aspiration. Aspiration of oral or gastric contents does not always lead to coughing, but it increases the risk of:
- airway obstruction
- pneumonia
- abscess formation
- pulmonary fibrosis
- adult respiratory distress syndrome (non-cardiogenic pulmonary oedema).

Box C Causes of dysphagia in advanced cancer

Cancer
Mass lesion between mouth and
  stomach
Damage to cranial nerves
Bulbar palsy (cerebral metastatic
  disease)
Paraneoplastic

Debility
Dry mouth
Candidosis
Pharyngeal infection
Anxiety → oesophageal spasm
Extreme weakness
Hypercalcaemia (rare)

Treatment
Surgery
Chemotherapy/radiotherapy-induced
  mucositis/oesophagitis
Post-radiation fibrosis
Displacement of endo-oesophageal tube
Drugs (dystonic reaction)
  antipsychotics
  metoclopramide

Concurrent
Reflux oesophagitis
Benign stricture
Iron deficiency

A reduced level of consciousness increases the risk of aspiration. Aspiration of larger quantities of fluids or food while eating may result in episodes of choking from acute obstruction of the pharynx, larynx or trachea (see p.233).

Physiology

Swallowing is a complex phenomenon, comprising four distinct phases, two voluntary and two reflexive:
- *oral preparatory phase*: food is mixed with saliva and chewed to reduce particle size
- *oral swallowing phase*: the lips are closed to prevent leakage and the anterior tongue retracts and elevates in a wave which pushes the bolus into the oropharynx
- *pharyngeal phase*: this is triggered by the bolus reaching the posterior tongue. The larynx closes, breathing stops, and a peristaltic wave moves the bolus into the oesophagus in less than 1 second. These complex actions are necessary to protect the airway because the pharynx is a shared passage for air and food
- *oesophageal phase*: reflex peristalsis carries the bolus into the stomach.

Evaluation

The history together with clinical observation will generally indicate if the problem lies in the mouth or pharynx, or more distally in the oesophagus, and help to distinguish between dysphagia and odynophagia (painful swallowing). Remember:
- obstructing lesions cause dysphagia for solids initially with later progression to liquids
- neuromuscular disorders cause dysphagia for both solids and liquids at about the same time
- patients can almost always accurately identify the level of an obstruction.

For problems arising within the mouth and pharynx, difficulties will arise *before, during or immediately after* a swallow. Clinical features may include:
- food loss from the mouth
- food sitting in the mouth
- food coming down the nose.

Coughing/choking *before, during and/or immediately after a swallow* suggests a pharyngeal problem.

With oesophageal problems, *symptoms occur after a normal swallow;* endoscopy is generally indicated.

Explanation

Aspiration of food or saliva leading to distressing episodes of coughing or choking will make the patient extremely fearful of a recurrence. This fear should be validated and a strategy developed to give the patient confidence that they will not choke to death. Emphasize that:
- although aspiration leading to coughing is relatively common, the patient and family should be assured that it is *extremely rare* for aspiration to cause fatal choking
- there are measures which will reduce the frequency and intensity of aspiration or choking attacks.

Management

Aspiration of water alone is well tolerated if it does not cause bouts of coughing, and patients should not be denied sips of water or ice chips to relieve a dry mouth or thirst.

Correct the correctable

When cancer is causing obstruction, possible ways to improve the lumen include:
- oesophageal stent
- radiotherapy ± chemotherapy
- dexamethasone, e.g. 12–16mg/24h (continue with a reduced dose only if definitely helpful).

Non-drug treatment

Seek agreement between the patient, family and staff about feeding goals and treatment plans based on an explanation of what is possible and what is not.

Ideally, a speech and language therapist should be involved before aspiration or choking becomes a major problem. They can advise the patient and carers about techniques to help prevent and manage episodes of aspiration/choking:
- about 'safe swallowing' (individualized to the specific swallowing problem)
- about keeping calm
- how to remove any obstructing material from the mouth
- emergency treatment of choking (see p.233).

Specific input from a dietitian may also be helpful:
* how to maximize calorie intake in small volume meals, e.g.:
  ▷ adding cream to soup
  ▷ eating cold sour cream by the spoonful
  ▷ oral nutritional supplements
* recommending suitable soft food cookbooks
* use of a liquidizer/blender
* general advice about mealtimes.

Support for the patient and carers will also be required to help them cope with the psychosocial consequences of dysphagia: disruption at meal times of the normal pattern of eating, drinking, and social interaction.

Feeding tubes

The provision of artificial nutrition or hydration is regarded as a medical treatment and is *not* part of basic care.

Certain patients may benefit more than others, e.g. with cancer localized to the neck or in MND/ALS. Ideally, there should be discussion about artificial nutrition and hydration well in advance of the patient becoming unable to swallow (see p.18).

Sensitive discussion is required around the decision to commence enteral tube feeding. Much depends on both the speed of deterioration and the opinion of the patient and family, together with those of the professional carers.

Note: some patients are relieved when a doctor sensitively confirms that they will not be forced to have a nasogastric tube or gastrostomy.

If in doubt it is better to delay several days, or even weeks, before deciding to go ahead. It is easier not to start a treatment than to stop it.

Complications of tube feeding include:
* pain (post-insertion)
* haemorrhage
* pneumoperitoneum
* peritonitis
* peristomal infection
* mechanical obstruction
* tube migration
* peritubal leakage
* gastrocolonic fistula
* GI upset: vomiting, diarrhoea, constipation.

Ethical and practical guidelines on artificial nutrition and hydration are available.[12–14]

Drug treatment

Dysphagia and odynophagia caused by oesophagitis and oesophageal spasm can be treated with glyceryl trinitrate 400microgram SL 15min before food.

If total obstruction leads to drooling, prescribe an antimuscarinic (antisecretory) drug (see p.349).

Oral morphine has been used as an antitussive to reduce the likelihood of coughing from aspiration, e.g. of saliva, in patients with MND/ALS or similar neurological dysfunction. Generally begin with small doses, e.g. morphine solution 5–6mg t.d.s. before meals and at bedtime, and titrate the dose as necessary.

Patients who have difficulty in clearing matter from the trachea can also be supplied with hyoscine hydrobromide 0.3mg SL to help reduce excessive saliva and/or coughing when drinking or eating.

DYSPEPSIA

Dyspepsia (literally 'bad digestion'; synonym: indigestion) refers to a constellation of symptoms related to the upper GI tract particularly after meals, e.g. epigastric discomfort/pain, fullness or bloating, early satiety, nausea or vomiting.

Pathogenesis

Functional dyspepsia (without apparent organic cause) is common, affecting about 1/4 of the population. There are many potential causes of dyspepsia (Box D).

Box D Causes of dyspepsia in advanced disease

Cancer
Small stomach capacity
   unresected stomach cancer
   massive ascites
Gastroparesis (paraneoplastic neuropathy)

Treatment
Postsurgical
   postgastrectomy
   reflux oesophagitis
Radiotherapy
   lumbar spine
   epigastrium
Drugs
   physical irritant → gastritis,
     e.g. iron, tranexamic acid
   acid stimulant → gastritis,
     e.g. NSAIDs, corticosteroids
   delayed gastric emptying,
     e.g. antimuscarinics, opioids, cisplatin

Debility
Oesophageal candidiasis
Minimal food and fluid intake
Anxiety → aerophagia

Concurrent
Organic dyspepsia
   peptic ulcer
   reflux oesophagitis
   cholelithiasis
   renal failure
Non-ulcer dyspepsia
   dysmotility
   aerophagia

In functional dyspepsia, symptoms may relate to:
- hypersensitivity → normal gastric distension is uncomfortable
- gastric dysmotility: gastric emptying generally delayed but sometimes accelerated
- duodenal hypersensitivity to fat or acid
- psychological factors, e.g. stress, personality.

There are similarities with irritable bowel syndrome which may co-exist.

Evaluation

When appropriate, identify the underlying cause in order to provide specific treatment. Identify symptoms of reflux (heartburn, regurgitation) and treat appropriately (e.g. with a PPI).

Functional dyspepsia can be grouped by the predominant symptoms to help guide treatment:
- epigastric fullness or bloating, early satiety: postprandial distress syndrome
- epigastric pain/burning, generally unrelated to meals: epigastric pain syndrome.[15]

There may be associated nausea, vomiting and belching.

Management

Treat the underlying organic cause when appropriate.

Correct the correctable

For example, if possible, stop or reduce the dose of causal drugs drain ascites.

Non-drug treatment

Anecdotally, patients may benefit from:
- eating 'small and often', i.e. 5–6 small meals/snacks during the day rather than 2–3 big meals
- avoiding drinking a lot of fluid at meal times
- avoiding late evening meals
- a low fat diet
- avoiding certain foodstuffs, e.g. onions, peppers, citrus fruits, coffee, carbonated drinks, spices.[16]

Drug treatment

Postprandial distress syndrome (epigastric fullness or bloating, early satiety, nausea and vomiting)

Possible disordered gastric accommodation, motility and emptying:
- prescribe a prokinetic anti-emetic, e.g. metoclopramide, domperidone
- if symptoms worsen with a prokinetic, accelerated gastric emptying may be the underlying cause; discontinue the prokinetic and consider an antimuscarinic drug, e.g. amitriptyline 10–25mg at bedtime.[17]

Patients with a small stomach capacity may benefit from an antiflatulent after meals, to help clear space in an overfull stomach (see below).

Epigastric pain syndrome (epigastric pain/burning)

Possible hypersensitivity:

- acid suppression, e.g. with a PPI:
  ▷ most likely to benefit patients with concurrent heartburn
  ▷ also used in NSAID-related gastritis[18]
- TCAs.[17]

Excessive belching (eructation)

- prescribe simeticone, an antifoaming agent (antiflatulent) available in several proprietary antacids, e.g. Altacite plus®
- depending on a patient's individual needs, give p.r.n., q.d.s., or both.

GASTRIC STASIS

Gastric stasis (delayed gastric emptying) is common in advanced cancer.

Clinical features

The clinical features of gastric stasis range from mild dyspepsia and anorexia to persistent severe nausea and large-volume vomiting (Box E). Gastric stasis is normally functional and causes include:

- functional dyspepsia (see p.116)
- constipation
- drugs (e.g. opioids, antimuscarinics, levodopa)
- cancer of the head of the pancreas (disrupts duodenal transit)
- paraneoplastic autonomic neuropathy
- retroperitoneal disease (→ nerve dysfunction)
- spinal cord compression
- diabetic autonomic neuropathy
- Parkinson's disease
- post-surgical (e.g. gastric or oesophageal).

Management

Correct the correctable

For example:
- treat constipation
- stop or reduce the dose of causal drugs if possible.

> **Box E** Clinical features of gastric stasis
>
> **Symptoms**
>
> | | |
> |---|---|
> | Early satiety | Belching |
> | Post-prandial fullness | Hiccup |
> | Epigastric bloating | Nausea |
> | Epigastric discomfort | Retching |
> | Heartburn | Vomiting |
>
> **Signs**
> Epigastric distension
> Succussion splash } not invariable
>
> *A succussion splash requires >400–500mL of fluid in the stomach and plenty of gas.*
>
> Bowel sounds, generally normal but may be decreased if the stasis is drug-induced.
>
> If associated with autonomic neuropathy, there is often evidence of other autonomic abnormalities, e.g. orthostatic hypotension without a compensatory tachycardia.
>
> **Drug treatment**
> The use of metoclopramide generally leads to improvement and the resolution of the succussion splash.

Non-drug treatment

Provide dietary advice, e.g.:
- eat 'small and often', i.e. 5–6 small meals/snacks during the day rather than 2–3 big meals
- avoid carbonated drinks which will increase stomach gas.

Drug treatment

Prescribe a prokinetic anti-emetic, e.g. metoclopramide (p.342), domperidone (p.344).

Try to avoid the concurrent use of prokinetics and antimuscarinics; the latter block cholinergic receptors on intestinal muscle fibres, and thus will tend to antagonize the effect of prokinetic anti-emetics.

Erythromycin has a motilin-receptor agonist effect and can be tried if metoclopramide and domperidone fail to relieve.

There are case reports of benefit from antidepressants with anti-emetic properties, e.g. mirtazapine. It is unknown how these work, other than by breaking the vicious cycle whereby nausea exacerbates gastric stasis.

NAUSEA AND VOMITING

Nausea is an unpleasant feeling of the need to vomit, often accompanied by autonomic symptoms, e.g. pallor, cold sweat, salivation, tachycardia and diarrhoea.

Retching is rhythmic, laboured, spasmodic movements of the diaphragm and abdominal muscles, generally occurring in the presence of nausea and often culminating in vomiting.

Vomiting is the forceful expulsion of gastric contents through the mouth.

Pathogenesis

The pathogenesis of nausea and vomiting is complex (Figure 1). Nausea is an expression of autonomic stimulation, whereas retching and vomiting are mediated via somatic nerves. Nausea is associated with atony of the stomach, lower oesophageal sphincter and pylorus, which facilitates the retrograde expulsion of the contents of the upper GI tract.

Vomiting involves the co-ordinated activities of the GI tract, diaphragm and abdominal muscles. The expulsive effort of vomiting is produced by the primary and accessory muscles of respiration, notably the abdominal muscles, which pump out the contents of a flaccid upper GI tract.

The emetic pattern generator co-ordinates the process, receiving and integrating input from several sources.

Causes

There are many causes of nausea and vomiting (Box F), but gastric stasis (see p.117), bowel obstruction (see p.131), drugs and bio-chemical abnormalities probably account for most cases.

Evaluation

The sequence of events, together with an appropriate level of suspicion, often suggests the probable cause, which dictates the management strategy.

Management

Correct the correctable

For example, consider stopping gastric irritant drugs, treat hypercalcaemia.

Non-drug treatment

- a calm environment away from the sight and smell of food
- snacks rather than big meals.

Drug treatment

In practice, the choice of an anti-emetic in palliative care is guided by the probable cause of the nausea and vomiting and the mechanism by which the drug acts

---

Box F Causes of nausea and vomiting in advanced cancer

Cancer	**Treatment**
Gastroparesis (paraneoplastic visceral neuropathy)	Chemotherapy
Blood in stomach	Radiotherapy
Constipation	Drugs, e.g.
Bowel obstruction	antibiotics
Hepatomegaly	corticosteroids
Gross ascites	iron
Raised intracranial pressure	irritant mucolytics
Cough	lithium
Pain	NSAIDs
Anxiety	opioids
Hypercalcaemia	
Hyponatraemia	**Concurrent**
Renal failure	Functional dyspepsia
	Peptic ulcer
Debility	Alcohol gastritis
Constipation	Renal failure
Cough	Ketosis
Infection	

(Figure 1 and Table 3). This 'mechanistic approach' is successful in most patients (see QCG, p.123). For more information about anti-emetics, see p.342.

Other factors to consider include:

- response to anti-emetics already given
- relative merits of alternatives, e.g.:
  - ▷ effects on GI motility (e.g. antimuscarinics slow motility)
  - ▷ undesirable effects
  - ▷ cost
- when more than one anti-emetic drug is considered:
  - ▷ use combinations with different receptor affinities (e.g. cyclizine and haloperidol)
  - ▷ avoid combinations with antagonistic actions (e.g. cyclizine and metoclopramide)
  - ▷ consider a single broader spectrum drug; levomepromazine and olanzapine have affinity at many receptors and may well be as effective as, and easier for patients to handle than, two or more different anti-emetics simultaneously
- adjuvant use of:
  - ▷ antisecretory drugs (e.g. hyoscine *butylbromide*, glycopyrronium, octreotide)
  - ▷ corticosteroids (e.g. dexamethasone)
  - ▷ benzodiazepines (e.g. lorazepam, midazolam)
  - ▷ anti-epileptics (e.g. valproate)
- non-drug treatments.

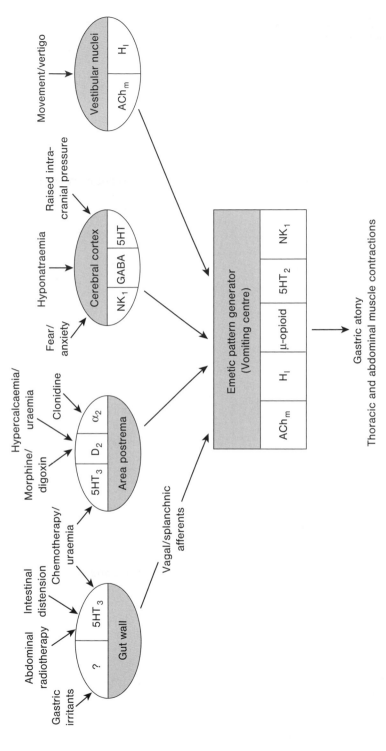

Figure I Diagram of the neural mechanisms controlling vomiting.

Abbreviations refer to receptor types:ACh_m = muscarinic cholinergic;α_2 = α_2-adrenergic;D_2 = dopamine type 2;GABA = gamma-aminobutyric acid; 5HT,$5HT_2$,$5HT_3$ = 5-hydroxytriptamine (serotonin) type undefined, type 2, type 3; H_1 = histamine type 1;NK_1 = neurokinin 1. Anti-emetics act as antagonists at these receptors, whereas the central anti-emetic effects of clonidine and opioids are agonistic.

Table 3 Classification of drugs used to control nausea and vomiting

Putative site of action	Class	Example
Central nervous system		
Vomiting centre	Antimuscarinic	Hyoscine *hydrobromide*[a]
	Antihistaminic antimuscarinic[b]	Cyclizine
	Broad-spectrum antipsychotic	Levomepromazine, olanzapine
	NK$_1$ antagonist	Aprepitant
Area postrema (chemoreceptor trigger zone)	D$_2$ antagonist	Haloperidol, metoclopramide, domperidone
	5HT$_3$ antagonist	Granisetron, ondansetron
Cerebral cortex	Benzodiazepine	Lorazepam
	Cannabinoid	Nabilone
	Corticosteroid	Dexamethasone
	NK$_1$ antagonist	Aprepitant
GI tract		
Prokinetic	5HT$_4$ agonist	Metoclopramide
	D$_2$ antagonist	Metoclopramide, domperidone
	Motilin agonist	Erythromycin
Antisecretory	Antimuscarinic	Hyoscine *butylbromide*, glycopyrronium
	Somatostatin analogue	Octreotide, lanreotide
Vagal 5HT$_3$-receptor blockade	5HT$_3$ antagonist	Granisetron, ondansetron, (metoclopramide at high doses)
Anti-inflammatory	Corticosteroid	Dexamethasone

a. although also has a GI tract antisecretory effect, higher doses risk undesirable CNS effects (unlike hyoscine *butylbromide* or glycopyrronium which do not cross the blood brain barrier)
b. antihistamines and phenothiazines both have H$_1$ antagonistic and antimuscarinic properties.

QUICK CLINICAL GUIDE: NAUSEA AND VOMITING

1   From the patient's history and physical examination, decide what is the most likely cause (or causes) of the nausea and vomiting. Take a blood sample if biochemical derangement is suspected. For bowel obstruction, see QCG: Inoperable bowel obstruction.

2   Correct correctable causes/exacerbating factors, e.g. drugs, severe pain, cough, infection, hypercalcaemia. *(Remember: antibacterial treatment and correction of hypercalcaemia are not always appropriate in a dying patient).*

3   Prescribe the most appropriate anti-emetic regularly and p.r.n.

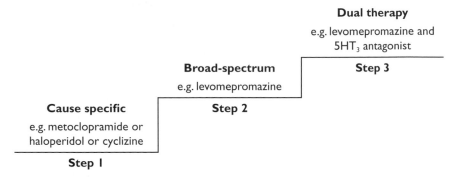

Cause specific	Broad-spectrum	Dual therapy
		e.g. levomepromazine and 5HT$_3$ antagonist
	e.g. levomepromazine	**Step 3**
e.g. metoclopramide or haloperidol or cyclizine	**Step 2**	
Step 1		

Commonly used Step 1 (cause-specific) anti-emetics

For gastritis, gastric stasis, functional bowel obstruction (peristaltic failure)
Prokinetic anti-emetic:
- metoclopramide
  ▷ PO 10mg t.d.s.–q.d.s. & 10mg p.r.n.
  ▷ CSCI 30–40mg/24h & 10mg SC p.r.n.
  ▷ PO/CSCI usual maximum 100mg/24h
- domperidone
  ▷ PO 10mg b.d.–t.d.s.

For most chemical causes of vomiting, e.g. morphine, hypercalcaemia, renal failure
Anti-emetic acting principally in chemoreceptor trigger zone:
- haloperidol
  ▷ PO 500microgram–1.5mg at bedtime & p.r.n.
  ▷ SC/CSCI 2.5–5mg/24h & 1mg SC p.r.n
  ▷ PO/SC/CSCI usual maximum 10mg/24h.
Metoclopramide also has a central action.

Commonly used Step 1 (cause-specific) anti-emetics (Contd.)

For raised intracranial pressure (in conjunction with dexamethasone) or motion sickness
Anti-emetic acting principally in the vomiting centre:
- cyclizine
  - ▷ PO 50mg b.d.–t.d.s. & 50mg p.r.n.
  - ▷ CSCI 100–150mg/24h & 50mg SC p.r.n.
  - ▷ PO/CSCI usual maximum 200mg/24h.

For mechanical bowel obstruction with colic (see inoperable bowel obstruction QCG) and/or need to reduce GI secretions
Antispasmodic and antisecretory anti-emetic:
- hyoscine *butylbromide*
  - ▷ CSCI 60–120mg/24h & 20mg SC p.r.n.
  - ▷ usual maximum 300mg/24h.

---

4 Give by SC injection or CSCI if continuous nausea or frequent vomiting.

5 Start with a stat p.r.n. dose to cover the period before the first regular dose or the delay in reaching therapeutic levels by CSCI.

6 Initially, review anti-emetic dose each day; take note of p.r.n. use, and adjust the regular dose accordingly.

7 If little benefit despite upward titration of the dose, reconsider the likely cause(s), and review the choice of anti-emetic and route of administration.

Sometimes it is necessary to convert to a broad-spectrum anti-emetic, and occasionally dual therapy will be needed.

Commonly used Step 2 and 3 anti-emetics

Step 2: Broad-spectrum
- levomepromazine
  - ▷ PO/SC: 6–6.25mg at bedtime & p.r.n.
  - ▷ usual maximum 50mg/24h either all at bedtime or 25mg b.d.
  - ▷ at home, consider CSCI if a bedtime SC injection is impractical.

Step 3: Dual therapy (combining anti-emetics with different mechanisms)
- levomepromazine + a $5HT_3$ antagonist, e.g. granisetron 1–2mg SC once daily or CSCI, or ondansetron 16mg/24h CSCI, *when there is a massive release of 5HT/serotonin from enterochromaffin cells or platelets,* e.g. with chemotherapy, abdominal radiation, bowel distension, renal failure
- levomepromazine + a benzodiazepine, e.g. lorazepam 0.5–1mg SL b.d. or midazolam 10mg/24h CSCI, *particularly when anxiety or anticipatory nausea*
- levomepromazine + dexamethasone 8–16mg PO/SC stat & once daily *when all else fails*; stop dexamethasone if no benefit after one week; otherwise taper by 2mg/week to the minimum effective dose.

---

8 Prokinetics act through a cholinergic system which is competitively antagonized by antimuscarinics; concurrent use is best avoided.

9 Seizures occasionally present as nausea (e.g. with meningeal carcinomatosis); this responds to anti-epileptic drugs or benzodiazepines.

10 Continue the anti-emetic(s) unless the cause is self-limiting. Except in mechanical bowel obstruction (see QCG: Inoperable bowel obstruction), consider changing to PO after 3 days of good control with CSCI.

11 With successful dual therapy, it may be possible to simplify the regimen after 1–2 weeks by tapering the dose of one of the two anti-emetics.

CONSTIPATION

Constipation is defined as the passage of small hard faeces infrequently with difficulty. It is common in advanced illness and is generally caused by multiple factors, e.g. poor food and fluid intake, weakness, the underlying disease, drugs (particularly opioids).

Constipation may be asymptomatic, but in some patients it can lead to:
- anorexia, nausea, vomiting, bowel obstruction
- abdominal distension, discomfort, pain
- rectal pain (constant or spasmodic)
- urinary dysfunction, e.g. hesitancy, retention, overflow incontinence
- rectal discharge, faecal leakage, overflow diarrhoea
- delirium.

Evaluation

Enquire about the patient's normal (pre-morbid) bowel habit and present status.

Examine the abdomen for faecal masses in the descending colon, possibly in the transverse colon, and occasionally in the ascending colon. Constipation can cause caecal distension and tenderness, or a more classical picture of bowel obstruction.

Rectal examination can be done selectively, if indicated by the history and the abdominal examination. However, all patients with a rectal discharge, faecal leakage or diarrhoea should automatically have a digital rectal examination.

Management

For most patients constipation responds to laxatives. However, sometimes constipation remains difficult to manage.

Non-drug treatment

General measures
- when possible stop or reduce the dose of constipating drugs
- mobilize the patient if possible

- a prompt response to the patient's request for a commode or for help to get to the toilet
- use of a commode rather than a bedpan
- advise a position which increases abdominal pressure and aids defaecation:
  ▷ place feet on a foot stool to elevate the knees above the hips
  ▷ lean forward keeping the spine straight with elbows rested on the knees
- raise the toilet seat and install hand rails in the patient's home to increase toilet independence.

Diet

In patients well enough to tolerate an increased intake of food:
- add bran to diet
- increase fluid intake (at least 1.5L/24h, i.e. about 8 cupfuls)
- encourage fruit juices.

Drug treatment

See Quick Clinical Guide: Opioid-induced constipation (below) and EPCF (p.369). Because of anorexia and physical debility, laxatives are the mainstay of treatment of constipation in advanced disease.

Laxative choice is guided by an appreciation of the pathophysiology of constipation (particularly opioid-induced), how different laxatives work (see p.369), and their cost. Stimulant laxatives are generally preferable, e.g. bisacodyl and senna.

Dantron is another popular stimulant laxative. However, danthron-containing laxatives cost more and can lead to contact skin burns in patients with urinary or faecal incontinence.

QUICK CLINICAL GUIDE: OPIOID-INDUCED CONSTIPATION

Generally, all patients prescribed an opioid should also be prescribed a stimulant laxative, with the aim of achieving a bowel movement without straining every 1–3 days. A standardized protocol aids management.

Sometimes, rather than automatically changing to the local standard laxative, it may be appropriate to optimize a patient's existing regimen.

This guidance can also be followed in patients who are not on opioids, although smaller doses may well suffice.

1   Ask about the patient's past and present bowel habit and use of laxatives; record the date of last bowel action.

2   Palpate for faecal masses in the line of the colon; examine the rectum digitally if the bowels have not been open for ≥3 days or if the patient reports rectal discomfort or has diarrhoea suggestive of faecal impaction with overflow.

3   For inpatients, keep a daily record of bowel actions.

4   Encourage fluids generally, and fruit juice and fruit specifically.

5   When an opioid is prescribed, prescribe bisacodyl or senna and titrate the dose according to response:

Bisacodyl

If *not* constipated:
• generally start with 5mg at bedtime
• if no response after 24–48h, increase to 10mg at bedtime.

If already constipated:
• generally start with 10mg at bedtime
• if no response after 24–48h, increase to 20mg at bedtime
• if no response after a further 24–48h, consider adding a second daytime dose
• if necessary, consider increasing to a maximum of 20mg t.d.s.

Senna

If *not* constipated:
• generally start with 15mg at bedtime
• if no response after 24–48h, increase to 15mg at bedtime and each morning

If already constipated:
• generally start with 15mg at bedtime and each morning
• if no response after 24–48h, increase to 22.5mg at bedtime and each morning
• if no response after a further 24–48h, consider adding a third daytime dose
• if necessary, consider increasing to a maximum of 30mg t.d.s.
An oral solution (7.5mg/5mL) is an alternative to tablets; it is tasteless and generally cheaper.

6 During dose titration and subsequently, if ≥3 days since last bowel action, give suppositories, e.g. bisacodyl 10mg and glycerol 4g, or a micro-enema. If these are ineffective, administer a phosphate enema and possibly repeat the next day.

7 If the maximum dose of the stimulant laxative is ineffective and/or there has been no bowel evacuation within 3–4 days of commencing a stimulant, add a faecal softener laxative and titrate as necessary, e.g.
- macrogols (e.g. Movicol®) 1 sachet each morning *or*
- lactulose 15mL once daily–b.d.

8 In a patient receiving opioids, if adequately titrated oral laxatives + rectal interventions fail to produce the desired response, consider SC methylnaltrexone.

Methylnaltrexone

Methylnaltrexone is a peripherally acting opioid antagonist administered as a SC injection. It is relatively expensive and should be considered in patients with opioid-induced constipation only when the optimum use of laxatives is ineffective. In patients with advanced disease, because constipation is generally multifactorial in origin, methylnaltrexone is added to the existing laxative regimen.

- dose recommendations:
  ▷ for patients weighing 38–61kg, start with 8mg on alternate days
  ▷ for patients weighing 62–114kg, start with 12mg on alternate days
  ▷ outside this range, give 150microgram/kg on alternate days
  ▷ the interval between administrations can be varied, either extended or reduced, but not more than once daily
- in severe renal impairment (creatinine clearance <30mL/min) reduce the dose:
  ▷ for patients weighing 62–114kg, reduce to 8mg
  ▷ outside this range, reduce to *75microgram/kg*, rounding up the dose volume to the nearest 0.1mL
- methylnaltrexone is contra-indicated in cases of known or suspected bowel obstruction. It should be used with caution in patients with conditions which may predispose to perforation
- common undesirable effects include abdominal pain/colic, diarrhoea, flatulence, and nausea and vomiting; these generally resolve after a bowel movement; postural hypotension can also occur
- about 1/3–1/2 of patients given methylnaltrexone have a bowel movement within 4h. The bowel movement can occur rapidly, consider having pads and a commode in place, particularly in those with poor mobility.

---

9 If the stimulant laxative causes bowel colic, divide the total daily dose into smaller more frequent doses or change to a faecal softener (see above), and titrate as necessary.

10 As initial treatment, a faecal softener is preferable in patients with a history of colic with stimulant laxatives.

DIARRHOEA

Diarrhoea is an increase in the frequency of defaecation and/or fluidity of the faeces. Sometimes defined as the passage of more than three unformed stools in 24h.[19] It is generally associated with an increase in faecal water and electrolyte excretion, and sometimes the passage of blood and pus. If severe, diarrhoea may manifest as faecal incontinence.

Causes

There are many potential causes (Box G) but the most common are:

- laxative overdose
- faecal impaction with overflow
- partial bowel obstruction
- gastro-enteritis, mainly viral
- radiation enteritis
- drugs
- steatorrhoea.

Box G Causes of diarrhoea ('LOOSED')

Length of bowel (shortened)
Bowel resection, colostomy
Ileostomy, ileocolic fistula

Overflow
Faecal impaction (see p.371)
Obstruction (see p.131)

Osmotic
Non-absorbable sugars, e.g.
    lactulose, sorbitol-containing solutions
Enteral feeds
Magnesium salts

Secretory
Infective, e.g. gastro-enteritis, *C.difficle*
    diarrhoea, cholera, bacterial overgrowth
Injury, e.g. radiotherapy, chemotherapy,
    ulcerative colitis
Cholegenic

Enhanced motility
Diet
Constitutional
Anxiety
Irritable bowel syndrome
Hyperthyroidism
Steatorrhoea
Carcinoid syndrome
Islet cell tumours, e.g. VIPoma
Visceral neuropathy, e.g. diabetic,
    paraneoplastic
Coeliac plexus block
Lumbar sympathectomy

Drugs, e.g.
Antacids, e.g. magnesium salts
Antibacterials
Chemotherapy, e.g. 5-fluoro-uracil
Iron
Laxatives
SSRIs

Steatorrhoea is excess fat in faeces (>20g/24h). Generally, the faeces are pale in colour, bulky and float making them difficult to flush away. Causes of steatorrhoea include pancreatic cancer, chronic pancreatitis and obstructive jaundice.

Radiation enteritis generally occurs within 6 weeks of therapy and it settles after 2–6 months. Occasionally the onset is months or years after exposure, and results in ulceration, fibrosis and stricture or fistula formation. There may be associated malabsorption and bacterial overgrowth.

Diarrhoea, along with fever, abdominal pain, nausea and vomiting, is also a feature of neutropenic enterocolitis (synonyms: necrotizing enterocolitis, typhlitis), a life-threatening complication of chemotherapy. There is bacterial or fungal infection of the bowel wall associated with necrosis. Urgent treatment is required to avoid death from sepsis or perforation.

Diarrhoea is common in AIDS; pathogens are identifiable in about 1/2 the cases.

Clostridium difficile diarrhoea

This is a complication of antibacterial therapy, particularly broad-spectrum antibacterials, e.g. amoxicillin, cephalosporins, clindamycin, ciprofloxacin, clarithromycin, erythromycin. It is caused by colonization of the bowel by C. difficile and the production of toxins which cause the mucosal damage.

Symptoms of watery diarrhoea (+ mucus ± blood), abdominal pain, fever and malaise, dehydration ± delirium generally begin within 1 week of starting antibacterial therapy or shortly after stopping, but may occur up to 1 month later.[20]

A pseudomembranous colitis is present in severe cases, with sloughing of the inflamed colonic epithelium, manifesting as foul-smelling diarrhoea mingled with mucus and blood. C. difficile diarrhoea has a mortality of up to 25% in elderly frail patients.

Evaluation

A carefully elicited history and clinical examination is often sufficient to determine the most likely cause (see Box G).

A careful review of medication is important, and will generally indicate whether too much laxative is the cause.

If appropriate, consider blood tests, abdominal radiograph and faecal microscopy and culture, including C. difficile toxin.

Management

Prevention of C.difficile diarrhoea

Adhere to local guidelines concerning environmental measures and antibacterial prescribing.

Correct the correctable

- review diet, and avoid laxative foods if possible, e.g. beans, lentils, raw fruit. Stop alcohol and high-osmolar dietary supplements
- review medication, including laxatives, and modify if indicated. If diarrhoea is due to laxative overdose, reduce the dose but do not prescribe an anti-diarrhoeal drug
- consider antibacterial treatment if infective cause or if bacterial overgrowth seems likely
- if patient has *C. difficile* diarrhoea, stop causal antibacterial if possible, and treat according to local guidelines.

Non-drug treatment

If diarrhoea is severe or persistent, it is important to prevent dehydration. Options include an oral rehydration solution, e.g. Dioralyte® 200–400mL or, if unavailable, flat Coke or lemonade after each loose motion. If the patient is nauseated, vomiting or dehydrated, parenteral rehydration may be necessary.

Drug treatment

For the treatment of *C.difficile* refer to local guidelines.

A non-specific antidiarrhoeal drug, e.g. loperamide (p.341), is used after excluding faecal impaction, obstruction, colitis (ulcerative, infective or antibacterial-related) and other causes requiring specific treatment.

Morphine (p.329) may sometimes be necessary to achieve control (e.g. in AIDS). This has both peripheral and central constipating effects, whereas loperamide acts only peripherally.

Octreotide 250–1,500microgram/24h CSCI may also be necessary in chemotherapy- or radiotherapy-induced diarrhoea:

- used first-line in severe cases (i.e. an increase of ≥ 7 stools/day over baseline, need for hospital admission, IV fluids)
- used second-line in mild-moderate cases not responding to loperamide 24mg/24h.

BOWEL OBSTRUCTION

Obstruction of the alimentary tract can occur at any level. Clinically, it is useful to think in terms of four syndromes, reflecting obstruction at high (proximal) or low (distal) levels:

- oesophageal, commonly the gastro-oesophageal junction
- gastric outlet and proximal small bowel
- distal small bowel
- large bowel.

Patients with disseminated intra-abdominal cancer, e.g. from colon or ovarian cancer, commonly have multiple sites of obstruction involving both small and large bowel. At each level, the obstruction can be functional (peristaltic failure) or mechanical (organic), or both. It can also be:

- partial or complete
- transient (acute) or persistent (chronic).

Some patients with mechanical bowel obstruction experience recurrent episodes which settle within a few days of resting the GI tract, i.e. nil by mouth and IV fluids. The frequency and duration of such episodes tend to increase, and eventually the obstruction may become complete and irreversible.

The prognosis is generally poor with a median survival of 1–3 months.[21,22]

Causes

Bowel obstruction in advanced cancer may be caused by one or more of the following:
- the cancer itself, e.g.:
  - ▷ mechanical obstruction
  - ▷ functional obstruction (retroperitoneal disease → visceral neuropathy)
- past treatment, e.g. adhesions, post-radiation ischaemic fibrosis
- drugs, e.g. opioids, antimuscarinics
- debility, e.g. faecal impaction, electrolyte abnormalities
- unrelated benign condition, e.g. strangulated hernia.

Clinical features

The predominant symptoms will depend on the level of the obstruction.

Mechanical oesophageal obstruction generally manifests as dysphagia for solids first and liquids second.

In gastric outlet and proximal small bowel obstruction there may be vomiting with even a small oral intake, and retrosternal and epigastric discomfort from gastro-oesophageal reflux and gastric distension. Even with no oral intake, the stomach needs to clear:
- swallowed saliva (~ 1500mL/24h)
- basal gastric juices (~ 1500mL/24h).

Thus, if a patient is vomiting less than 2–3L/24h, something is getting past the obstruction. Nausea may be intermittent or constant.

In distal small bowel and large bowel obstruction, vomiting is generally less frequent (1–2 per day) and can be foul smelling/faeculent.

Abdominal pain from the underlying cancer is common, often a constant deep ache. Colic is common with mechanical obstruction.

Distension is variable (more likely with distal obstruction) and bowel habit ranges from absolute constipation to diarrhoea secondary to bacterial liquefaction of retained faeces.

Bowel sounds vary from absent in functional obstruction to hyperactive and audible (borborygmi) in mechanical obstruction. Tinkling bowel sounds are uncommon.

Evaluation

Evaluation is based on the patient's history and abdominal examination, together with information gleaned from surgical records, e.g. past laparotomy findings. Further investigations, e.g. abdominal radiograph, CT scan, endoscopy, can help to identify the level and nature of the obstruction and should be considered in all patients with an obstruction of unknown cause.

Management

High obstruction

Oesophageal obstruction

Correct the correctable

Self-expanding metal stents coated with a plastic membrane are used to relieve dysphagia, and also to close tracheo-oesophageal fistulas in patients with cancer of the oesophagus or proximal stomach.

Most patients obtain rapid benefit. Mortality from the procedure is low, but morbidity is relatively high, e.g.:
- chest pain requiring additional analgesia; generally settles after a 2–3 days
- bleeding
- oesophageal perforation
- fistula formation
- gastro-oesophageal reflux, aspiration
- airway compression.

Recurrent dysphagia, occurs in 1/4–1/3 of patients due to:
- continued growth of the cancer around or within the stent
- overgrowth of granulation tissue
- food bolus impaction
- stent migration.

For recurrent obstruction due to cancer, repeat stent placement can be considered. For patients with a reasonable prognosis, brachytherapy is an option.

Because of the relatively high rate of recurrent dysphagia, the use of metal stents as the *only* treatment for dysphagia is best suited to patients with a short prognosis, or other situations when anticancer therapies are inappropriate.

Pylorus/duodenum

Correct the correctable

- self-expanding metal stent
- gastrojejunostomy (open or laparoscopic surgery).

Correct any electrolyte imbalances which may contribute to peristaltic failure, e.g. low potassium, low magnesium.

Non-drug treatment

If the obstruction is partial, dietary advice may help, e.g.:

* take small amounts of a liquid or sloppy diet throughout much or all of the day, e.g. sips of a nutritional supplement drink
* avoid carbonated drinks which will fill the stomach with gas.

If a gastrojejunostomy or a stent is not appropriate or possible, a venting procedure is occasionally necessary:

* nasogastric tube
* gastrostomy.

Drug treatment

Functional obstruction:

* metoclopramide 30mg/24h CSCI; if beneficial, optimize the dose up to 100mg/24h
* if the vomiting is made worse, this indicates mechanical obstruction; discontinue the metoclopramide.

Mechanical obstruction:

With a high obstruction, it is generally not possible to stop vomiting completely with drugs; a practical goal is minimizing the frequency, e.g. to 2–3 times/24h. Where a venting procedure is not possible, drug treatment will be necessary, e.g. antimuscarinics (see p.136).

Low obstruction

Distal small bowel/large bowel

Correct the correctable

Surgical intervention, e.g. palliative resection, bypass or colostomy, may be of benefit in a carefully selected group of patients and should be considered if the following criteria are all fulfilled:

* a single discrete mechanical obstruction seems likely, e.g. postoperative adhesions or an isolated cancer, e.g. carcinoid of the terminal ileum
* the patient's general performance status is good (i.e. independent and active) and disease is not widely disseminated
* the patient is willing to undergo surgery.

Diffuse intra-abdominal carcinomatosis is a contra-indication to surgical intervention as evidenced by, e.g. diffuse palpable intra-abdominal tumours, rapidly accumulating ascites.

Correct any electrolyte imbalances which may contribute to peristaltic failure, e.g. low potassium, low magnesium.

Non-drug treatment

Initially, resting the GI tract for several days may allow a mechanical obstruction to settle (see Quick Clinical Guide: Inoperable bowel obstruction, p.136). This helps break the vicious cycle of increased GI distension → increased secretion and reduced reabsorption → increased distension accompanied by reduced motility. Generally, the approach is combined with drug treatment.

When apparent that an obstruction is irreversible and chronic, the aim of drug treatment is to minimize vomiting so as to avoid the need for a nasogastric tube and to permit sufficient oral fluids to maintain hydration without an IVI. *This may not always be possible.*

Patients in chronic obstruction should be encouraged to drink small amounts and to rely more on oral liquid nutritional supplements for calories. Although small amounts of their favourite foods can be taken, those difficult to digest, e.g. high in fibre, are best avoided.

Antimuscarinics and diminished fluid intake often result in a dry mouth and thirst; these are generally relieved by conscientious mouth care.

In left-sided colorectal obstruction, self-expanding metal stents ± subsequent surgery may be an option. Complications are similar to oesophageal stents (see above).[23]

Drug treatment

See Quick Clinical Guides: Inoperable bowel obstruction, p.136, and Nausea and vomiting, p.123.

Drug treatment focuses primarily on the relief of pain and nausea and vomiting. Administration is generally by CSCI or SC. Dose titration over several days may be necessary before optimum relief is achieved.

In one series where bowel rest, dexamethasone and ranitidine were part of a standardized approach, vomiting was completely controlled in about one third of patients.[24]

An attempt can be made to reduce the obstruction with corticosteroids, but evidence is limited and their use is controversial.[25] In addition to reducing oedema around a tumour and thereby improving the patency of the bowel lumen, corticosteroids also have a specific anti-emetic effect.

QUICK CLINICAL GUIDE: INOPERABLE BOWEL OBSTRUCTION

Initial management

1 Resting the GI tract for several days may allow an obstruction to settle spontaneously:
   - restrict PO intake to sips of fluid to keep the mouth comfortable, and hydrate IV/SC, e.g. 10–20mL/Kg/24h
   - a nasogastric tube can be reserved for patients experiencing large volume vomits more than 2–3 times/24h
   - correct electrolyte imbalances which may contribute to peristaltic failure, e.g. low potassium, low magnesium
   - a combination of analgesics (opioids and antispasmodics), anti-emetics and antisecretory drugs should be used to manage abdominal pain, colic, and nausea and vomiting (see below)
   - some centres add dexamethasone, e.g. 6.6mg once daily SC for 5–7 days (evidence suggests only a trend towards benefit) with ranitidine 50mg t.d.s.–q.d.s. IV/SC or 150–200mg/24h CSCI as antacid cover; ranitidine, unlike PPIs, reduces gastric secretions and can be mixed with most other drugs used in a syringe driver.

Ongoing management (≥1 week)

2 If the obstruction does not settle with the above measures, the aim (*although not always achieved*) is to:
   - control pain and nausea *and*
   - minimize vomiting so as to avoid the need for a nasogastric tube *and*
   - permit sufficient oral fluids to maintain hydration.

Symptom management

3 For constant background cancer pain, morphine should be given regularly by the clock and p.r.n. For those with colic, an antispasmodic antisecretory anti-emetic should be given (see below).

4 Drugs for inoperable bowel obstruction are best given by CSCI (for more information on anti-emetic doses, see QCG: Management of nausea and vomiting), but some, e.g. dexamethasone, levomepromazine, can be given as a single SC daily dose.

5 The ladder shows a general approach; dose titration over several days may be necessary before optimum relief is achieved:
   - start on Step 1 if *no* colic: probable functional obstruction (i.e. peristaltic failure):
     ▷ metoclopramide 30–40mg/24h CSCI & 10mg SC p.r.n.
     ▷ if beneficial, optimize the dose up to 100mg/24h
   - start on Step 2 if colic: probable mechanical obstruction:
     ▷ hyoscine *butylbromide* 60–120mg/24h CSCI & 20mg SC p.r.n.
     ▷ usual maximum 300mg/24h.

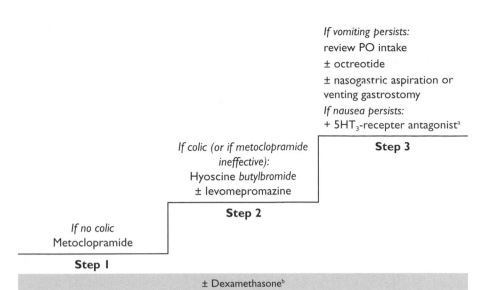

If vomiting persists:
review PO intake
± octreotide
± nasogastric aspiration or
venting gastrostomy
If nausea persists:
+ 5HT$_3$-recepter antagonist[a]

Step 3

If colic (or if metoclopramide
ineffective):
Hyoscine butylbromide
± levomepromazine

Step 2

If no colic
Metoclopramide

Step 1

± Dexamethasone[b]

a. e.g. granisetron 1–2mg SC once daily, ondansetron 16mg/24h CSCI
b. see point 1 above.

6 Instead of levomepromazine, some centres use:
- cyclizine 100–150mg/24h CSCI & 50mg SC p.r.n. or
- haloperidol 2.5–5mg/24h CSCI & 1mg SC p.r.n.

Note: cyclizine mixed with hyoscine butylbromide may be incompatible.

7 If levomepromazine is too sedative, consider giving both cyclizine and haloperidol; or olanzapine 1.25–2.5mg SC (not UK) at bedtime instead.

8 If hyoscine butylbromide is inadequate to control vomiting, or to obtain more rapid relief, consider octreotide (a somatostatin analogue and antisecretory agent):
- if colic, add to hyoscine butylbromide
- if no colic, substitute or use instead of hyoscine butylbromide:
  ▷ octreotide 100microgram SC stat
  ▷ CSCI 500microgram/24h
  ▷ usual maximum 1,000microgram/24h, occasionally higher.

9 If vomiting persists, review the patient's oral intake. Antisecretory drugs cannot fully alleviate the vomiting of ingested fluid and food; consider nasogastric aspiration or venting gastrostomy.

10 In partial obstruction, there may be passage of flatus and faeces. When a laxative is required, use a stool softener that does not distend the bowel, i.e. sodium docusate 100–200mg b.d.

Nutrition

11 Some patients and carers are concerned about a restricted oral caloric intake, and need sensitive counselling. Note:
- a patient may manage small amounts of oral fibre-free nutritional supplements and/or readily digestible food

- sometimes a patient chooses a long-term nasogastric tube or considers a venting gastrostomy to permit unrestricted oral intake
- parenteral nutrition generally has no role in patients with limited options for anti-cancer treatment or poor performance status.

ASCITES

Ascites is the excessive accumulation of fluid in the peritoneal cavity as a result of excessive production (from capillaries) and/or reduced resorption of fluid (by lymphatics). Severe ascites causes a range of symptoms (Box H).

Box H Clinical features of ascites	
Abdominal distension	Nausea and vomiting
Abdominal discomfort/pain	Breathlessness
Early satiety, anorexia	Inability to sit upright
Dyspepsia, acid reflux	Leg oedema

Ascites can be complicated by bacterial peritonitis, either spontaneous or secondary.

Ascites is associated with a poor prognosis. In cancer, mean survival is about 5 months, worse in patients with an unknown primary and with GI cancer. In cirrhosis, median survival is about 2 years.

Causes

Cancer accounts for about 10% of all cases of ascites. Other causes include cirrhosis (commonest overall), heart failure, kidney disease and pancreatitis. The two main underlying mechanisms are:
- obstruction of the lymphatics in the peritoneum or regional lymph nodes by cancer
- portal hypertension and hypo-albuminaemia.

Evaluation

Clinical signs include increased abdominal girth, bulging of the flanks, shifting dullness and ankle oedema. Useful investigations include:
- *ultrasound*: can identify ≥100mL fluid, loculations and distinguish between distension due to fluid, cancer, organomegaly or bowel distension
- cytological, microbiological and biochemical examination: carried out when there is diagnostic uncertainty.

The ascitic total protein content is a reflection of the serum protein concentration and portal pressure. The difference between the level of albumin in the serum and ascitic fluid (serum:ascites albumin gradient) along with other features can help identify the main underlying mechanism (Table 4).

Table 4 Differential diagnosis of ascites

Serum:ascites albumin gradient			
<11g/L		≥11g/L	
Total ascitic fluid protien		**Jugular venous pressure**	
≥25g/L	**<25g/L**	**Normal or reduced**	**Elevated**
Peritoneal carcinomatosis	Protein-losing enteropathy	Liver metastases	Heart failure
TB	Nephropathy	Cirrhosis	Constrictive pericarditis
Pancreatic ascites	Malnutrition	Alcoholic hepatitis	Pulmonary hypertension
Bacterial peritonitis		Hepatic failure	
		Budd-Chiari syndrome	
		Portal vein thrombosis	
		Hypothyroidism	

When infection is suspected, diagnostic paracentesis should be undertaken to obtain a Gram stain, cell count, and culture to guide antibacterial management.

Management

Correct the correctable

If appropriate and successful, chemotherapy will control ascites. This can be either systemic or intraperitoneal.

Non-drug treatment

Paracentesis

Paracentesis is appropriate for patients with:
- an unknown diagnosis
- a tense distended abdomen in need of rapid relief
- ascites which is unlikely to respond to diuretic therapy, i.e. predominantly peritoneal (an *exudate* with relatively high albumin concentration) or chylous ascites
- ascites that has failed to respond to diuretic therapy
- intolerance to diuretic therapy
- possible bacterial peritonitis.

The only absolute contra-indications to paracentesis are clinically evident fibrinolysis or disseminated intravascular coagulation.

Most patients (90%) obtain symptom relief from paracentesis, sometimes after the removal of a relatively small volume, e.g. 1–2L. Ultrasound-guided paracentesis is increasingly used.[26]

Complications of paracentesis include:
- abdominal discomfort; may require additional analgesics
- bleeding, sufficient to require transfusion (<1%)
- bowel or bladder puncture
- persistent leak at the site of puncture (<1%)
- hypotension: risk minimized by limiting paracentesis to ≤5L in patients with cirrhosis receiving diuretics, and any patient with serum creatinine >250micromol/L (indicative of renal failure)), albumin <30g/L or sodium <125mmol/L
- pulmonary embolism; possibly due to the release of pressure from abdominal veins
- local infection or peritonitis; the risk is minimal with an aseptic technique.

With cirrhotic ascites, if drainage of >5L is required:
- stop diuretics used for ascites 48h before procedure, during paracentesis, and immediately afterwards
- administer volume expanders, e.g. IV albumin 200mg/L (20%), 100mL for every 2.5L of ascites drained
- monitor pulse and blood pressure every 30min during paracentesis, then hourly for 6h.

With cancer-related ascites, removal of >5L is less problematic.[27] However, in the presence of abnormal creatinine, albumin or sodium (see above), it makes sense to take a similar approach as in cirrhotic ascites.

Indwelling catheters

For patients requiring frequent paracentesis and a prognosis of >1 month, an indwelling tunnelled drain can be considered, e.g. Pleurx® catheter. This will reduce the frequency of hospital visits, of particular benefit to frail patients.

Patients are taught to drain off fluid using special drainage sets with vacuum bottles, initially up to 2L every day for 1–2 weeks, and then as required, generally alternate days. The overall complication rate (i.e. infection, loculation, persistent leakage) is similar to intermittent drainage (<10%).[28]

Peritoneovenous shunts

Shunts with a one-way valve allowing fluid to be drained from the peritoneal cavity into the superior vena cava are a potential alternative to frequent intermittent drainage, with the advantage of avoiding protein and fluid depletion.[29] However, they are prone to occlusion and other complications, and their use has been largely superseded by the increasing use of indwelling catheters.

Drug treatment

Diuretics

Hyperaldosteronism often occurs with ascites associated with portal hypertension (producing a *transudate* with a serum:ascites albumin gradient ≥11g/L):
- cirrhosis
- hepatocellular cancer
- extensive liver metastases.

Spironolactone, an aldosterone antagonist, either alone or in combination with furosemide is successful in the majority of patients with these conditions.[30] Elimination of ascites takes 10–28 days (Box 1).

In peritoneal carcinomatosis or chylous ascites, a response to spironolactone is less likely. Consider its use only when secondary hyperaldosteronism is also present (suggested by ankle oedema).

Corticosteroids

In peritoneal carcinomatosis, after a preliminary paracentesis, depot corticosteroids have been instilled to reduce the rate of ascitic fluid formation, e.g.:
- triamcinolone acetonide 8mg/kg, up to a maximum of 520mg (13 vials) *or*
- methylprednisolone 10mg/kg, up to a maximum of 640mg (8 vials).

Evidence is limited, but in an open study, mean interval between paracenteses increased from 9 days to 18 days.[31,32]

Box 1 Diuretic treatment for ascites

Monitor body weight and renal function.

Start with spironolactone 100–200mg each morning with food; give in divided doses if it causes nausea and vomiting.

If necessary, increase by 100mg every 3–7 days to achieve a weight loss of 0.5–1kg/24h (<0.5kg/24h when peripheral oedema absent).

A typical maintenance dose is 200–300mg once daily; maximum dose 400–600mg once daily.

If not achieving the desired weight loss with spironolactone 300–400mg once daily, consider adding furosemide 40–80mg each morning.

In cirrhosis, furosemide is generally increased in 40mg steps every 3 days to a maximum of 160mg once daily.

If Na^+ falls <120mmol/L, temporarily stop diuretics.

If K^+ falls to <3.5mmol/L, temporarily stop or decrease the dose of furosemide.

If K^+ rises to >5.5mmol/L, halve the dose of spironolactone; if >6mmol/L, temporarily stop spironolactone.

If creatinine rises >150micromol/L, temporarily stop diuretics.

Even if paracentesis becomes necessary, diuretics should be continued as they reduce the rate of recurrence.

Renal function must be monitored as a diuretic-induced reduction in plasma volume and renal perfusion can result in increased Na^+ and water resorption. These changes reduce the effect of the diuretic and contribute to renal impairment.

Octreotide

Octreotide is reported to reduce the rate of formation of malignant ascites, increasing the time between paracentesis.[33] It may interfere with ascitic fluid formation through a reduction in splanchnic blood flow and/or blood vessel permeability.

Octreotide could be considered in patients with rapidly accumulating ascites due to peritoneal carcinomatosis or massive liver metastases failing to respond to diuretic therapy. Octreotide may also help resolve chylous ascites.[34]

JAUNDICE

Jaundice is a yellowish discolouration of the skin, mucous membranes and eyes caused by elevated levels of bilirubin in the blood (hyperbilirubinaemia).

Clinical features

The principle features include:
- change in the colour of the skin (requires serum bilirubin >35mmol/L)
- anorexia
- nausea
- pruritus
- fatigue
- dark urine and pale faeces (when biliary obstruction).

Patients are at increased risk of bleeding (reduced levels of clotting factors) and renal impairment (hepato-renal syndrome).

Causes

In advanced cancer jaundice may be caused by one or more of the following:
- cancer obstructing the biliary system, e.g. cancer of the head of the pancreas, lymph nodes at the porta hepatis, liver metastases
- drugs, e.g. phenothiazines, valproate
- concurrent disorders, e.g. cirrhosis, gallstones, haemolysis, viral hepatitis.

Evaluation

A careful history and examination will help identify the most likely cause. Routine bloods tests should include LFTs and coagulation studies. An ultrasound scan will help identify potentially reversible biliary obstruction.

Management

Correct the correctable

Specific management will depend on the cause, e.g. stopping potentially causal drugs.

Non-drug treatment

Biliary stent

Stop and think! Will the benefits outweigh the burdens of the procedure? A stent is generally inappropriate for patients with a prognosis of only 1–2 weeks.

Stents can be placed radiologically either endoscopically or percutaneously.

Most patients experience symptom relief, but overall prognosis is poor, an average of 2–3 months.[35]

Complications of the procedure include perforation, biliary sepsis and pancreatitis. Complications of stents include blockage (less with metal than plastic stents), migration and sepsis (cholangitis).

Surgical procedures

There may be a limited role for surgical relief of bile duct obstruction in carefully selected patients, when less invasive options are not feasible.

Treatment of cholestatic pruritus

See p.228.

REFERENCES

1   Finlay I and Davies A (2005) Fungal infections. In: A Davies and I Finlay (eds) *Oral Care in Advanced Disease.* Oxford University Press, Oxford, pp. 55–71.

2   Pappas PG *et al.* (2009) Clinical practice guidelines for the management of candidiasis: 2009 update by the Infectious Diseases Society of America. *Clinical Infectious Diseases.* **48:** 503–535.

3   Bruera E *et al.* (1985) Action of oral methylprednisolone in terminal cancer patients: a prospective randomized double-blind study. *Cancer Treatment Reports.* **69:** 751–754.

4   Vadell C *et al.* (1998) Anticachectic efficacy of megestrol acetate at different doses and versus placebo in patients with neoplastic cachexia. *American Journal of Clinical Oncology.* **21:** 347–351.

5   Ruiz Garcia V *et al.* (2013) Megestrol acetate for treatment of anorexia-cachexia syndrome. *Cochrane Database Systematic Reviews.* **3:** CD004310. www.thecochranelibrary.com

6   Laviano A *et al.* (2003) Cancer anorexia: clinical implications, pathogenesis, and therapeutic strategies. *Lancet Oncology.* **4:** 686–694.

7   Fearon K *et al.* (2010) Definition and classification of cancer cachexia: an international consensus framework. *Lancet Oncology.* **12:** 489–495.

8   Davis MP *et al.* (2004) Appetite and cancer-associated anorexia: a review. *Journal of Clinical Oncology.* **22:** 1510–1517.

9   Arends J *et al.* (2006) ESPEN guidelines on enteral nutrition: non-surgical oncology. *Clinical Nutrition.* **25:** 245–259.

10 Baldwin C and Weekes C (2008) Dietary advice for illness-related malnutrition in adults. *Cochrane Database of Systematic Reviews.* **1:** CD002008. www.thecochranelibrary.com

11 Bosaeus I and Bosaeus I (2008) Nutritional support in multimodal therapy for cancer cachexia. *Supportive Care in Cancer.* **16:** 447–451.

12 National Council for Palliative Care and The Association of Palliative Medicine for Great Britain & Ireland (2007) *Artificial nutrition and hydration - guidance in end of life care for adults.* www.ncpc. org.uk/publications/index.html

13 General Medical Council (2002) *Withholding and withdrawing life-prolonging treatments: good practice in decision making.* www.gmc-uk.org

14 British Medical Association (2007) *Withholding and withdrawing life-prolonging medical treatment. Guidance for decision making (3e).* Blackwell Publishing, Oxford.

15 Geeraerts B and Tack J (2008) Functional dyspepsia: past, present, and future. *Journal of Gastroenterology.* **43:** 251–255.

16 Sigterman KE *et al.* (2013) Short-term treatment with proton pump inhibitors, H2-receptor antagonists and prokinetics for gastro-oesophageal reflux disease-like symptoms and endoscopy negative reflux disease. *Cochrane Database of Systematic Reviews.* **5:** CD002095. www. thecochranelibrary.com

17 Cherny N (2008) Evaluation and management of treatment-related diarrhea in patients with advanced cancer: a review. *Journal of Pain and Symptom Management.* **36:** 413–423.

18 Saad RJ and Chey WD (2006) Review article: current and emerging therapies for functional dyspepsia. *Alimentary Pharmacology and Therapeutics.* **24:** 475–492.

19 Camilleri M (2007) Functional dyspepsia: mechanisms of symptom generation and appropriate management of patients. *Gastroenterology Clinics of North America.* **36:** 649–664.

20 Shannon-Lowe J *et al.* (2010) Prevention and medical management of Clostridium difficile infection. *British Medical Journal.* **340:** c1296.

21 Laval G *et al.* (2006) Protocol for the treatment of malignant inoperable bowel obstruction: a prospective study of 80 cases at Grenoble University Hospital Center. *Journal of Pain and Symptom Management.* **31:** 502–512.

22 Chakraborty A *et al.* (2011) Malignant bowel obstruction: natural history of a heterogeneous patient population followed prospectively over two years. *Journal of Pain and Symptom Management.* **41:** 412–420.

23 Watt AM *et al.* (2007) Self-expanding metallic stents for relieving malignant colorectal obstruction: a systematic review. *Annals of Surgery.* **246:** 24–30.

24 Currow DC *et al.* (2015) Double-blind, placebo-controlled, randomized trial of octreotide in malignant bowel obstruction. *Journal of Pain and Symptom Management.* **49:** 814–821.

25 Mercadante S *et al.* (2007) Medical treatment for inoperable malignant bowel obstruction: a qualitative systematic review. *Journal of Pain and Symptom Management.* **33:** 217–223.

26 McGibbon A *et al.* (2007) An evidence-based manual for abdominal paracentesis. *Digestive Diseases and Sciences.* **52:** 3307–3315.

27 Stephenson J and Gilbert J (2002) The development of clinical guidelines on paracentesis for ascites related to malignancy. *Palliative Medicine.* **16:** 213–218.

28 Rosenberg S *et al.* (2004) Comparison of percutaneous management techniques for recurrent malignant ascites. *Journal of Vascular Interventional Radiology.* **15:** 1129–1131.

29 Osterlee J (1980) Peritoneovenous shunting for ascites in cancer patients. *British Journal of Surgery.* **67:** 663–666.

30 Becker G *et al.* (2006) Malignant ascites: systematic review and guideline for treatment. *European Journal of Cancer.* **42:** 589–597.

31 Mackey J *et al.* (2000) A phase II trial of triamcinolone hexacetanide for symptomatic recurrent malignant ascites. *Journal of Pain and Symptom Management.* **19:** 193–199.

32 Jenkin RP *et al.* (2008) The use of intraperitoneal triamcinolone acetonide for the management of recurrent malignant ascites in a patient with non-Hodgkin's lymphoma. *Journal of Pain and Symptom Management.* **36:** e4–5.

33 Jatoi A *et al.* (2012) A pilot study of long-acting octreotide for symptomatic malignant ascites. *Oncology.* **82:** 315–320.

34 Yildirim AE *et al.* (2011) Idiopathic chylous ascites treated with total parenteral nutrition and octreotide. A case report and review of the literature. *European Journal of Gastroenterology and Hepatology.* **23:** 961–963.

35 Dy SM *et al.* (2012) To stent or not to stent: an evidence-based approach to palliative procedures at the end of life. *Journal of Pain and Symptom Management.* **43:** 795–801.

9. SYMPTOM MANAGEMENT: RESPIRATORY

BREATHLESSNESS

Breathlessness is the subjective experience of breathing discomfort. It comprises qualitatively distinct sensations which vary in intensity. The experience derives from interactions among multiple physiological, psychological, social and environmental factors and may induce secondary physiological and behavioural responses.[1]

Breathlessness on exertion is a normal (physiological) experience, occurring at lower levels of exertion with physical deconditioning and increasing age. It becomes pathological when it limits activities of daily living or is associated with mood disturbance, e.g. anxiety.

Breathlessness commonly:
- is intermittent, occurring in episodes lasting 5–15min precipitated, for example, by exertion, bending over, talking, anxiety, and associated with feelings of exhaustion
- restricts general activities of daily living and social functioning leading to a loss of independence and of role, resulting in frustration, anger and depression
- induces feelings of anxiety, fear, panic (see p.187), hopelessness and impending death.[2,3]

Breathlessness is common in patients with advanced cancer, particularly those with involvement of the lungs. About 50% of the patients with incurable lung cancer report breathlessness.

Explanations for breathlessness in the absence of lung involvement include limb ± respiratory muscle weakness related to physical deconditioning or cachexia. Even in patients who are breathless on exertion, limb muscle fatigue is frequently reported as contributing to the limitation of activities of daily living.[4]

The prevalence of breathlessness in other advanced diseases ranges between 90–95% (COPD), 60–90% (heart disease) and 10–60% (AIDS and renal disease).[5]

The incidence of breathlessness increases as death nears; it is present in 70% of patients with cancer in the last few weeks before death, and is severe in 25% of patients in their last week of life.[6] Breathlessness is an independent predictor of survival second only to performance status.[7]

Causes

Breathlessness in advanced disease is often multifactorial (Box A). For example, in cancer, most patients will have one or more of the following:

- parenchymal or pleural disease
- a history of smoking
- abnormal spirometry (mixed > restrictive > obstructive pattern)
- weak inspiratory muscles.[8]

About half are hypoxic and about one fifth have evidence of concurrent cardiac ischaemia or arrhythmia.[8] However, anxiety is the only feature to consistently correlate with breathlessness.[8–10]

Box A Causes of breathlessness

Primary condition
Anaemia
Asthma
Atelectasis
Cancer (see below)
COPD
Empyema
Heart failure
Pneumonia
Pneumothorax
Pulmonary embolism

Cancer
Abdominal distension
Ascites (massive)
Cachexia
    respiratory muscle weakness
Cancer micro-emboli in the pulmonary
    vascular bed
Cardiac metastases or direct invasion
Lymphangitis carcinomatosa
Obstruction of a large airway
Pericardial effusion
Phrenic nerve palsy
Pleural effusion
Replacement of lung by cancer
SVC obstruction

Treatment
Chemotherapy-induced
    pneumonitis
    fibrosis
    cardiomyopathy
Pneumonectomy
Radiation-induced fibrosis

Psychological
Anxiety
    panic attack
    panic disorder
Depression

Evaluation

The history, examination and appropriate investigation(s) will identify pulmonary, cardiac or neuromuscular abnormalities (Box B).

Box B Evaluation of the breathless patient

History
Speed of onset.
Associated symptoms, e.g. pain, cough, haemoptysis, sputum, stridor, wheeze.
Exacerbating and relieving factors.
Symptoms suggestive of hyperventilation:
- poor relationship of dyspnoea to exertion
- presence of hyperventilation attacks
- breathlessness at rest
- rapid fluctuations in breathlessness within minutes
- fear of sudden death during an attack
- breathlessness varying with social situations.

Past medical history, e.g. history of cardiovascular disease.
Drug history, e.g. drugs precipitating fluid retention or bronchospasm.
Symptoms of anxiety or depression.
Social circumstances and support networks.
Level of independence:
- ability to care for themselves
- coping strategies.

What does the breathlessness mean to the patient?
How do they feel when they are breathless?

Examination
Central cyanosis (a bluish tinge to the tongue and oral mucous membranes) indicates arterial hypoxaemia. *Note. Cyanosis may be absent in severe anaemia despite hypoxaemia, and conversely be present in polycythaemia despite normal arterial oxygen.*
Observe the patient walking a set distance or carrying out a specific task.
Does hyperventilation reproduce symptoms?

Investigations
Common
Chest radiograph.
Haemoglobin concentration.
Less common
Ultrasound scan (useful for differentiating between pleural effusion and solid tumour).
Oxygen saturation (may be useful if evaluating value of oxygen).
Peak flow/simple spirometry (evaluating response to bronchodilators or corticosteroids).
ECG.
Echocardiography.
CT pulmonary angiography.

Evaluation should also include an exploration of the patient's knowledge, beliefs and behaviours associated with their breathlessness, and its impact on them.

Try to determine the cause of any recent deterioration because *rapid changes* often provide an opportunity for corrective treatment, e.g. antibacterials, pleural drainage.

Management

For pragmatic purposes, breathlessness can be divided into three categories:
- breathlessness on exertion (prognosis = months–years)
- breathlessness at rest (prognosis = weeks–months)
- terminal breathlessness (prognosis = days–weeks).

The categories have prognostic significance, illustrated above for patients with cancer, e.g. median survival when breathless at rest is 6–8 weeks; but probably longer in other advanced diseases.

The relative importance of the three treatment categories (correct the correctable, non-drug treatment, drug treatment) changes as the patient's condition deteriorates (Figure 1). For the management of terminal breathlessness, see p.277.

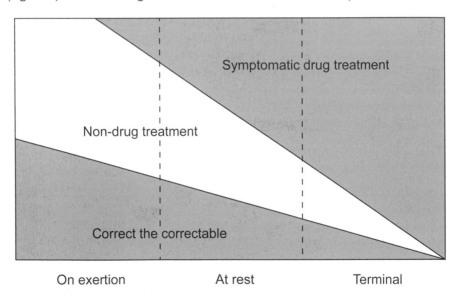

Figure 1 Management approach for severe breathlessness.

Correct the correctable

Particularly while the patient is still ambulant, consideration should be given to the identification and correction of correctable causes (Table 1), including anxiety, panic and/or depression.

Non-drug treatment

Exploration and explanation are essential aspects of non-drug treatment (Box C).[11,12]

Table I Correctable causes of breathlessness

Cause	Treatment
Respiratory infection	Antibacterials
	Physiotherapy
COPD/asthma	Bronchodilators
	Corticosteroids
	Physiotherapy
Hypoxia	Trial of oxygen
Obstruction of trachea, bronchus	Corticosteroids
	LASER
	Radiotherapy
	Stent
SVCO	See p.239
Lymphangitis carcinomatosa	Corticosteroids
	Diuretics
	Bronchodilators
Pleural effusion	Thoracocentesis
	Drainage and pleurodesis
	See p.162
Ascites	Diuretics
	Paracentesis
Pericardial effusion	Pericardiocentesis
	Pericardotomy/pericardial window
Anaemia	Blood transfusion
Heart failure	Diuretics
	ACE inhibitors
Pulmonary embolism	Anticoagulation
Respiratory muscle weakness	Assisted ventilation, e.g. in selected patients with MND/ALS

Simple models (Figure 2) enable patients and carers to understand the vicious cycles which exacerbate breathlessness, particularly anxiety–panic, and the rationale behind non-drug approaches (Box C).

Any health professional with an interest can be trained to offer these techniques, although generally nurses, occupational therapists and physiotherapists have taken the lead. In some areas, specific breathlessness services exist.

> **Box C** Non-drug treatment of breathlessness
>
> **Exploring the perception of the patient and carers**
> What is the meaning of the breathlessness to the patient and to the carers?
> Explore anxieties, particularly fear of sudden death when breathless.
> Inform the patient and carers that breathlessness in itself is not life-threatening.
> State what is/is not likely to happen, e.g. 'You won't choke or suffocate to death'.
> Agree realistic goals; help the patient and carers adjust when progressive
> deterioration is inevitable.
> Help the patient to cope with and adjust to loss of role, abilities, etc.
>
> **Maximizing the feeling of control over breathlessness**
> Breathing control (see text).
> Relaxation techniques.
> Plan of action for acute episodes:
> • simple written instructions outlining a step-by-step plan
> • increase confidence in coping with acute episodes.
> Use of an electric fan (see text).
> Complementary therapies benefit some patients.
>
> **Maximizing functional ability**
> Encourage exertion to breathlessness to maintain fitness/reverse deconditioning
> (see text).
> Walking aids.
> Evaluation by district nurse, occupational therapist, physiotherapist and social
> worker may all be necessary to identify where additional support is required.
>
> **Reduce feelings of personal and social isolation**
> Meet others in a similar situation.
> Attendance at a day centre.
> Respite admissions.

Breathing control

Shallow, rapid breathing is an ineffective and inefficient pattern of breathing that contributes to anxiety and panic. In breathing control the patient is encouraged to take normal tidal breaths and to relax the neck, shoulders and upper chest, in order to:
• promote a relaxed and calming breathing pattern: 'Float the air in, relax the breath out'
• minimize the work of breathing
• establish a sense of control over breathing that aids confidence in coping with breathless episodes.

The main aim is to use the diaphragm rather than the accessory muscles. Ideally, patients should nose breathe and allow expiration to be passive (taking 1.5–2 times longer than inspiration) with an end expiratory pause. It can be taught as the 3 R's:

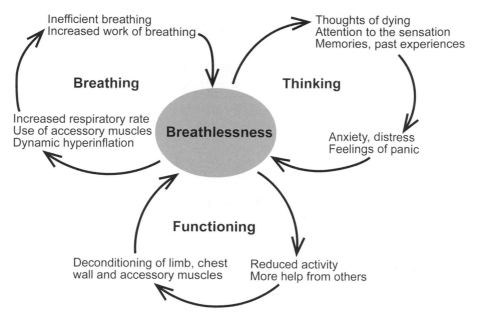

Figure 2 The 'breathing, thinking, functioning' model illustrating the vicious cycles which exacerbate breathlessness (© Cambridge Breathlessness Intervention Service, reproduced with permission)

- *Rise:* Let the tummy rise as you breathe in; take in just the air that you need
- *Relax:* Relax the tummy, relax the breath out
- *Rest:* Don't rush into the next breath, let it come naturally.

The technique is mostly used to help recover from breathlessness, but can also be used during exertion. It should be practiced for 10min each day, to aid recall when required, and as an opportunity to promote general relaxation.

Breathing control can be combined with pursed lip breathing in patients with severe COPD prone to dynamic hyperinflation. It is performed as nasal inspiration followed by expiratory blowing against partially closed lips. Some patients adopt this instinctively.

Breathing control is *not* suitable for patients with severe hyperinflation of the lungs with a flattened, weak diaphragm dependent on their accessory muscles for breathing at rest.

Positioning

Particular positions may help breathlessness in specific circumstances. Patients can be encouraged to try these out, if not already adopted instinctively. For example, patients with:
- COPD: lean forward with arms/elbows resting on the knees or a table; this increases abdominal pressure improving the efficiency of the flattened diaphragm. Bracing of the arms fixes the shoulder girdle improving the efficacy of the accessory muscles

- unilateral bronchopulmonary disease (e.g. collapse, consolidation, pleural effusion): lie on their side with the normal lung down; this maximizes ventilation–perfusion matching (this advantage is lost with a large pleural effusion).

Any patient using accessory muscles to breathe may find bracing the arms helpful. Other options include placing the arms behind the head or against a wall, and resting hands on hips, in pockets, on belt loops or a waistband.

Use of an electric fan

Many patients report benefit from a cooling draft of air directed against the face, possibly via stimulation of facial and nasopharyngeal cold-sensitive receptors.[13–15] Mostly, the fan is used in conjunction with the above techniques to ease breathlessness after exertion. It should be held about 15–20cm away from the face and directed towards the nose and mouth.

Maximizing functional ability

Breathlessness may lead to a vicious cycle of reduced activity → skeletal muscle deconditioning → increased breathlessness. Regular activity and exercise can help to reverse this, thereby improving breathlessness and function.

Explanation that, although unpleasant, breathlessness is *not* dangerous is important and that activity which induces breathlessness is to be encouraged and not avoided.

What constitutes appropriate activity and exercise is tailored according to the patient's goals, illness, performance status and prognosis, and can range from increasing the time spent walking each day to taking part in relatively intensive rehabilitation programmes, e.g. cardiac, pulmonary.

Drug treatment

Generally, symptomatic drug treatments for breathlessness are used after appropriate corrective and non-drug treatments have been fully exploited.

Bronchodilators

COPD is a major cause of breathlessness, either alone or as a co-morbidity, notably in lung cancer. However, COPD may be unrecognized, and so go untreated.

National and international guidelines for the use of bronchodilators in patients with COPD are available and generally, should be followed.[16,17] However, in palliative care, when airflow obstruction is suspected, evaluating the impact on symptoms of a 1–2 week trial of a bronchodilator is probably a more pragmatic and relevant approach than undertaking objective tests of ventilatory function.

A β_2 agonist ± an antimuscarinic, inhaled via a spacer or nebulizer, improves breathlessness in most lung cancer patients with COPD.[18,19] Both classes of drug improve breathlessness by airway bronchodilation and/or reducing air-trapping at rest (static hyperinflation) and on exertion (dynamic hyperinflation). A reduction in hyperinflation probably explains the clinical benefit even with little or no change in the FEV_1. Patients should be encouraged to take a p.r.n. dose of a short-acting β_2 agonist prior to exertion.

For patients in the last weeks or days of life, particularly those having difficulties with metered-dose inhalers, the regular use of short-acting nebulized bronchodilators may be preferable.

If a patient is receiving long-term corticosteroids for another indication (see p.365), it is often possible to discontinue inhaled corticosteroids.

Opioids

Generally, opioids are more beneficial in patients who are breathless at rest than in those who are breathless only on exertion. Even with maximal exertion, breathlessness generally recovers within a few minutes, much quicker than it takes to administer and benefit from an opioid. Thus, non-drug measures are of primary importance for exertional breathlessness (see p.148).

Systematic reviews consistently support the use of opioids by oral and parenteral routes, but *not* by nebulizer.[20–22]

Morphine and other opioids reduce the ventilatory response to hypercapnia, hypoxia and exercise, decreasing respiratory effort and breathlessness. Improvements are seen at doses that do *not* cause respiratory depression. In opioid-naïve patients:
- start with small doses of morphine, e.g. 2.5–5mg PO p.r.n.; larger doses can be poorly tolerated
- if ≥2 doses/24h are needed, prescribe morphine regularly and titrate the dose according to response, duration of effect and undesirable effects
- relatively small doses may suffice, e.g. 20–60mg/24h.[22–24]

In patients already taking morphine for pain and with:
- severe breathlessness (i.e. ≥7/10), a dose that is 100% or more of the q4h analgesic dose may be needed
- moderate breathlessness (i.e. 4–6/10), a dose equivalent to 50–100% of the q4h analgesic dose may suffice
- mild breathlessness (i.e. ≤3/10), a dose equivalent to 25–50% of the q4h analgesic dose may suffice.

However, as with pain, individual titration is required for optimal benefit. In some patients, morphine by CSCI is better tolerated and provides greater relief, possibly by avoiding the peaks (with undesirable effects) and troughs (with loss of effect) of oral medication. If using an alternative opioid to morphine, adopt the same approach as above.

Opioids are also used in patients with severe COPD who have distressing breathlessness despite usual treatments. A low-dose and slow titration is generally advocated, e.g.:[25]
- start with morphine 1mg PO b.d., increasing to 1–2.5mg q4h over one week
- thereafter, increase dose by 25% each week until satisfactory relief obtained
- when a stable dose is found, consider switching to a m/r formulation.

Oxygen

Despite the widespread use of oxygen to relieve breathlessness, most studies show *no* additional benefit from oxygen compared with medical air delivered by nasal prongs.[26]

This suggests that a sensation of airflow is an important determinant of benefit. Thus, patients should be encouraged to test the benefit of a cool draught from a portable or hand-held fan (see p.152).

National guidelines recommend that, in palliative care patients, oxygen should be restricted to those with severe hypoxaemia (e.g. SpO_2 ≤90%) or those who report significant relief of breathlessness from oxygen. In non-hypoxaemic patients, non-drug approaches and opioids should be tried before oxygen.[27]

The appropriate concentration varies with the underlying condition and the dose is generally titrated to achieve near normoxaemia (SpO_2 of 94–98%) which is associated with better outcomes than hyperoxaemia.[27]

Inappropriate prescription can have serious or fatal effects, e.g. in patients with hypercapnic ventilatory failure who are dependent upon hypoxia for their respiratory drive a lower target SpO_2 should be used (88–92%). These patients should *not* be given a high concentration.

When death is imminent, in the absence of respiratory distress, oxygen should *not* be routinely used even for severe hypoxaemia. Further, in most of those already receiving oxygen, it is possible to discontinue it without causing distress.[28]

Anxiolytics

If a patient is severely disabled by anxiety or panic attacks, consider if a pathological anxiety, panic or depression disorder exists, which requires more specific therapy, e.g. an antidepressant.

Because of the association between breathlessness and anxiety, reducing anxiety is likely to help a patient cope better.

Non-drug approaches to managing anxiety ± panic attacks should be considered before drug approaches (see p.189), particularly as:

- unlike opioids, anxiolytics probably do not have a specific anti-breathlessness effect[29]
- panic attacks generally settle within minutes, much quicker than the time it takes to administer and benefit from an anxiolytic.

If, despite non-drug approaches and morphine, the patient remains very anxious, either a benzodiazepine or an SSRI is used depending on prognosis:

- benzodiazepine, if prognosis is <2–4 weeks, e.g. diazepam 2–10mg PO at bedtime and p.r.n. or lorazepam 0.5–1mg PO b.d. and p.r.n.
- SSRI (± a benzodiazepine initially), if prognosis is >2–4 weeks, e.g. citalopram 10mg PO each morning.

Midazolam with an opioid is of particular benefit in relieving terminal breathlessness (see p.277).

Antipsychotics have an anxiolytic (but not a specific anti-panic effect) as well as an antipsychotic effect. They are helpful in patients who are anxious and delirious. Haloperidol is the antipsychotic of choice and is without significant respiratory depressant effects.

COUGH

Coughing helps clear the central airways of foreign matter, secretions or pus and should generally be encouraged. It is pathological when:
- ineffective, e.g. dry or unproductive
- it adversely affects sleep, rest, eating, or social activities
- it causes other symptoms such as muscle strain, rib fracture, vomiting, syncope, headache, or urinary incontinence.

Cough effectiveness is reduced by factors which:
- decrease expiratory pressure and airflow, i.e. respiratory or abdominal muscle weakness
- increase mucus tenacity, i.e. reduce the water content of secretions
- decrease mucociliary function, e.g. smoking, infection.

In patients with cancer, the prevalence of cough is 50–80%, and is highest in patients with lung cancer. An acute cough is defined as one lasting <3 weeks, a chronic cough >8 weeks.

Pathogenesis

Cough is caused by mechanical and/or chemical stimulation of:
- rapidly adapting myelinated stretch ('irritant') and C-fibre receptors in the airway
- other structures innervated by the vagi, trigeminal and phrenic nerves.

Afferent input terminates in the brain stem. Input from higher centres allows cough to be voluntarily induced or suppressed.

Gastric reflux can cause cough via a vagally-mediated bronchoconstrictor reflex or by aspiration into the airways. Typical symptoms of reflux are often absent and coughing may occur predominantly during the day when upright.

In COPD, cough is caused by inflammation and/or the need to eliminate large volumes of bronchial secretions. Because ciliary clearance of mucus is slow in COPD, coughing helps to clear secretions even if it seems non-productive.

ACE inhibitors cause a dry cough in <10% of patients either immediately or after weeks–months of use. Confirmation of the diagnosis is by resolution of the cough within 4 weeks of discontinuing the ACE inhibitor.

Sensitization of the cough reflex appears important in chronic cough of various causes.

Evaluation

The commonest cause of acute cough is respiratory tract infection (Box D). In advanced cancer, chronic cough is most likely caused by endobronchial tumour within the central airways.

Box D Causes of cough

Cardiopulmonary
Asthma
Chest infection
COPD
Heart failure
Smoking
Tracheo-oesophageal fistula
Tumour
   endobronchial
      airway infiltration, distortion,
      obstruction
   lung parenchyma
      airway distortion, obstruction
      lymphangitis carcinomatosis
   mediastinum
   pleura, pericardium
   pleural effusion
Upper airway cough syndrome
   (post-nasal drip)
Vocal cord paralysis

Oesophageal
Gastro-oesophageal reflux

Aspiration
Bulbar muscle weakness
Gastro-oesophageal reflux
Neuromuscular inco-ordination

Treatment
ACE inhibitors
ß-Blockers
Chemotherapy, e.g.
   bleomycin, methotrexate,
   cyclophosphamide
Nitrofurantoin
Radiotherapy, dose-related
   pneumonitis in 5–15% (early onset)
   fibrosis (late onset, >6 months)

Is the cough wet or dry?

A wet cough generally serves a physiological purpose and expectoration should be encouraged. A dry cough serves no purpose and should be suppressed. A wet cough distressing a dying patient who is too weak to expectorate should also be suppressed with antitussives.

Is the cough caused by the cancer?

It is generally obvious when the cough is caused by the cancer. Associated features such as episodic wheezing (asthma) or heartburn (gastro-oesophageal reflux) suggest an alternative cause. Appropriate investigations may include:
- chest radiograph
- sputum culture
- induced sputum to detect airway eosinophilia
- spirometry (pre- and post-bronchodilator)

- laryngoscopy
- bronchoscopy
- CT of thorax.

Common causes, alone or in combination, include:
- upper airway cough syndrome (post-nasal drip)
- asthma
- gastro-oesophageal reflux
- COPD.

Can the cancer be modified?

Radiotherapy (teletherapy or endobronchial brachytherapy) improves cough in 50–60% of patients. Other options may include chemotherapy, hormone therapy or surgery. If in doubt, seek advice from an oncologist.

Can the impact of the cancer be modified?

For example, by draining a pleural effusion.

Management

Correct the correctable (cause-specific treatment)

Ideally, treatment should be directed at the underlying cause (Table 2).

Non-drug treatment (wet cough)

- advise how to cough efficiently; it is impossible to cough effectively lying on your back
- physiotherapy
- steam inhalations.

A forced expiration (a huff) from a low–medium lung volume:
- is effective in clearing secretions
- is better tolerated than the assisted cough manoeuvre (involves compressing the lower thorax and abdomen with the hands)
- requires less effort for the patient
- can be augmented by postural drainage.

Drug treatment

Protussives (expectorants) make coughing more effective and less distressing by making secretions less tenacious; antitussives reduce the intensity and frequency of coughing by suppressing the cough reflex.

Wet cough

Various types of protussives are available:
- *nebulized saline* 0.9%: 2.5mL q.d.s. and p.r.n., and before physiotherapy
- *irritant mucolytic*: produces a greater volume of less tenacious secretions, e.g. guaifenesin, ipecacuanha
- *chemical mucolytic*: reduces the viscosity of secretions, e.g. carbocisteine 750mg t.d.s., reduced to b.d. once satisfactory response obtained.

Table 2 Correctable causes of cough

Cause	Treatment
Smoking	Stop smoking; median time to improvement is 4 weeks
Post-nasal drip	
allergic rhinitis	Nasal corticosteroid ± sodium cromoglicate
	Antihistamine; second-generation antihistamines are non-sedating but are less drying than the older sedative antimuscarinic antihistamines
perennial and post-infection rhinitis	Antihistamine ± decongestant
vasomotor rhinitis	Nasal ipratropium bromide
bacterial sinusitis	Antibacterial ± decongestant ± nasal corticosteroid (acute) ± antihistamine (chronic)
Asthma	Bronchodilators ± corticosteroids
COPD	Stop smoking
	Bronchodilators, e.g. ipratropium bromide
	Corticosteroids (specific circumstances)
Gastro-oesophageal reflux	Avoid coffee, smoking or drugs which decrease lower oesophageal sphincter tone
	Prokinetic agent, increases oesophageal sphincter tone
	PPI to reduce gastric acid
ACE inhibitor	Discontinue the ACE inhibitor; if not possible, substitute an angiotensin-II receptor antagonist, e.g. losartan

Nebulized hypertonic saline (3–7%) is used in cystic fibrosis, and this is extending to other conditions, e.g. bronchiectasis. Further specialist options are authorized for use in cystic fibrosis, e.g. dornase alpha, mannitol.

With a wet cough, an antitussive may be necessary to ensure sleep at night and to prevent exhaustion during the day. When used during the day (in conjunction with a protussive), the aim is to make expectoration more effective and less tiring.

Dry cough

Antitussives can be divided into peripherally-acting demulcents and centrally-acting opioids. Treatment typically starts with a demulcent, adding an opioid if necessary.

Demulcents contain soothing substances such as glycerol or syrup (e.g. simple linctus BP 5mL t.d.s.–q.d.s.). The high sugar content stimulates the production of saliva and soothes the oropharynx. The associated swallowing may also interfere with the cough reflex.

Opioids act primarily by suppressing the cough reflex centre in the brain stem. They are less effective for cough due to upper airway disorders, e.g. upper respiratory tract infection, possibly because laryngeal cough involves opioid-insensitive central mechanisms and/or reflects a different reflex (i.e. an expiration reflex).

Codeine, pholcodine and dextromethorphan are common ingredients in combination antitussive products but often in small and probably ineffective doses. Thus, the benefit of combination products may reside mainly in the sugar content (a demulcent effect).

For opioid-naïve patients, consider:
- codeine (linctus or tablet) 15–30mg (5–10mL) t.d.s.–q.d.s.
- if not effective, switch to morphine, starting with:
  ▷ an *immediate-release* formulation 5–10mg q.d.s.–q4h (but 2.5–5mg q.d.s.–q4h if not switching from codeine) *or*
  ▷ a *modified-release* formulation 10–20mg b.d. (but 5–10mg b.d. if not switching from codeine)
- if necessary, increase the dose until the cough is relieved or until undesirable effects prevent further escalation.

If a patient is already receiving a strong opioid for pain relief it is a nonsense to prescribe codeine or a second strong opioid as well. If opioid antitussives are unsatisfactory, specialist advice should be obtained.

For analgesia in palliative care, strong opioids are increasingly preferred over weak opioids; the same rationale can be applied to antitussives (see p.326).

The MHRA has advised against the use of OTC cough products containing codeine for the under 18s, and dextromethorphan and pholcodine for the under 6s.

If opioid antitussives are unsatisfactory, other possible treatments include:
- sodium cromoglicate 10mg inhaled q.d.s. improves cough in patients with lung cancer within 36–48h[30]
- gabapentin 300mg PO t.d.s. increased up to 600mg PO t.d.s is more effective than placebo in idiopathic chronic cough;[31] case reports have used smaller starting doses, e.g. 100mg PO b.d.[32]
- diazepam e.g. 5mg PO once daily/at bedtime is reported to have an effect in intractable cough associated with lung metastases[33]
- baclofen 10mg PO t.d.s. or 20mg PO once daily has an antitussive effect in healthy volunteers and in patients with ACE inhibitor cough; maximum effect is seen after 2–4 weeks.[34]

Amitriptyline and pregabalin are also effective in idiopathic chronic cough. Thus, drugs with CNS inhibitory effects probably act by interfering with the cough reflex and/or central sensitization which leads to cough hypersensitivity, present in most patients with chronic cough.

HAEMOPTYSIS

Haemoptysis is the expectoration of blood originating from the lower respiratory tract. Generally, it is self-limiting and small volume. Rarely, massive haemoptysis occurs which may be life-threatening, generally because of suffocation rather than exsanguination (see p.249).[35]

The lungs have two blood supplies:
- low-pressure pulmonary circulation which supplies blood for gas exchange
- high-pressure bronchial circulation which supplies blood to the structures of the respiratory tract; this is more important in haemoptysis.

Causes

There are many potential causes of haemoptysis (Box E). Common causes of massive haemoptysis include:
- lung cancer
- bronchiectasis
- fungal infections
- tuberculosis.

Box E Causes of haemoptysis

Cancer	**Cardiovascular**
Primary lung	Aortobronchial fistula
Lung metastases	Arteriovenous malformation
Haematological	Congestive heart failure
	Mitral stenosis
Lung disease	Pulmonary embolus
COPD	Pulmonary hypertension
Cystic fibrosis	Vasculitis, e.g. polyangiitis
Pneumoconiosis	
Pulmonary fibrosis	**Other**
Sarcoidosis	Anticoagulation
	Bleeding disorders
Lung infection	Immune disorders
Abscess	Trauma
Bronchiectasis	
Bronchitis	
Fungal, e.g. aspergilloma	
Pneumonia	
Tuberculosis	

About 20% of patients with lung cancer experience haemoptysis at some point; in 3% it is fatal. Massive haemoptysis is most likely with squamous cell cancer lying centrally or causing cavitation.

In haematological cancers, haemoptysis is associated with fungal infection.

Evaluation

The history and examination generally indicate the probable source of the bleeding. It is important to differentiate haemoptysis from bleeding from the pharynx or upper GI tract. When necessary, confirmatory tests include chest radiograph, CT thorax, CT angiography, bronchoscopy.

Management

Validate the patient's concern, i.e. never say, 'Don't worry about it', but 'I'm glad you mentioned it, I imagine you must be very concerned about it'.

With mild–moderate haemoptysis, assure patients that, although upsetting and unpleasant, it is rarely life-threatening.

Correct the correctable

When possible, treatment should be cause-specific. Consider if there are aggravating factors which can be modified:
- exclude a bleeding diathesis (check PT, APTT, FBC)
- review use of anticoagulants: stop if possible
- switch from a non-selective NSAID to paracetamol or an NSAID which does not impair platelet function (see p.324).

Non-drug treatment

Radiotherapy leads to prolonged relief in about 70% of patients with cancer-related haemoptysis. Palliative external beam radiation is generally given as 1–2 treatments, which permits retreatment if necessary. Patients with a good performance status may be offered a higher dose.

For patients with unrelieved or recurrent haemoptysis in whom further external beam radiation is not possible, other options will vary according to local availability and include:
- brachytherapy (endobronchial radiation)
- cryotherapy
- LASER therapy
- radiofrequency ablation.

Arterial embolization (e.g. of the bronchial artery) is used as a first-line treatment, e.g. for massive haemoptysis and arteriovenous malformation, and also for recurrent haemoptysis which does not settle with other treatments.[36,37]

Drug treatment

Tranexamic acid is an antifibrinolytic which may reduce the volume and duration of mild–moderate haemoptysis:[38]
- 1.5g PO stat and 1g t.d.s.
- if bleeding not subsiding after 3 days, increase dose to 1.5–2g t.d.s.
- manufacturer's recommended maximum dose = 1.5g t.d.s.

- in practice, doses of ≤2g q.d.s. have been used
- discontinue I week after cessation of bleeding or reduce to 500mg t.d.s.
- restart if bleeding occurs, and possibly continue indefinitely.

Other options include nebulized tranexamic acid, e.g. use standard undiluted 500mg/5mL ampoule for injection t.d.s–q.d.s.[39,40]

PLEURAL EFFUSION

A small amount of fluid (20–30mL) is present in the pleural space for lubrication. It is produced by capillaries and removed by lymphatics at a rate of 100–200mL/24h. A pleural effusion forms as a result of excess production and/or reduced resorption of fluid.

Effusions are classified as exudates or transudates (Table 3). Exudates develop when permeability of the pleural surface and/or capillaries is increased; transudates when hydrostatic forces favour pleural fluid accumulation.

Lung and breast cancer account for 2/3 of malignant pleural effusions.[41] Over 95% are exudates. Haemorrhagic effusions generally result from invasion of blood vessels or cancer-related angiogenesis.

Pleural effusions are present in up to 50% of patients with pulmonary emboli. About 90% are small (i.e. <1/3 of the hemithorax) and ipsilateral, contralateral or bilateral to the embolus. A high index of clinical suspicion is required, with CT pulmonary angiography the investigation of choice.

Table 3 Classification of pleural fluid (Light's criteria)[42]

	Exudate	Transudate
Distinguishing features		
Pleural fluid:serum protein ratio	>0.5	<0.5
Pleural fluid LDH	>2/3 the upper limit of normal serum concentration	<2/3 the upper limit of normal serum concentration
Pleural fluid:serum LDH ratio	>0.6	<0.6
Common causes		
	Cancer Pneumonia Tuberculosis	Cirrhosis Left ventricular failure

Pleural effusions cause breathlessness as a result of lung compression, causing ventilation–perfusion mismatch and hypoxia. There may also be associated cough and chest pain.

Evaluation

The history, physical examination and chest radiograph help to indicate when a diagnostic pleural fluid aspiration is needed to confirm the cause of a probable exudate.

For bilateral effusions in the presence of a known cause of a transudate, e.g. left ventricular failure, diagnostic pleural fluid aspiration is *not* needed unless there are atypical features or a failure to respond to treatment of the underlying cause.

Note: exudative effusions have been reported with commonly used drugs, e.g. amiodarone, ß-blockers, methotrexate, nitrofurantoin and phenytoin.

Diagnostic imaging includes:
- *chest radiograph*: detects an effusion >200mL
- *ultrasound*: increasingly undertaken at the bedside to:
  ▷ distinguish pleural fluid from thickening, exudates from transudates and malignant from benign effusions
  ▷ guide pleural fluid aspiration; safer and higher success rate than 'blind' aspiration
- *CT scan*: contrast-enhanced undertaken:
  ▷ in undiagnosed exudative pleural effusion (before complete fluid drainage)
  ▷ to help distinguish malignant from benign pleural thickening
  ▷ in complicated pleural infection, i.e. failed tube drainage and requiring surgery.

Pleural fluid aspiration is undertaken with a fine-bore (21G) needle and a 50mL syringe. As a minimum, samples are sent for:
- cytology (20–40mL); diagnostic in about 60% of malignant effusions
- Gram stain and microbiological culture (5mL)
- biochemistry: protein, LDH (2–5mL).

Serum total protein and LDH are also measured to apply Light's criteria to distinguish between a transudate and an exudate (Table 3).

Note: diuretic therapy increases pleural protein and LDH, and can result in a transudate being wrongly classified as an exudate. A raised BNP will help to confirm heart failure as the cause of the effusion.

Depending on the suspected cause of the effusion, additional tests may be undertaken on the pleural fluid, e.g.:
- pancreatitis → amylase
- haemothorax → haematocrit
- infection (when fluid non-purulent) → pH
- rheumatoid arthritis → glucose.[42]

The predominance of certain cells in the effusion, e.g. lymphocytes, neutrophils, eosinophils, may help narrow the differential diagnosis, but none are disease-specific. The appearance and odour of the pleural fluid can also be diagnostically helpful (Table 4).

Table 4 Diagnostically useful pleural fluid characteristics

Characteristic	Probable diagnosis
'Anchovy sauce' appearance	Ruptured amoebic abscess
Bile-stained	Biliary fistula
Contains food particles	Perforated oesophagus
Milky appearance	Chylothorax/pseudochylothorax
Putrid odour	Anaerobic empyema

When cancer is suspected but pleural aspiration is inconclusive, thoracoscopy under local or general anaesthetic is the investigation of choice; it has a high diagnostic yield and is therapeutic, e.g. drainage ± talc pleurodesis.

Management

Treatment should be cause-specific and advice sought from the relevant specialists.

The focus of this section is malignant pleural effusion; advice should be sought from the thoracic cancer multidisciplinary team.

Treatment options (Table 5) are influenced by the:
- severity of symptoms
- patient's performance status/prognosis
- likelihood of response to systemic therapy (e.g. chemo-, biological and hormonal therapies)
- degree of lung re-expansion following drainage of pleural fluid.

Pleural aspiration and drain insertion should be undertaken under ultrasound guidance, unless the clinical situation contra-indicates, e.g. severe symptoms in a frail patient too unwell to move. However, portable scanners for use at the bedside are increasingly available.

Both pleural aspiration and drain insertion may lead to pneumothorax, haemothorax, empyema, fluid loculation (making further intervention difficult) and cancer seeding in the chest wall. Complications of indwelling catheters include cellulitis and cancer seeding along the catheter tract.

As soon as a chest radiograph confirms fluid drainage and lung re-expansion, pleurodesis should be undertaken (Box F). Suction may rarely be required for incomplete lung expansion and a persistent air leak. A high-volume, low-pressure system is used with gradual increase in pressure to about −20mmHg. Persistent incomplete lung re-expansion may relate to trapped lung, caused by:
- a thick visceral peel
- pleural loculations
- proximal large airway obstruction
- a persistent pneumothorax.

Patients with persistent incomplete lung re-expansion should be considered for thoracoscopy (see below). Fibrinolytic agents (e.g. streptokinase) are sometimes instilled to break down pleural loculations and improve drainage.

In patients with mesothelioma, prophylactic radiotherapy should be given to the site of thoracoscopy, surgery or large-bore chest tube insertion to reduce the likelihood of seeding and local recurrence.

Table 5 Treatment options for malignant pleural effusion[41]

Treatment	Indication	Comments
Monitor only	Small, asymptomatic effusion	
Pleural aspiration	Prognosis <4 weeks and/or patient frail. Widely available, well tolerated and can be undertaken as an outpatient.	Repeat treatments likely because 1.5L is maximum removed (stop if cough, chest pain develop) and short time to recurrence (50% within 4 days; 97% within 4 weeks).
Intercostal small-bore (10–14F) tube drainage + talc slurry	Prognosis >4 weeks. Requires inpatient admission.	To avoid re-expansion pulmonary oedema, drainage of a large pleural effusion is done incrementally; a maximum of 1.5L is removed at 2h intervals, stopping if cough, chest pain or vasovagal symptoms develop. Following drainage, talc is instilled to cause pleurodesis and achieve long-term control (>80%). Pleurodesis is unlikely to succeed when trapped lung results in incomplete re-expansion and >50% of unopposed pleura.
Thoracoscopy + talc poudrage	Patients with a good performance status, prognosis >4 weeks, and who still require a diagnosis. Requires inpatient admission and either sedation or general anaesthesia depending on technique used.	Following drainage, atomized talc is applied (poudrage) to cause pleurodesis and achieve long-term control (>80%). Loculations, blood clots and adhesions can be removed to aid lung re-expansion and optimize success from talc poudrage. Conversely, can identify instances of trapped lung unlikely to respond to pleurodesis which will require an indwelling catheter.
Ambulatory long-term indwelling pleural catheter, e.g. Pleurx®	Preferred option for patients unsuitable for pleurodesis (e.g. trapped lung preventing re-expansion) and those with recurrent effusion following 1–2 episodes of drainage and pleurodesis.	Inserted under local anaesthesia, and patients and carers instructed on how to drain off small amounts at regular intervals using vacuum bottles. Symptoms controlled in 90%. The irritant effect of the tube may contribute to a 'spontaneous' pleurodesis seen in ≤75% of patients after 1–2 months, allowing removal.

Box F Pleurodesis with talc slurry following tube drainage[41]

Talc is a cheap, widely available and effective sclerosant. It induces inflammation and activation of the coagulation system in the pleural space producing fibrin. This leads to adhesion of the pleural layers, thereby obliterating the pleural space.

Undesirable effects include chest pain and fever.

Undertake pleurodesis as soon as a chest radiograph confirms fluid drainage and lung re-expansion (irrespective of the amount of pleural fluid draining/24h).

If lung re-expansion is incomplete, pleurodesis can be attempted provided <50% of unapposed pleura.

Pain should be managed by:
• premedication with a systemic opioid ± benzodiazepine 10min before the pleurodesis, to achieve a level of sedation which does not interfere with the patient's ability to communicate or co-operate (monitor with pulse oximetry, ensure resuscitation equipment available), together with
• the instillation into the pleural space of lidocaine solution (3mg/kg; up to a maximum of 250mg, i.e. 25mL of lidocaine 1%) just before the talc.

Instil sterile graded talc 4–5g in 50mL 0.9% normal saline (the 'slurry').

Clamp tube for 1h. It is not necessary to rotate the patient.

Remove tube within 24–48h provided:
• a chest radiograph confirms the lung remains re-expanded and satisfactory fluid drainage
• pleural fluid drainage is <250mL/24h.

If the effusion subsequently recurs, either repeat tube drainage and pleurodesis or insert an indwelling pleural catheter depending upon the presence of trapped lung (see text).

HICCUP

A hiccup is a spontaneous myoclonic contraction of the diaphragm (unilateral > bilateral) ± intercostal muscles. This causes sudden inspiration and the associated abrupt closure of the glottis produces the characteristic sound.

The components of the hiccup reflex arc include:
• phrenic, vagal and sympathetic nervous system afferents
• diffuse 'hiccup centre' in midbrain, brainstem and proximal cervical cord
• phrenic, intercostal and vagal efferents.

Although generally transient (<48h), hiccup can be persistent (<1 month) or intractable (>1 month) and result in significant distress from disturbed sleep, exhaustion and increased debility.[43]

Causes

A wide range of conditions stimulate the reflex arc to produce hiccup (Box G). Most cases probably relate to:

- gastric distension   most common
- gastro-oesophageal reflux   ↓
- diaphragmatic irritation   ↓
- phrenic nerve irritation.   less common

Box G Causes of hiccup (selected list)[43,44]

CNS
Epilepsy
Multiple sclerosis
Parkinson's disease
Psychological
Stroke
Trauma
Tumour

Head and neck
Goitre
Inflammation/infection
Tumour (e.g. cancer, cyst)
Tympanic membrane irritation

Thoracic
Aortic aneurysm
Infection/pneumonia
Myocardial infarction
Pericarditis
Phrenic nerve irritation
Tumour

Abdominal
Bowel obstruction
Cholecystitis
Diaphragmatic irritation
Gastric distension
Gastro-oesophageal reflux
Gastritis/peptic ulceration
Pancreatitis
Tumour

Metabolic
Biochemical derangement
Hyperglycaemia
Hypo-adrenalism
Hypocapnia

Drugs
Alcohol
Benzodiazepines
Corticosteroids (e.g. IV dexamethasone)
Dopamine agonists (e.g. apomorphine)
Opioids

Evaluation

On the basis of probability and pattern recognition, after explanation to the patient, it generally makes sense to proceed to a trial of therapy (see below).

Rarely, a more thorough diagnostic evaluation may be necessary, e.g.:

- CT of thorax and abdomen
- upper GI endoscopy
- oesophageal manometry and pH monitoring
- MRI of head and neck.

Management

There is limited high-quality evidence to guide management.[43,45]

Correct the correctable

Identify and treat the underlying cause when possible.

Advise patients with possible gastric distension or delayed gastric emptying to consider adopting the equivalent of a 'small stomach' or post-gastrectomy approach to eating and drinking, i.e. 'small and often', separating the main food from the main fluid intake.

Non-drug treatment

This includes traditional 'folk' remedies and other manoeuvres which interrupt or suppress the hiccup reflex by stimulating the pharynx (Box H).[43] They may be worth considering for transient hiccup.

Box H Non-drug treatment of transient hiccup

Nasal or oropharyngeal stimulation
- inhalation of 'smelling salts'
- rapidly ingest two heaped teaspoons of granulated sugar or two glasses of liqueur
- swallow dry bread or crushed ice
- massage of the junction between hard and soft palate with a cotton bob
- forceful tongue traction sufficient to induce a gag reflex.

Indirect stimulation of the pharynx (via hyperextension of the neck):
- drink from the wrong side of a cup (or sitting 'doubled up' and drinking water)
- a cold key dropped inside the back of the person's shirt or blouse.

Vagal stimulation
- cold compress to face
- carotid sinus massage
- induced fright.

Respiratory manoeuvres
- breath holding
- rebreathing from a paper bag (hypercapnia)
- Valsalva manoeuvres.

Drug treatment

When possible this should be cause-specific. When the cause is unknown, or extensive evaluation is not appropriate (e.g. frail patient with a poor prognosis), proceed on the basis of common things occur commonly and prescribe metoclopramide and an antiflatulent or PPI for possible gastric distension or acid reflux.

If the above fails, consider a switch to a central suppressant (Table 6). Based on available evidence and tolerability, baclofen or gabapentin are reasonable first-line central suppressants.[43]

Table 6 Drug treatment of hiccup (PO unless stated otherwise)

Class of drug	Drug	Acute relief	Maintenance regimen
Reduce gastric distension ± gastro-oesophageal reflux			
Antiflatulent (carminative)	Peppermint water[a,b]	10mL	Probably best used p.r.n. only
Antiflatulent (defoaming agent)	Simeticone, e.g. in Altacite Plus®	10mL	10mL q.d.s.
Prokinetic	Metoclopramide[b,c]	10mg	10mg t.d.s.–q.d.s.
PPI	Lansoprazole	30mg	30mg each morning
Central suppression of the hiccup reflex			
First-line options			
GABA agonist	Baclofen	5mg	5–20mg t.d.s., occasionally more
Anti-epileptic	Gabapentin	'Burst gabapentin', i.e. 400mg t.d.s. for 3 days, then 400mg once daily for 3 days, then stop; repeat if necessary[d]	400mg t.d.s.
Second-line option			
Dopamine antagonist	Metoclopramide	As above	As above
Third-line options			
Calcium-channel blocker	Nifedipine	10mg PO/SL	10–20mg t.d.s., occasionally more
Anti-epileptic	Sodium valproate	200–500mg	15mg/kg/24h in divided doses
Dopamine antagonist	Haloperidol	5–10mg PO or IV if no response	1.5–3mg at bedtime
Benzodiazepine	Midazolam	2mg IV, followed by 1–2mg increments every 3–5min	10–60mg/24h by CSCI if patient in last days of life

a. facilitates belching by relaxing the lower oesophageal sphincter; an old-fashioned remedy; can result in gastro-oesophageal reflux
b. peppermint water and metoclopramide should not be used concurrently because of their opposing actions on the gastro-oesophageal sphincter
c. tightens the lower oesophageal sphincter and hastens gastric emptying
d. a smaller dose advisable in elderly frail patients and those with renal impairment, e.g. start with 100mg t.d.s.

The choice of central suppressant may be influenced by other symptoms the patient may be experiencing, e.g.:

- nausea $\rightarrow$ metoclopramide
- nerve pain $\rightarrow$ gabapentin
- muscle spasm $\rightarrow$ baclofen.

Although chlorpromazine and haloperidol are licensed for the treatment of hiccup, other options with potentially fewer undesirable effects, particularly long-term, should be used in preference.

REFERENCES

1 American Thoracic Society (2012) Update on the mechanisms, assessment and management of dyspnea. *American Journal of Respiratory and Critical Care Medicine*. **185:** 435–452.
2 O'Driscoll M *et al.* (1999) The experience of breathlessness in lung cancer. *European Journal of Cancer Care*. **8:** 37–43.
3 Henoch I *et al.* (2008) Dyspnea experience and management strategies in patients with lung cancer. *Psychooncology*. **17:** 709–715.
4 Wilcock A *et al.* (2008) Symptoms limiting activity in cancer patients with breathlessness on exertion: ask about muscle fatigue. *Thorax*. **63:** 91–92.
5 Solano J *et al.* (2006) A comparison of symptom prevalence in far advanced cancer, AIDS, heart disease, chronic obstructive pulmonary disease and renal disease. *Journal of Pain and Symptom Management*. **31:** 58–69.
6 Reuben DB and Mor V (1986) Dyspnoea in terminally ill cancer patients. *Chest*. **89:** 234–236.
7 Reuben DB *et al.* (1988) Clinical symptoms and length of survival in patients with terminal cancer. *Archives of Internal Medicine*. **148:** 1586–1591.
8 Dudgeon D and Lertzman M (1999) Dyspnea in the advanced cancer patient. *Journal of Pain and Symptom Management*. **16:** 212–219.
9 Bruera E *et al.* (2000) The frequency and correlates of dyspnea in patients with advanced cancer. *Journal of Pain and Symptom Management*. **19:** 357–362.
10 Dudgeon DJ *et al.* (2001) Physiological changes and clinical correlations of dyspnea in cancer outpatients. *Journal of Pain and Symptom Management*. **21:** 373–379.
11 Thompson E *et al.* (2005) Non-invasive interventions for improving well-being and quality of life in patients with lung cancer–a systematic review of the evidence. *Lung Cancer*. **50:** 163–176.
12 Zhao I and Yates P (2008) Non-pharmacological interventions for breathlessness management in patients with lung cancer: a systematic review. *Palliative Medicine*. **22:** 693–701.
13 Farquhar MC *et al.* (2014) Is a specialist breathlessness service more effective and cost-effective for patients with advanced cancer and their carers than standard care? Findings of a mixed-method randomised controlled trial. *BMC Medicine*. **12:** 194.
14 Bausewein C *et al.* (2010) Effectiveness of a hand-held fan for breathlessness: a randomised phase II trial. *BMC Palliative Care*. **9:** 22.
15 Galbraith S *et al.* (2010) Does the use of a handheld fan improve chronic dyspnea? A randomized, controlled, crossover trial. *Journal of Pain and Symptom Management*. **39:** 831–838.
16 NICE (2010) Chronic obstructive pulmonary disease: management of chronic obstructive pulmonary disease in adults in primary and secondary care. *Clinical Guideline*. CG101. www.nice.org.uk

17 NHLBI/WHO (2013) Global Initiative for Chronic Obstructive Lung Disease. Global strategy for the diagnosis, management and prevention of chronic obstructive pulmonary disease. www.goldcopd.com

18 Congleton J and Muers MF (1995) The incidence of airflow obstruction in bronchial carcinoma, its relation to breathlessness, and response to bronchodilator therapy. *Respiratory Medicine.* **89:** 291–296.

19 Janssens J-P *et al.* (2000) Management of dyspnea in severe chronic obstructive pulmonary disease. *Journal of Pain and Symptom Management.* **19:** 378–392.

20 Jennings A *et al.* (2002) A systematic review of the use of opioids in the management of dyspnoea. *Thorax.* **57:** 939–944.

21 Brown SJ *et al.* (2005) Nebulized morphine for relief of dyspnea due to chronic lung disease. *Annals of Pharmacotherapy.* **39:** 1088–1092.

22 Vargas-Bermudez A *et al.* (2015) Opioids for the management of dyspnea in cancer patients: evidence of the last 15 years-A systematic review. *Journal of Pain and Palliative Care Pharmacotherapy.* **29:** 341–352.

23 Abernethy AP *et al.* (2003) Randomised, double blind, placebo controlled crossover trial of sustained release morphine for the management of refractory dyspnoea. *British Medical Journal.* **327:** 523–528.

24 Poole PJ *et al.* (1998) The effect of sustained-release morphine on breathlessness and quality of life in severe chronic obstructive pulmonary disease. *American Journal of Respiratory and Critical Care Medicine.* **157:** 1877–1880.

25 Rocker G *et al.* (2009) Palliation of dyspnoea in advanced COPD: revisiting a role for opioids. *Thorax.* **64:** 910–915.

26 Johnson MJ *et al.* (2013) The evidence base for oxygen for chronic refractory breathlessness: issues, gaps, and a future work plan. *Journal of Pain and Symptom Management.* **45:** 763–775.

27 British Thoracic Society (2015) Guidelines for oxygen use in adults in healthcare and emergency settings (v30 released for public consultation).

28 Campbell ML *et al.* (2013) Oxygen is nonbeneficial for most patients who are near death. *Journal of Pain and Symptom Management.* **45:** 517–523.

29 Awan S and Wilcock A (2015) Nonopioid medication for the relief of refractory breathlessness. *Current Opinion in Supportive and Palliative Care.* **9:** 227–231.

30 Moroni M *et al.* (1996) Inhaled sodium cromoglycate to treat cough in advanced lung cancer patients. *British Journal of Cancer.* **74:** 309–311.

31 Ryan NM *et al.* (2012) Gabapentin for refractory chronic cough: a randomised, double-blind, placebo-controlled trial. *Lancet.* **380:** 1583–1589.

32 Mintz S and Lee JK (2006) Gabapentin in the treatment of intractable idiopathic chronic cough: case reports. *American Journal of Medicine.* **119:** e13–15.

33 Estfan B and Walsh D (2008) The cough from hell: diazepam for intractable cough in a patient with renal cell carcinoma. *Journal of Pain and Symptom Management.* **36:** 553–558.

34 Dicpinigaitis PV (2006) Current and future peripherally-acting antitussives. *Respiratory Physiology and Neurobiology.* **152:** 356–362.

35 Larici AR *et al.* (2014) Diagnosis and management of hemoptysis. *Diagnostic and Interventional Radiology.* **20:** 299–309.

36 Mejia ARR Radiological evaluation and endovascular treatment of haemoptysis. *Current Problems in Diagnostic Radiology* (in press).

37 Fujita T *et al.* (2014) Immediate and late outcomes of bronchial and systemic artery embolization for palliative treatment of patients with nonsmall-cell lung cancer having hemoptysis. *American Journal of Hospice and Palliative Care.* **31:** 602–607.

38 Moen CA et al. (2013) Does tranexamic acid stop haemoptysis? Interactive Cardiovascular and Thoracic Surgery. 17: 991–994.
39 Solomonov A et al. (2009) Pulmonary hemorrhage: A novel mode of therapy. Respiratory Medicine. 103: 1196–1200.
40 Hankerson MJ et al. (2015) Nebulized tranexamic acid as a noninvasive therapy for cancer-related hemoptysis. Journal of Palliative Medicine. 18: 1060–1062.
41 Roberts ME et al. (2010) Management of a malignant pleural effusion: British Thoracic Society Pleural Disease Guideline 2010. Thorax. 65: ii32–40.
42 Hooper C et al. (2010) Investigation of a unilateral pleural effusion in adults: British Thoracic Society Pleural Disease Guideline 2010. Thorax. 65: ii4–17.
43 Steger M et al. (2015) Systemic review: the pathogenesis and pharmacological treatment of hiccups. Alimentary Pharmacology and Therapeutics. 42: 1037–1050.
44 NICE (2012) Clinical knowledge summaries. Hiccups _ management. http://cks.nice.org.uk/hiccups#!scenario
45 Moretto EN et al. (2013) Interventions for treating persistent and intractable hiccups in adults. Cochrane Database of Systematic Reviews. 1: CD008768. www.thecochranelibrary.com

FURTHER READING

Booth S et al. (eds) (2014) Managing breathlessness in clinical practice. Springer-Verlag, London.
British Thoracic Society & Association of Chartered Physiotherapists in Respiratory Care (BTS & ACPRC) (2009) Guidelines for the physiotherapy management of the adult, medical, spontaneously breathing patient. Thorax. 64 (Suppl 1): i1–i51.
Gibson PG and Vertigan AE (2015) Management of chronic refractory cough. British Medical Journal. 351: h5590.
Kloke M et al. (2015) Treatment of dyspnoea in advanced cancer patients: ESMO Clinical Practice Guidelines. Annals of Oncology. 26 (Suppl 5): v169–v173.
Mahler DA et al. (2010) American College of Chest Physicians consensus statement on the management of dyspnea in patients with advanced lung or heart disease. Chest. 137:674–691.
Wee B et al. (2012) Management of chronic cough in patients receiving palliative care: review of evidence and recommendations by a task group of the Association for Palliative Medicine of Great Britain and Ireland. Palliative Medicine. 26: 780–787.

10. SYMPTOM MANAGEMENT: GENITO-URINARY

URINARY SYMPTOMS

The management of urinary symptoms is aided by an understanding of definitions, syndromes and bladder innervation (Table 1).

Table 1 Useful definitions[1]

Symptom/syndrome	Definition
Frequency	Voiding too often (>8 times in 24h).
Nocturia	Waking at night to void.
Urgency	A sudden compelling desire to void which is difficult to delay.
Urge incontinence	The involuntary leakage of urine associated with urgency.
Overactive bladder syndrome	Urgency ± urge incontinence, frequency, and nocturia in the absence of urinary tract infection or other obvious pathological cause, generally caused by detrusor overactivity. *Second most common cause of urinary incontinence in women.*
Stress incontinence	The involuntary loss of urine associated with coughing, sneezing, laughing or lifting.
Genuine stress incontinence (urethral sphincter incompetence)	The involuntary leakage of urine when the intravesical pressure exceeds maximum urethral pressure in the absence of detrusor activity. The fault always lies in the sphincter mechanisms of the bladder, and is associated with multiparity, after the menopause and after hysterectomy. *Most common cause of urinary incontinence in women.*
Dysuria	Pain during and/or after voiding. Often urethral in origin (a burning sensation) but may be caused by bladder spasm (intense suprapubic and urethral pain), or both.
Hesitancy	A prolonged delay between attempting and achieving micturition.

'You **p**ee with your **p**arasympathetics; you **s**top with your **s**ympathetics'

The bladder sphincter relaxes when the detrusor (bladder muscle) contracts, and vice versa (Table 2). The urethral sphincter is an additional voluntary mechanism innervated by the pudendal nerve (S2–4).

Table 2 Autonomic innervation of the bladder

Innervation	Neurotransmitter	Sphincter	Detrusor
Sympathetic (T10–12, L1)	Noradrenaline (norepinephrine)	Contracts (α-receptors)	Relaxes (β-receptors)
Parasympathetic (S2-4)	Acetylcholine	Relaxes	Contracts

Several classes of drugs have an impact on bladder function:
- α-adrenergic receptor antagonists, e.g. tamsulosin: relaxes bladder neck sphincter
- antimuscarinics, e.g. oxybutynin: contraction of the bladder neck sphincter and relaxation of the detrusor
- morphine and other opioids:
  ▷ bladder sensation decreased
  ▷ sphincter tone increased
  ▷ detrusor tone increased
  ▷ ureteric tone and amplitude of contractions increased.

Although these effects may help certain bladder symptoms, they can be undesirable in other situations, e.g. antimuscarinics and opioids can cause hesitancy and occasionally retention.

FREQUENCY, URGENCY AND URGE INCONTINENCE

Causes

The causes of frequency overlap with those of urgency and urge incontinence (Box A). The precipitating factor in urge incontinence is delayed voiding relative to need. Delay is associated with:
- weakness and difficulty in getting to a commode
- disinterest:
  ▷ dejection
  ▷ depression
- lack of awareness:
  ▷ confusion
  ▷ drowsiness.

The differential diagnosis includes:
- genuine stress incontinence
- retention with overflow
- urinary fistula
- flaccid sphincter (presacral plexopathy).

Box A Causes of urgency and urge incontinence

Cancer
Bladder spasms
Extravesical ⎫
Intravesical ⎭ mechanical irritation
Hypercalcaemia (causes polyuria)
Pain
Sacral plexopathy

Treatment
Drugs
   cyclophosphamide
   diuretics
Radiation cystitis

Debility
Infective cystitis

Concurrent causes
Central neurological disease
   dementia
   multiple sclerosis
   poststroke
Idiopathic detrusor instability

Uraemia
Diabetes insipidus ⎫
Diabetes mellitus ⎭ cause polyuria

Management

Correct the correctable
- stop causative drug if possible
- treat infective cystitis with the appropriate antibiotic
- treat hypercalcaemia, diabetes mellitus, etc.

Non-drug treatment

Patients with mild symptoms may respond to regular time-contingent voiding, e.g. every 1–3h. They will also be helped by:
- proximity to the toilet
- ready availability of a bottle or commode
- a rapid response by nurses to requests for help
- avoiding excessive fluid intake
- abstaining from caffeine and alcohol (both are diuretics).

Drug treatment

Antimuscarinics are the drugs of choice, although treatment can be limited by undesirable effects (see p.349). Some are relatively selective for muscarinic receptors in the urinary tract, and should be used in preference. It may take four weeks to see the full response:
- oxybutynin 5mg b.d. increased progressively to q.d.s.; halve dose in the elderly:
  - ▷ if not tolerated, consider m/r or TD oxybutynin
  - ▷ also has a topical anaesthetic effect on the bladder mucosa
- fesoterodine m/r 4mg once daily increased to 8mg once daily if necessary.

If an antimuscarinic drug is contra-indicated, poorly tolerated or ineffective, consider:
- a β_3-agonist, e.g. mirabegron 50mg once daily;[2] dose adjustments are required with hepatic or renal impairment, and concurrent use of a strong CYP3A4 inhibitor (see SPC).

For postmenopausal women, with vaginal atrophy, consider intravaginal oestrogen.

For persistent nocturia without daytime urgency or frequency, consider:
- a loop diuretic, e.g. furosemide 40mg once daily around 1700–1800h
- in patients <65 years, a vasopressin analogue, e.g. desmopressin, although hyponatraemia is a possible complication.

BLADDER SPASMS

Bladder (detrusor) spasms are transient, often excruciating sensations felt in the suprapubic region and urethra/penis. They are generally secondary to irritation or hyperexcitability of the trigone.

Causes

Bladder spasms may relate to local cancer or other factors (Box B).

Box B Causes of bladder spasms	
Cancer	**Debility**
Intravesical ⎫	Anxiety
Extravesical ⎭ irritation	Infective cystitis
	Indwelling catheter
Treatment	mechanical irritation by catheter balloon
Radiation fibrosis	catheter sludging with partial retention

Management

Correct the correctable

Treatment options for reversible causes are listed in Table 3.

Drug treatment

Systemic analgesics should be used to control any constant background pain and an antimuscarinic given to reduce or prevent the spasms (see p.349). When relatively selective antimuscarinics are inadequate or inappropriate, consider less selective ones:
- hyoscine (Kwells®) 300microgram SL b.d.–q.d.s.
- hyoscine *butylbromide* 60–120mg/24h CSCI & 20mg SC p.r.n.; usual maximum 200mg/24h.

Table 3 Management of reversible causes of bladder spasms

Cause	Treatment options
Catheter irritation	Change catheter Reduce volume of balloon
Catheter sludging	Encourage oral fluids Bladder washouts, e.g. 100mL 0.9% normal saline Continuous bladder irrigation
Blood clots (haematuria)	Treat underlying cause, e.g. antimicrobials for infection, cystodiathermy for bladder cancer Tranexamic acid Continuous bladder irrigation

Infection (cystitis)	Antimicrobials
	Encourage oral fluids
	If catheterized
	    bladder washouts
	    change catheter
	    switch to intermittent catheterization q6h–q4h

If still not adequate, consider intravesical treatments:
- morphine (10–20mg t.d.s. or diamorphine 10mg t.d.s. diluted in 0.9% saline to 20mL); instil through an indwelling catheter and clamp for 30min
- bupivacaine t.d.s. (0.5% bupivacaine 10mL diluted in 0.9% saline to 20mL) used alone or with intravesical morphine.

VOIDING DIFFICULTIES

Voiding difficulties is a term encompassing three closely associated symptoms, namely, hesitancy, slow stream and terminal dribble. Voiding difficulties may be associated with urinary storage symptoms, e.g. frequency, nocturia, urgency, retention.

Causes
Voiding difficulties have many possible causes (Box C).

Management
Correct the correctable
Treatment options for reversible causes of hesitancy are listed in Table 4.

Non-drug treatment
In most patients with chronic symptoms, drug treatment should take precedence over non-drug treatment, i.e. catheterization. However, in debilitated bedbound

---

Box C Causes of voiding difficulties

Cancer
Cauda equina or sacral nerve root compression
Infiltration of bladder neck
Malignant enlargement of prostate
Presacral plexopathy
Spinal shock

Treatment
Antimuscarinics
Intrathecal nerve blocks
Morphine (occasionally)
Spinal analgesia (particularly with bupivacaine)

Debility
Generalized weakness
I nability to stand to void
Loaded rectum

Concurrent
Benign prostatic hyperplasia

Table 4 Management of reversible causes of hesitancy

Cause	Treatment options
Antimuscarinics	Stop if possible, or replace with a less antimuscarinic alternative
Loaded rectum	Suppositories Enema $\Big\} \rightarrow$ oral laxative regimen Digital removal
Inability to void lying down	Assistance to enable more upright posture
Benign prostatic hyperplasia	Transurethral resection

patients, a trial of catheterization may be preferable. In such patients, per urethral catheterization will be the norm. For patients who have several months to live, suprapubic catheterization should be considered.

Catheterization is generally required to relieve the discomfort of acute retention. If the patient is not in great distress and is well enough, the following may aid voiding:
• privacy
• standing
• the sound of running water
• a warm bath
• analgesia for pain.

If these fail, or are impractical, catheterization will be necessary.

Drug treatment

For the treatment of symptoms suggestive of benign prostatic hyperplasia options include:

- an α_1-adrenoceptor antagonist, e.g. m/r tamsulosin 400microgram once daily, for moderate-severe voiding lower urinary tract symptoms and a moderately enlarged prostate gland; *benefit seen within days*
- a 5α-reductase inhibitor, e.g. finasteride 5mg once daily (± an α_1-adrenoceptor antagonist), when there are greater degrees of prostatic enlargement; *benefit takes 3–6 months*
- an antimuscarinic, e.g. oxybutynin (see p.175); occasionally added to an α_1-adrenoceptor antagonist when significant persistent frequency, urgency and urge incontinence.

An alternative approach to the management of urinary hesitancy when urinary obstruction has been excluded is to use either a muscarinic drug, e.g. bethanechol 10–25mg t.d.s., or an anticholinesterase, e.g. distigmine bromide (not UK) 5mg once daily to stimulate bladder contraction. Because their mechanisms of action differ, they can be used concurrently with tamsulosin.

CATHETER CARE

Indications for a urinary catheter in patients with advanced illness include:
- acute urinary retention
- impaired bladder emptying
- urinary incontinence, particularly in the last days of life
- management of symptoms provoked by voiding, e.g. severe pain on movement.

Treatment options for common problems are listed in Table 5.

In catheterized patients:
- bacterial colonization is common (30% after 7 days, almost 100% after 28 days); it should not be investigated or treated unless symptomatic because generally bacteriuria does not progress to a urinary tract infection
- a urinary tract infection is unlikely to present with specific urinary tract symptoms or with fever; non-specific symptoms are more common, e.g. rigors and new-onset delirium
- a urine dipstick test is unreliable; when a urinary tract infection is clinically suspected send urine for culture, and then start empirical antimicrobial treatment
- changing a long-term catheter before starting an antibacterial improves bacteriological cure rates
- because of the risk of increasing antibacterial resistance, continuous prophylaxis against urinary tract infection is *not* recommended.

Table 5 Management of common urinary catheter problems

Problem	Treatment options
Bladder irritation ± spasms	Change catheter Reduce volume of balloon
Catheter sludging or blocking	Encourage oral fluids Bladder washouts, e.g. 100mL 0.9% normal saline Continuous bladder irrigation Change catheter
Catheter bypassing	Exclude blockage Reduce volume of balloon Consider larger gauge catheter Treat bladder spasm (see Bladder spasm, p.176)
Infection (cystitis) ± systemic symptoms	Antimicrobials Encourage oral fluids Bladder washouts Change catheter Switch to intermittent catheterization q6h–q4h Generally, do not use a prophylactic antimicrobial

SEXUAL ISSUES

Sexuality is a fundamental and integral part of being human. It is a multi-faceted phenomenon of which sexual *behaviour* is only one aspect. It encompasses psychological and sociological aspects of how a person relates to themselves and to others. Sexuality includes concerns about body image and self-esteem, and is influenced by cultural and religious factors.

Any chronic illness and many treatments can impact negatively on aspects of a person's sexuality. If not addressed, sexual concerns can add to the patient's distress.

Lesbian, gay, bisexual and transgender people may fear a lack of understanding and discrimination from health professionals. Consequently, they may 'suffer in silence', particularly if previously they have not felt able to be open about their sexual orientation.[3,4]

How intimacy is expressed is likely to change as the illness progresses; this might place greater emphasis on ways which do not involve sexual intercourse. Nonetheless, a fatal condition associated with physical deterioration, reduced stamina, altered body image and increasing dependency can be a major strain on relationships.[5]

When one partner takes on the role of care-*giver*, the other can become a dependent care-*receiver*. This can alter the sense of reciprocity in the couples' relationship. When one partner is dying, the couple's relationship is also dying.[6] This can to lead to physical and/or emotional 'disconnection', with both partners experiencing a deep sense of loss.

Some couples adapt positively to the changes, and are able to 'reconnect' (Figure 1). However, with others, disconnection is deep and seemingly intractable, particularly when fuelled by feelings of disgust and fear.

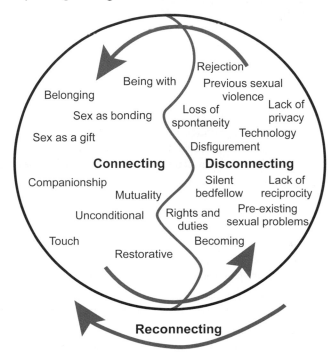

Figure 1 The changing dynamic of a couple's relationship when one of them is dying. Modified from Taylor 2014 with permission.[6]

It is important to be aware of the dynamics, and to provide opportunities for both partners to express their concerns and share the distress caused by the changed and changing circumstances.

Causes
Specific sexual problems can include:
- reduced libido (lack of sexual desire and inability to become physically aroused)
- erectile dysfunction/absent orgasm
- vaginal dryness/discharge/dyspareunia
- reduced fertility
- early menopause.

In addition to the psychosocial distress caused by a loss of reciprocity and spontaneity in the relationship, major contributory factors reducing libido and arousal include:
- the cancer itself, e.g. disfigurement, perineal erosion, spinal cord compression
- cancer treatment, e.g. radiotherapy, hormone therapy, mutilating radical surgery, ostomy bags

- uncontrolled symptoms and general debility, e.g. pain, breathlessness, nausea, fatigue
- concurrent morbidities, e.g. diabetes mellitus, multiple sclerosis, renal failure, depression
- drugs, e.g. psycho-active drugs, lithium, anti-epileptics, antihypertensives, thiazide diuretics, NSAIDs.

Management

There is consistent evidence that health professionals avoid addressing the sexual information and support needs of people with cancer and other advanced diseases.[7] This is mainly because of embarrassment and the unwarranted assumption that the patient will have 'lost interest'.

In consequence, a model has been developed to help overcome barriers in communication in this area. Originally labelled by the acronym PLISSIT, it has been recast as Ex-PLISSIT.[8] It comprises four levels of intervention:

1. *P*ermission-giving
2. *L*imited *I*nformation
3. *S*pecific *S*uggestions
4. *I*ntensive *T*herapy.

The Ex-PLISSIT variant extends the original model by emphasizing that permission-giving must be integral to *all four levels*, and by highlighting the importance of review.[8]

Permission-giving not only gives the patient (or partner) an invitation to raise sexuality-related topics but also gives the professional permission to delve (albeit sensitively) into this area.

In essence, the communication skills needed do not differ from communication skills generally (see Chapter 3, p.35). As always, it is important not to make assumptions, particularly because of the patient's age, culture and sexual orientation.

However, the embarrassment factor means it is crucial that you are aware of your own feelings, and how these can impact on your interaction with the patient. For this reason, professionals are encouraged to reflect, either alone or with a colleague, after any in-depth discussion around sexuality.[8]

1. *Permission-giving*

There are numerous possible 'opening gambits'. Going from the less direct to the more direct, these might include:

'How has your illness affected you as a couple?'

'Has your illness made it more difficult to be intimate with your partner?'

'Many people with your condition find it affects their intimate relationships and sexual activity. How is it for you? Is this something you'd like to talk about?'

'Have you any sexual concerns or problems you'd like to discuss?'

Then, depending on the reply:

'Would you like to talk about this?'

Note: even if a patient shares concerns, do not assume that they have disclosed everything. Thus, when you next meet, it is important to return to the subject by further permission-giving:

'When we last spoke, you mentioned how your relationship with your husband had been affected by your illness... and we talked about... How have things been since then?'

'Do you have other concerns or worries about your relationship with your partner?'

Note: even if the patient indicates they have no concerns, do not assume that all is well. They may subsequently feel able to share their concerns; and permission needs to be given for this:

'I mentioned intimacy last time we met... Is this something you'd like to discuss today?'

2. Limited Information

It is important not to assume that patients will want or need further information or a 'solution'. For many, the opportunity to talk about their experience and to have their feelings of loss validated is all that is needed.

However, patients and their partners benefit by confirmation that, for example, cancer is *not* transmitted by sexual intercourse, and that abstinence is *not* necessary during radiotherapy. A range of information is available from patient support websites, e.g. www.macmillan.org.uk.

Although some patients benefit by reading literature,[9] it is important not to use this as a 'cop out'. Offering literature – certainly immediately – could be a distancing tactic which prevents the patient from cathartically unburdening themselves by sharing their own (unique) concerns.

Acknowledge that sexuality remains important despite their illness. Patients should have privacy and permission to express their sexuality physically if this is important to them, e.g. a single room, a double bed if available, and time without interruptions by staff.

3. Specific Suggestions

Palliative care professionals should aim to become proficient at Levels 1 and 2. However, specific suggestions are generally best delegated to someone with experience in this area, possibly one of your colleagues.

Suggestions will relate to specific problems, e.g. lubricants or moisturizers for vaginal dryness, long-term catheters (see www.bladderandbowelfoundation.org.uk). If sexual intercourse is no longer possible, helping patients explore other forms of intimacy, e.g. body contact, touching, hugging, holding hands, kissing. Occasionally, medication for erectile dysfunction may be appropriate.

4. Intensive Therapy

A small number of patients may benefit from referral to sexual health specialists or counsellors.[10] However, most patients experiencing sexual problems can resolve them if told that it is all right to desire sexual activity and to discuss sexuality, and if they receive *limited information* about sexual matters and *specific suggestions* about ways to address sexual problems.

For those with sexual concerns which cannot be resolved, the opportunity to discuss their loss, and how they have adjusted to it, can in itself be cathartic.

REFERENCES

1 International Continence Society (2005) Factsheet 2: Overactive Bladder. www.icsoffice.org
2 NICE (2013) Mirabegron for treating symptoms of overactive bladder. *Technology Appraisal 290.* www.nice.org.uk
3 Harding R *et al.* (2012) Needs, experiences, and preferences of sexual minorities for end-of-life care and palliative care: a systematic review. *Journal of Palliative Medicine.* **15:** 602–611.
4 Fuller A *et al.* (2011) *Open to all? Meeting the needs of lesbian, gay, bisexual and transgender people nearing the end of life.* National Council for Palliative Care and the Consortium of Lesbian, Gay, Bisexual and Transgendered Voluntary and Community Organisations, London.
5 Taylor B (2015) Does the caring role preclude sexuality and intimacy in coupled relationships? *Sexuality and Disability.* **33:** 365–374.
6 Taylor B (2014) Experiences of sexuality and intimacy in terminal illness: a phenomenological study. *Palliative Medicine.* **28:** 438–447.
7 Ussher JM *et al.* (2013) Talking about sex after cancer: a discourse analytic study of health care professional accounts of sexual communication with patients. *Psychology and Health.* **28:** 1370–1390.
8 Taylor B and Davis S (2007) The extended PLISSIT model for addressing the sexual wellbeing of individuals with an acquired disability or chronic illness. *Sexuality and Disability.* **25:** 135–139.
9 Ussher JM *et al.* (2013) Information needs associated with changes to sexual well-being after breast cancer. *Journal of Advanced Nursing.* **69:** 327–337.
10 Penson RT *et al.* (2000) Sexuality and cancer: conversation comfort zone. *Oncologist.* **5:** 336–344.

11. SYMPTOM MANAGEMENT: PSYCHOLOGICAL & NEUROLOGICAL

PSYCHOLOGICAL SYMPTOMS

For most people, learning that they have a life-limiting illness is devastating, and is associated with a range of strong emotions. With time and appropriate support (see p.52), most patients adjust to their altered circumstances, but some develop a recognizable psychiatric disorder, notably depression.

For those already suffering from dementia, the physical and psychological stress of a superadded terminal condition can cause the dementia to rapidly worsen.

Further, particularly near the end of life, many patients experience episodes of delirium, including those with underlying dementia. Precipitating/exacerbating factors include biochemical derangement, organ failure, drugs, brain tumours and paraneoplastic syndromes.

ANXIETY

Severe anxiety typically manifests as a complex of physical and psychological symptoms, reflecting fear, worry and apprehension (Box A).[1]

Severe anxiety impacts on every aspect of personhood; not only psychological but also physical, social and spiritual. The physical symptoms may overshadow the psychological ones, and are often the ones the patient presents with – a reminder that all physical symptoms are 'somatopsychic' phenomena (see p.81).

Anxiety often stems from uncertainty, fear about the future, and the threat of separation from loved ones. Many anxious terminally ill patients sleep badly, have frightening dreams, and may be reluctant to be alone at night, or even left alone during the day. However, a high level of anxiety is *not* inevitable in those with terminal illness.

Box A Manifestations of anxiety	
Insomnia, nightmares	Dry mouth
Dizziness	Dysphagia
Tremor	Anorexia
Apprehension, jitteriness	Nausea and vomiting
Poor concentration, rumination	Diarrhoea
Headache	Urinary frequency
Sweating	Muscle tension
Palpitations	Fatigue
Chest tightness	Weakness
Breathlessness	Non-adherence

In advanced disease, anxiety is commonly associated with depressive symptoms (see below) and delirium (see below). Unsurprisingly, palliative care patients with anxiety and/or depression report more severe physical symptoms, social concerns and existential issues.[2]

Anxiety may be associated with potentially reversible conditions such as uncontrolled pain, severe breathlessness, hypoxia, and sepsis. It may be caused or exacerbated by medication, e.g. corticosteroids.

Management
Correct the correctable
For example:
• review drug regimen
• relieve pain, breathlessness, and other distressing symptoms.

Non-drug treatment
Patients should be offered appropriate support (see Chapter 4, p.52). The aim is to give the patient an opportunity to talk openly about their concerns (see Chapter 3, p.35), and also to let them know that you are aware of the awfulness of what they are going though. Thus:
• facilitate the airing and sharing of worries and fears ('a trouble shared is a trouble halved')
• correct misconceptions
• develop a strategy for coping with uncertainty (see p.42).

This general approach can be augmented by various therapies, offered by different members of the multiprofessional team, e.g.:

- relaxation therapy (occupational therapist, complementary therapist)
- distraction therapy (occupational therapist, craft therapist)
- arts therapies (e.g. art, music therapist).

For patients responding well to this general approach, there may be no need to prescribe an anxiolytic.

For patients with severe anxiety (or panic attacks) not responding to the above, more specialist psychological approaches can be considered, e.g. cognitive behavioural therapy (CBT). The efficacy of CBT and drug therapy is comparable.[3] However, availability may be limited.

Drug treatment

In some patients, together with psychological support, it will be necessary to prescribe drugs. These are tailored to the likely duration of use:
- benzodiazepine, *if prognosis is <2–4 weeks*, e.g.:
  ▷ diazepam 2–10mg PO at bedtime and p.r.n.
  ▷ lorazepam 0.5–1mg PO b.d. and p.r.n.
- SSRI (± a benzodiazepine initially), *if prognosis is >2–4 weeks*, particularly if:
  ▷ anxiety-depression (see p.340)
  ▷ persistent panic attacks (see below)

Pregabalin (p.345) also acts quickly but response rates are lower than for SSRIs and benzodiazepines. Thus, it is generally reserved for patients not responding to antidepressants.

An antipsychotic is generally reserved for anxiety secondary to delirium or psychosis, or where benzodiazepines and antidepressants are ineffective.

PANIC ATTACKS

Panic is an episodic failure of the protective 'fight or flight' response to a major threat, in which all structure and reality checks are lost, and mental mayhem ensues.

In the dying, an overwhelming sense of doom or absolute despair often supervenes. Panic is associated with various autonomic symptoms (Box B). It is physiologically demanding and cannot be maintained indefinitely. Panic attacks may occur in clusters.

Evaluation

In life-threatening disease, panic may be:
- an exacerbation of a pre-existing anxiety disorder (in which case the onset of panic attacks may well predate the diagnosis of cancer)
- a reaction to the patient's current circumstances
- secondary to uncontrolled symptoms, particularly breathlessness (see below)
- a feature of agitated delirium
- precipitated by medication, e.g. corticosteroids
- a form of temporal lobe epilepsy in patients with brain tumours.

Box B Manifestations of a panic attack[4]

A discrete period of intense fear or discomfort in which four or more of the following symptoms develop abruptly and reach a peak within 10 minutes:
- palpitations, pounding heart, or accelerated heart rate
- sweating
- trembling or shaking
- sensations of shortness of breath or smothering
- feeling of choking
- chest pain or discomfort
- nausea or abdominal distress
- feeling dizzy, unsteady, lightheaded or faint
- derealization (feelings of unreality) or depersonalization (being detached from oneself)
- fear of losing control or going crazy
- fear of dying
- paraesthesias (numbness or tingling sensations)
- chills or hot flushes.

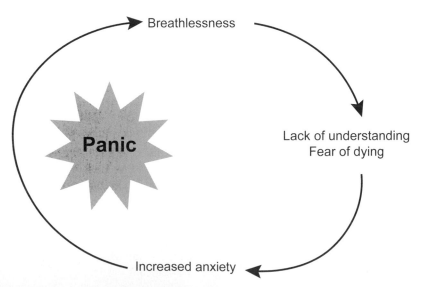

Figure 1 Breathlessness is a common trigger for panic

Patients with breathlessness are at increased risk of panic attacks (Figure 1). Indeed, all severely breathless patients should be 'screened' for panic attacks (see p.145).

A common feature is the persistent fear about the attacks and their consequences, e.g. fear of suffocation and death during an attack.[5] Other features of respiratory panic include:

- episodes of breathlessness occurring at rest
- poor relationship of breathlessness to exertion
- rapid fluctuations of breathlessness within minutes
- breathlessness associated with certain social situations.

Some patients with end-stage MND/ALS appear fearful at times but are unable to vocalize their feelings. Because such patients often have incipient respiratory failure, it is probable that the non-verbally expressed fear reflects episodes of panic.

Management

Correct the correctable

Use cause-specific treatments when possible, e.g. anti-epileptics for panic occurring as a manifestation of temporal lobe epilepsy.

Non-drug treatment

Also see anxiety, p.185.

With breathless patients, panic often responds to a calming presence and encouraging the hyperventilating patient to breathe more slowly by focusing on ensuring adequate expiration. Patients should also be taught about optimal breathing techniques, breathing control and relaxation (see p.150).

Whether or not associated with breathlessness, it is important to explore possible reasons for the panic attacks. In patients with a life-threatening condition, there is an obvious precipitating cause, namely the fear of impending death, disintegration and annihilation. Often such fears are only thinly disguised and empathic discussion can help by bringing them into the open.

For panic attacks which fail to decrease after open discussion, CBT is the treatment of choice.[6] However, availability may be limited.

Drug treatment

As for anxiety, p.187.

DEPRESSION

A major depression occurs in 5–20% of patients with advanced cancer.[1] An additional 15–20% experience less severe depression which is likely also to be a major source of suffering and despair.

Clinical depression is often not recognized because symptoms overlap with appropriate grief about dying (sadness), with demoralization (spiritual distress, hopelessness, 'no point in struggling on'),[7] and with the somatic symptoms of the cancer (anorexia, sleep disturbance, constipation, weight loss). Further, many patients try to ignore or hide their negative feelings ('I just have to accept it and get on with it').

It is important to identify depression particularly because conventional treatment achieves a good response in about 80% of cases. Untreated depression:
- intensifies other symptoms
- leads to social withdrawal
- prevents the patient from completing 'unfinished business'.

Clinical features and evaluation

Diagnosing depression can be difficult in the presence of a debilitating physical illness (see Quick Clinical Guide, p.192).

It is important to ask patients directly about their mood; do *not* rely just on the reports of others. Useful questions include:

'How are you coping?'

'How are you feeling?'

'What has your mood been like lately?'

'Are you depressed?'

'Have you had a serious depression before? Are things like that now?'[8]

Some patients are seemingly depressed but in reality are simply close to death with no residual energy and a corresponding loss of pleasure in life. In more robust patients, it is necessary to differentiate between:
- sadness provoked by the change in personal circumstances (adjustment reaction)
- loss of morale because of unrelieved severe pain or other distressing symptoms, anxiety, insomnia, and a sense of desolation
- depression (Box C and Figure 2).

Box C Features which help to distinguish a depressive illness from sadness (adjustment reaction) and demoralization (spiritual distress)

Features of all three conditions	Features more typical of depression
Loss of interest	Loss of all emotion and pleasure in life
Decreased concentration	Social withdrawal
Tearfulness	Not distractable (but with diurnal variation)
Anxiety	Irritability
Decreased sleep, tiredness	Excessive guilt
Anorexia	Intractable pain
Suicidal ideas	Suicide attempts

Evaluation is difficult because the somatic symptoms of depression overlap with the symptoms of cancer:
- anorexia
- weight loss
- constipation
- sleep disturbance
- loss of libido.

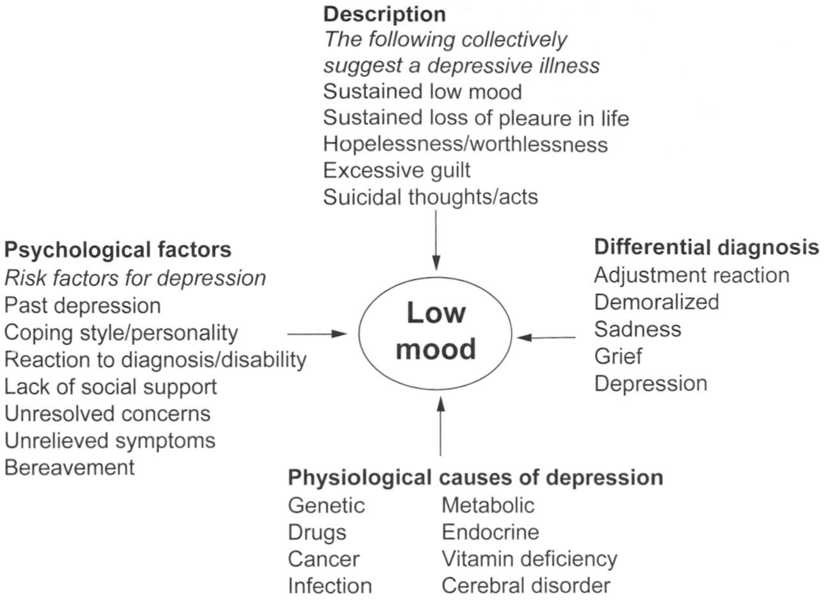

Description
*The following collectively
suggest a depressive illness*
Sustained low mood
Sustained loss of pleaure in life
Hopelessness/worthlessness
Excessive guilt
Suicidal thoughts/acts

Psychological factors
Risk factors for depression
Past depression
Coping style/personality
Reaction to diagnosis/disability
Lack of social support
Unresolved concerns
Unrelieved symptoms
Bereavement

Low mood

Differential diagnosis
Adjustment reaction
Demoralized
Sadness
Grief
Depression

Physiological causes of depression
Genetic   Metabolic
Drugs   Endocrine
Cancer   Vitamin deficiency
Infection   Cerebral disorder

Figure 2 The four dimensions of the evaluation of low mood.

When there is doubt, a decision can be delayed for 1–2 weeks. During this time, with the general support given by the palliative care service, morale may rise and adjustment reactions worked through.

Sometimes it may help to use a validated screening tool, e.g. the Edinburgh Depression Scale.[9,10] However, this is unlikely to clarify the situation in cases which are not clearcut. A psychiatric consultation should be requested when doubt persists.

Depression or other significant psychiatric disorder is the underlying cause in about half of those desiring to hasten death (see p.20).

Explanation

The nature of the explanation will vary according to the patient's physical and psychological state. Patients are often helped by being told that depression is not shameful. For example:

'It seems to me that you've developed a depressive illness … Being physically ill is hard work and emotionally exhausting. Ongoing stress reduces certain chemicals in the brain and this results in depression … Antidepressants are tablets which help the brain replenish these chemicals.'

Management

This is summarized in the Quick Clinical Guide (below). Also see Antidepressants (p.339).

QUICK CLINICAL GUIDE: DEPRESSION

Sadness and tears, even if associated with transient suicidal thoughts, do not justify the diagnosis of depression or the prescription of an antidepressant. Often they are part of an adjustment reaction, and improve with time. Other patients are demoralized rather than depressed and respond to symptom management and psychosocial support.

Evaluation

1   Screening: about 5–20% of patients with advanced cancer develop a major depression. Cases will be missed unless specific enquiry is made of all patients:
'What has your mood been like lately?… Are you depressed?'
'Have you had serious depression before? Are things like that now?'

2   Assessment interview: if depression is suspected, explore the patient's mood more fully by encouraging the patient to talk further with appropriate prompts. Symptoms suggesting clinical depression include:
    - sustained low mood (i.e. most of every day for several weeks) ⎫
    - sustained loss of pleasure/interest in life (anhedonia) ⎬ core symptoms
    - diurnal variation (worse in mornings and better in evenings)
    - waking significantly earlier than usual (e.g. 1–2h) and feeling 'awful'
    - feelings of hopelessness/worthlessness
    - excessive guilt
    - withdrawal from family and friends
    - persistent suicidal thoughts and/or suicidal acts
    - requests for euthanasia.

3   Differential diagnosis: the symptoms of depression and cancer, and of depression and sadness overlap. If in doubt whether the patient is suffering from depression, review after 1–2 weeks of general support and improved symptom management. If still undecided, seek advice from a psychologist/psychiatrist.

4   Medical causes: depression may be the consequence of:
    - a medical condition, e.g. hypercalcaemia, cerebral metastases
    - a reaction to severe uncontrolled physical symptoms
    - drugs, e.g. antineoplastics, benzodiazepines, antipsychotics, corticosteroids.

Management

5   Correct the correctable: treat medical causes, particularly severe pain and other distressing symptoms.

6   Non-drug treatment:
    - explanation and assurance that symptoms can be treated
    - depressed patients often benefit from the ambience of a Palliative Care Day Centre
    - specific psychological treatments (via a clinical psychologist, etc.)
    - other psychosocial professionals, e.g. chaplain and arts therapists, have a therapeutic role, but avoid overwhelming the patient with simultaneous multiple referrals.

7   Drug treatment:
    - if the patient is expected to live for >4 weeks, prescribe a conventional antidepressant; if <4 weeks, consider a psychostimulant
    - the starting and continuing doses of antidepressants are generally lower in debilitated patients than in the physically fit
    - all antidepressants can cause withdrawal symptoms if stopped abruptly; generally withdraw gradually over 4 weeks

- at usual doses, one SSRI can be directly substituted for another without cross-tapering or a washout period. Mirtazapine 15mg can be directly substituted for SSRIs (fluoxetine, citalopram or paroxetine 20mg; sertraline 50mg)
- taper higher SSRI doses before switching
- switching to or from a TCA or a MAOI requires additional care – seek advice.

PCF preferred antidepressants

First-line
Psychostimulant, e.g. methylphenidate
Particularly if prognosis <2–4 weeks:
- start with 2.5–5mg b.d. (on waking/breakfast time and noon/lunchtime)
- if necessary, increase using daily increments of 2.5mg b.d. up to 20mg b.d.
- occasionally higher doses are necessary, e.g. 30mg b.d. or 20mg t.d.s.

SSRI, e.g. sertraline or citalopram
Particularly if prognosis >2–4 weeks, and if associated anxiety:
- no antimuscarinic effects, but may cause an initial increase in anxiety
- if necessary prescribe diazepam at bedtime
- start with sertraline 50mg or citalopram 10mg once daily, increasing the latter to 20mg after 1 week
- if no improvement after 4 weeks, or only a partial improvement after 6–8 weeks, either:
  ▷ increase dose by sertraline 50mg or citalopram 10mg *or*
  ▷ switch to a second-line antidepressant
- maximum daily dose sertraline 200mg or citalopram 40mg (20mg in patients >60 years, those with hepatic impairment, and consider with patients also taking cimetidine, omeprazole or other inhibitors of CYP2C19)
- low likelihood of a withdrawal (discontinuation) syndrome.

Second-line
Alternative SSRI, e.g. sertraline or citalopram
Dose as above.
Mirtazapine
A good choice for patients with anxiety/agitation:
- start with 15mg at bedtime
- if little or no improvement after 2 weeks, increase to 30mg at bedtime
- concurrent H_1-receptor antagonism leads to sedation but this decreases at the higher dose because of noradrenergic effects.
- fewer undesirable effects than TCAs.
If no response after 4 weeks, consider third-line options.

Third-line options
- seek advice from a psychiatrist
- dose escalation
- switch antidepressant
- combine an SSRI or SNRI with mirtazapine, olanzapine or quetiapine.

SUICIDE RISK

Patients with advanced disease are at an increased risk of suicide. Risk factors include:
- poorly controlled pain/other symptoms
- advanced illness/poor prognosis
- delirium/disinhibition
- lack of social support
- substance abuse
- previous history/family history of psychiatric illness or suicide.

Suicidal ideation is defined as thoughts of taking one's own life.[1] Contrary to the fears of many clinicians, asking about suicidal ideation and planning does not increase suicidal thoughts in patients.

For most patients, any thoughts of suicide occur only as a fleeting consideration at a particularly distressing time. However, for a few, such thoughts are more persistent and may result in a definite plan to end one's life. When this is the case, *urgent psychiatric referral is critical.*

INSOMNIA

Insomnia is difficulty in falling or staying asleep, and leads to impaired daytime functioning. There are numerous causes of insomnia (Box D).

Management

Management focuses on identifying underlying causes and correcting them if possible, e.g. optimizing pain management by increasing the dose of analgesics at bedtime.

Non-drug interventions include:
- changing mattress/bed if uncomfortable
- sleep hygiene: avoiding caffeine and alcohol, and excessive volumes of fluid before bed, avoid having a bedroom TV, reducing light and noise at bedtime
- getting up at a regular time each day, regardless of how much sleep has been had
- increasing daytime activity to avoid daytime napping
- exploration of fears and anxieties, including those manifesting as recurrent unpleasant dreams/nightmares
- specific relaxation techniques e.g. meditation.

Drug treatments include:
- restrict corticosteroids and diuretics to morning dosing
- night sedative, e.g. zopiclone
- a sedative anti-depressant, e.g. amitriptyline or mirtazapine, if insomnia related to a clinical depression.

Box D Causes of wakeful nights

Physiological
Dementia with reversal of normal
sleep-wake cycle
Normal old age
Sleep during day
   long siesta
   catnaps
   sedative drugs
Wakeful stimuli
   light
   noise
   urinary frequency

Psychological
Anxiety
Depression
Fear of dying in the night
Withdrawal of night sedation

Sleep disorders
Sleep apnoea

Unrelieved symptoms
Breathlessness
Diarrhoea
Incontinence
Pain
Pruritus
Restless legs
Vomiting

Drugs
Alcohol (may cause rebound
wakefulness)
β-Blockers (can cause bad dreams)
Caffeine
Corticosteroids
Diuretics
Sympathomimetics
Withdrawal of night sedation

PRE-EXISTING PSYCHIATRIC DISEASE

Long-term and recurrent psychiatric illness is common. The lifetime prevalence of conditions such as bipolar disorder and schizophrenia is around 1–3%, and the prevalence of anxiety and depression much higher. With patients who have a history of psychiatric illness, it is important to:

- note previous treatment, hospital admissions (whether compulsory or voluntary), and any suicide attempts
- liaise with specialist psychiatric services
- check for drug interactions when prescribing new medication
- adhere to the monitoring requirements for high-risk medicines, e.g. lithium, clozapine
- ensure that those dependent on drugs and/or alcohol have access to appropriate replacement therapy; facilitate harm reduction measures such as supplying clean needles.

DELIRIUM

Delirium is the term used to describe acute confusion (acute brain failure) associated with a medical condition, intoxication or substance withdrawal (Box E). Mental clouding leads to a disturbance of comprehension and bewilderment which manifests with a wide range of neuropsychiatric abnormalities.

Box E Diagnostic criteria for delirium[4]

1. Disturbance in attention (i.e. reduced ability to direct, focus, sustain, and shift attention) and awareness.

2. Change in cognition (e.g. memory deficit, disorientation, language disturbance, perceptual disturbance) which is not better accounted for by a pre-existing, established, or evolving dementia.

3. The disturbance develops over a short period (generally hours–days) and tends to fluctuate during the course of the day.

4. There is evidence from the history, physical examination, or laboratory findings that the disturbance is caused by a direct physiological consequence of a general medical condition, an intoxicating substance, medication use, or more than one cause.

Delirium occurs in <30% of hospitalized patients, and in <85% at the end of life.[11] Despite it being the most common neuropsychiatric complication of end-stage disease, delirium is often undiagnosed (and thus untreated).

Delirium is generally reversible except in those close to death; in the latter, management will generally focus on controlling distressing symptoms and behaviour.

Clinical features

Despite many different causes, the clinical features of delirium are fairly stereotyped, with a set of core symptoms (Box F). The disordered level of arousal and cognition is typically of acute onset, developing over hours–days.

Delirium is commonly classified into three clinical subtypes based on the level of arousal and psychomotor activity:

- hyperactive: characterized by restlessness, agitation, hypervigilance, hallucinations and delusions (more associated with drug intoxication, and with alcohol and drug withdrawal)
- hypo-active: characterized by psychomotor retardation, lethargy, reduced awareness of surroundings, with hallucinations and delusions less common (more associated with hypoxia, metabolic disturbances and encephalopathy; carries a higher risk of death)
- mixed: alternating features of both agitation and lethargy.

Hyperactive delirium may be accompanied by overactivity of the autonomic nervous system: facial flushing, dilated pupils, injected conjunctivae, tachycardia, sweating.

Box F Clinical features of delirium

Prodromal symptoms (restlessness, anxiety, sleep disturbance and irritability)

Fluctuating course

Disorganized thinking

Rambling incoherent speech

Reduced attention span (easily distractible)
  perseveration (inability to shift attention onto a new subject)
  short-term memory impairment (cannot register new material)
  disorientation for time, place or person

Increased or decreased psychomotor activity
  altered arousal
  motor abnormalities (e.g. tremor, myoclonus)
  disturbance of the sleep–wake cycle

Affective symptoms (emotional lability, sadness, anger, euphoria, fear)

Agitation ± noisy aggressive behaviour

Altered perceptions
  misinterpretations (e.g. mistaking a stranger for one's dead mother)
  hallucinations (predominantly visual and tactile rather than auditory)
  psychosis and delusions (poorly formed)

Cortical abnormalities (dysgraphia, constructional apraxia, dysnomic aphasia)

Electro-encephalogram abnormalities (global slowing of activity)

Particularly in hypo-active delirium, clinical suspicion is helpful in recognizing the presence of hallucinations and delusions. For example, a hypo-active withdrawn lethargic patient may:
- 'pluck' at the bed-clothes or at empty space; this is an indication of hallucinosis
- look distressed with eyes frequently darting from side to side; an indication of possible hallucinosis and/or delusions.

Even though the patient is not overtly agitated, such signs indicate the need for an antipsychotic (see below).

Note: Patients manifesting the following are sometimes misdiagnosed as confused:
- not taking in what is said:
  ▷ deaf
  ▷ anxious
- muddled speech:
  ▷ poor concentration
  ▷ nominal dysphasia
- non-convulsive status epilepticus (see p.206).

Hypnagogic (going to sleep) and hypnopompic (waking up) hallucinations are normal phenomena; they are *not* pathological and do *not* indicate delirium.

Pathogenesis

Everybody is at risk of delirium. However, the risk varies from person to person depending on their vulnerability both physically and psychologically (Box G). Thus, it is useful to think in terms of an individual's 'delirium threshold'.

Risk factors tend to be synergistic. The use of opioids, and cognitive and organ impairment are major risk factors. In elderly patients, the prescription of a seemingly appropriate dose of a night sedative may be sufficient to precipitate delirium.

Box G Risk factors for delirium		
Delirium threshold lowered	**Precipitating factors for delirium**	
Extremes of age	Change of environment	Thiamine deficiency
Dementia	Unfamiliar excessive stimuli	Biochemical disturbance
Learning disability	too hot/too cold	hypercalcaemia
Visual impairment	crumbs in bed	hyponatraemia
Hearing impairment	wet sheets	Drug-induced
Previous episode of	General deterioration	opioids
delirium	fatigue	benzodiazepines
Alcohol abuse	Uncontrolled symptoms	antimuscarinics
Depression	pain	corticosteroids
Reduced physical	faecal impaction	chemotherapy
activity	urinary retention	polypharmacy
	infection	Withdrawal state
	dehydration	alcohol
	hypoxia	nicotine
	anxiety	psychotropics
	depression	Organ impairment
	Primary or secondary	hepatic
	brain tumours	renal
	Paraneoplastic syndromes	respiratory
		Sleep deprivation
		Surgery
		Trauma

Evaluation

The gold standard for diagnosing delirium is the clinician's evaluation based on the criteria in DSM5 in Box E, and elaborated in Box F. No laboratory test can diagnose delirium.

Provided the patient is not already cognitively impaired (e.g. from dementia), the inability to write one's name and address correctly or to draw a clock face correctly is possibly as sensitive an indicator of early delirium as some of the more lengthy and intrusive tests.[12]

In patients close to death, evaluation will largely be limited to a consideration of any easily reversible precipitating factors (see Box G), notably urinary retention, faecal impaction, uncontrolled pain, infection, drug-intoxication, acute alcohol or nicotine withdrawal.

In patients not close to death, the following may be useful if there is no obvious reason for the delirium:

- oxygen saturation
- blood tests: FBC, urea, creatinine, electrolytes, calcium, LFTs, glucose
- cultures: blood, urine, sputum
- imaging: chest radiograph.

Brain CT and/or MRI are indicated when specific intracranial pathology is suspected.

Management

Correct the correctable

For example:

- relieve bladder retention and/or disimpact the rectum
- reduce opioid, psychotropic, and antimuscarinic medication (if feasible)
- oxygen if hypoxic
- antibacterials for infection (if appropriate)
- dexamethasone if brain tumour (see p.365)
- a benzodiazepine for alcohol withdrawal
- nicotine replacement if withdrawal from smoking.

Non-drug treatment

The family should be provided with a clear explanation about the cause and fluctuations in the patient's mental state. They should be assured that the patient is not 'losing their mind', and advised not to be too forceful if and when they contradict the patient.

An attempt should be made to help the patient to express their distress. Misinterpretations, nightmares and hallucinations often reflect the patient's fears; and their content should be explored with the patient. In addition:

- continue to treat the patient with courtesy and respect
- explain what is happening and why
- stress that delirium is not madness, and that there may be lucid intervals
- state what can be done to help
- respond to the patient's comments
- keep calm and avoid confrontation
- repeat important and helpful information
- allay fear and suspicion, and reduce misinterpretations by:
  - ▷ use of a night light
  - ▷ limiting the number of staff caring for the patient
  - ▷ explaining every procedure in detail
- if indicated, prescribe an antipsychotic 'to let you relax and rest for a few hours'
- if mobile, the patient should be allowed to walk about accompanied.

As far as possible, avoid changes in the patient's environment; provide a single room with minimal sensory stimulation; and encourage a family member or close friend to be present as much as possible.

Patient restraint and hazards such as bed-rails should *not* be used. One-to-one nursing may be needed to ensure the patient's safety.

Drug treatment

Particularly when it is not possible to correct the underlying cause, consider an antipsychotic drug for both hyper- and hypo-active delirium (see p.355).

If the patient remains agitated, it may become necessary to add a benzodiazepine (see p.356). The impact of the combined use of an antipsychotic and a benzodiazepine in a dying patient will almost certainly lower the patient's level of consciousness, sometimes resulting in deep sedation until death.

DEMENTIA

Dementia, like delirium, is characterized by cognitive impairment and confusion (bewilderment). Cognitive deficits can be identified by formal tests such as the Mini-Mental State Examination.

Although dementia and delirium have a number of common features, and sometimes co-exist, it is important to distinguish between them because they:
• are distinct disease processes
• have different patterns of progression
• require different management (Table 1).

Table 1 Comparison of global cognitive impairment disorders

Delirium	Dementia
Mental clouding (information not taken in)	Brain damage (information not retained)
Acute or subacute onset	Chronic (but progress may appear to accelerate in end-stage disease)
Often fluctuating with periods of lucidity	Generally progressive
Reversible (less so at end of life)	Irreversible
Hallucinations common	Hallucinations less common
Speech rambling and incoherent	Speech stereotyped and limited
Often diurnal variation	Constant (in later stages)
Often aware and anxious	Unaware and unconcerned (in later stages)
Hyper- or hypo-active	Little or no motor disturbance (until late stage)
Fleeting systematized delusions	Delusions rare (except dementia with Lewy bodies, a post-mortem diagnosis)

Dementia is most commonly caused by Alzheimer's disease, and also by cerebral atherosclerosis and Lewy body disease. Cholinesterase inhibitors are used to reduce cognitive impairment.

Behavioural disturbances include agitation, physical aggression, culturally or sexually inappropriate behaviour, hoarding, and sleep disturbance.

Management of challenging behaviours in dementia

Correct the correctable

Patients with dementia may become agitated for many reasons, including an *appropriate* response to a distressing situation. Possible precipitants should be treated or modified:

- intercurrent infections
- pain and/or other distressing symptoms
- environmental factors.

Ensure that new carers are aware of the patient's daily routine. Consider the use of 'This is me' or a similar tool.[13]

If no cause for the agitation is found, consider an empirical trial of paracetamol. Pain can be difficult to identify. In an RCT, a stepwise trial of analgesia (paracetamol → opioid → pregabalin) reduced agitation in unselected patients (i.e. without any specific indicator of pain).[14]

Non-drug treatment

Structured behaviour management is the mainstay of treatment for the neuropsychiatric and behavioural features of dementia. Training in non-drug management of behavioural disturbance reduces the need for psychotropic medication.[15]

Drug-treatment

Psychotropic medication should be used only where other measures have failed. The efficacy of antipsychotics for challenging behaviour is marginal and generally outweighed by their undesirable effects (including increased risk of stroke and overall mortality).[16] Antidepressants, benzodiazepines and anti-epileptics are not consistently effective. Where drug treatment is required, consider seeking specialist advice. Options include:

- haloperidol (p.352)
- an atypical antipsychotic, e.g. olanzapine, quetiapine, risperidone (p.352)
- cholinesterase inhibitors (benefit is marginal, but may be better tolerated)
- trazodone (50mg at bedtime, where sleep disturbance predominates).[16]

Use the lowest effective dose for the shortest possible time. Attempt dose reduction every 2–3 months; many patients do *not* deteriorate when medication is withdrawn.[16,17]

RAISED INTRACRANIAL PRESSURE

Raised intracranial pressure is associated with intracranial mass lesions, cerebrospinal fluid circulation disorders, and more diffuse intracranial abnormalities. Onset may be acute or chronic. Specific examples include:
- primary and secondary brain tumours
- intracranial haemorrhage
- cerebral abscess
- drugs, e.g. lithium, tetracycline antibacterials.

Clinical features

Clinical features depend on the cause and the speed of onset:
- headache, classically worse on waking and when straining or coughing
- vomiting, worse in the morning
- change in behaviour
- visual disturbance
- pulsatile tinnitus
- seizures.

Clinical examination may reveal:
- papilloedema (not always apparent)
- focal neurological signs, e.g. cranial nerve lesions
- reduced level of consciousness
- reduced heart rate and raised blood pressure.

Evaluation

Contrast CT or MRI of the brain is undertaken to determine the cause and to guide management. If the patient is too unwell for a scan, a trial of corticosteroids can be given (see below). If the patient improves, further investigation can be considered.

Management

As always, management is preceded by explanation, and includes general support (see p.52).

For patients with a brain tumour, prescribe:
- corticosteroids, e.g. dexamethasone (p.365)
- appropriate analgesics (p.323) and anti-emetics (p.342).

Do *not* prescribe anti-epileptics unless seizures have occurred.

Other treatment options depend on location, number and size of the tumours, histological diagnosis, performance status, and include:
- surgical resection
- radiotherapy (whole brain, stereotactic).
- discuss with the appropriate site-specific cancer MDT.

SEIZURES

Causes

There are many potential causes of seizures in advanced disease (Box H).

Evaluation

Diagnosis is based largely on history from the patient, family and/or friends, and any eye-witnesses. There are two questions to answer:
- was it a seizure?
- is the cause correctable?

Was it a seizure?

Epilepsy is more likely if there are precipitating factors (e.g. television, sleep deprivation), prodrome/aura, unilateral symptoms (more likely in partial seizures):
- *during the seizure*:
  ▷ tongue biting, particularly at edge of tongue
  ▷ faecal incontinence (urinary incontinence is less specific)
  ▷ paroxysmal stereotypic movements, e.g. the body becomes rigid (tonic phase) possibly followed by regular muscle jerking (clonic phase)
  ▷ apnoeic episodes with cyanosis
- *after the seizure*:
  ▷ sleepiness
  ▷ confusion
  ▷ amnesia
  ▷ muscle aches.

The main differential diagnoses are syncope and psychogenic seizures. Syncope may be preceded by 'wooziness' but no aura or unilateral symptoms. Loss of consciousness is much briefer (<20sec), and the patient rapidly returns to normal. Muscle jerks may occur secondary to hypoxia.

In psychogenic seizures, the patient may have a psychiatric history. The patient may be motionless and have fluttering eye movements with forceful eye closure. Unusual or erratic movements may be seen, e.g. pelvic thrusting, out-of-phase limb thrashing. Breathing is more likely to be continuous and no cyanosis. Incontinence and tongue biting are uncommon. It is often refractory to treatment.

Is the cause correctable?

Unless imminently dying, the cause of the seizure should generally be sought (Box H). The drug history should consider poor adherence to and/or drug interactions with existing anti-epileptics, and the use of drugs which lower the seizure-threshold.

Possible investigations include:
- FBC
- urea, creatinine, electrolytes, LFTs, calcium, magnesium, glucose
- ECG and chest radiograph
- CT/MRI
- lumbar puncture
- EEG.

Box H Causes of seizures

Cancer
Brain metastases
Primary brain tumour

Drugs
Antipsychotics
Levodopa
TCAs
Theophylline
Tramadol
Withdrawal of
    anti-epileptics
    benzodiazepines

Infective
Brain abscess
Creutzfeld-Jacob disease
Encephalitis
HIV
Malaria
Meningitis
Septicaemia
Tuberculosis

Cardiac
Arrhythmias   } cause
Severe aortic stenosis } hypoxia

Substance abuse
Alcohol excess or withdrawal
Amphetamines
Cocaine

Metabolic
Hypo/hyperglycaemia
Hypo/hypernatraemia
Hypo/hypercalcaemia
Hypomagnesaemia
Uraemia

Neurological
Head trauma
Multiple sclerosis
Neurodegenerative diseases
    Alzheimer's
    multi-infarct dementia
Posterior reversible encephalopathy syndrome
Primary epilepsy
Stroke

Herbal remedies
Ginkgo bilboa

Other
Porphyria
Systemic lupus erythematosus
Sarcoid

Management

Initial management of seizures and status epilepticus

Generally, give a benzodiazepine:

- midazolam 10mg buccal/SC/IM/IV; if not settled, repeat after 10min *or*
- *if midazolam unavailable*: diazepam 10–20mg solution PR; if not settled, repeat after 10min.

A benzodiazepine can be withheld in a patient with known self-limiting seizures, i.e. lasting ≤5min without treatment, *unless* the seizure lasts ≥5min, or ≥3 seizures in 1h.

It is important to:

- check the blood glucose
- administer glucose solution 50% 50mL IV and thiamine 250mg IV (e.g. Pabrinex® 2 vials) if the patient is malnourished or if possibility of alcohol abuse.

Figure 3 is modified from NICE guidance.[18] IM midazolam may be more effective than IV lorazepam.[19] Phenobarbital has been given preference over phenytoin because it is more likely to be immediately available in many palliative care units. Status epilepticus is defined as a continuous seizure lasting more than 30min, or ≥2 discrete seizures between which the patient does not recover consciousness.

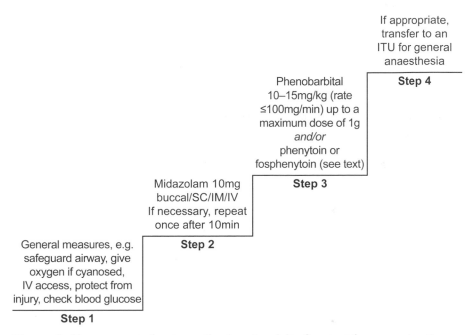

Figure 3 Management of status epilepticus in adults. See text for more detail.

Fosphenytoin is a pro-drug of phenytoin which can be given more rapidly than phenytoin. However, both require close monitoring of the patient, e.g. vital signs, ECG, and resuscitation facilities to be available, because of the risk of hypotension, cardiac arrhythmia and CNS depression.

If resuscitation facilities are poor, PR paraldehyde is a possible alternative because it causes little respiratory depression.

Ongoing management

After the seizures have been controlled, treatment should be continued with an appropriate maintenance regimen.

If the underlying cause of the seizure can be treated, e.g. meningitis or alcohol withdrawal, long term anti-epileptic drugs are unnecessary.

If the underlying cause (e.g. brain tumour, stroke) makes further seizures probable, an anti-epileptic is generally started (see p.345). Such seizures are partial onset (even if they rapidly generalise). Seek the advice of a neurologist if the diagnosis or the most appropriate anti-epileptic is in doubt.

Prophylactic anti-epileptics in those at risk of seizures

About 20% of patients with cerebral tumours will experience seizures, but the risk is *not* reduced by prophylactic anti-epileptics, except possibly immediately following neurosurgery.[20,21]

NON-CONVULSIVE STATUS EPILEPTICUS

Non-convulsive status epilepticus (NCSE) is characterized by seizure activity on an EEG but without associated tonic-clonic activity. NCSE occurs in about 5% of cancer patients with no evidence of brain metastases.[17]

The incidence is probably higher in patients with brain tumours. NCSE can be caused by any of the conditions which can provoke seizures (see Box H, p.204).

Because of its clinical features (Box I), NCSE can mimic dementia, delirium, other psychiatric disorders or coma. Presenting features may have a fluctuating course and persist over hours, days, or weeks.[22,23]

Box I Possible clinical features of non-convulsive status epilepticus	
Cognitive symptoms	**Motor signs**
Confusion	Automatisms
Dysphasia	Fluctuating pupil size (hippus)
Personality change	Nystagmus
Fear	Mild clonus of an extremity
Paranoid ideation	
Psychosis	

A high index of suspicion is needed to diagnose NCSE, and can be confirmed only by EEG.

Treatment for NCSE is less urgent than that for convulsive status epilepticus. In a case series, most responded to levetiracetam, but *not* valproate or phenytoin.[24] Also see Table 15, p.348.

MYOCLONUS

Myoclonus is sudden, brief, irregularly repetitive shock-like involuntary movements. Myoclonus may be:
- focal (a single muscle or group of muscles), regional or multifocal (generalized)
- unilateral or bilateral (either asymmetrical or symmetrical)
- mild (twitching) or severe (jerking).

Myoclonus is caused by either primary muscle activity or secondary to CNS stimulation. The latter is a central pre-epileptiform phenomenon and should not be ignored; it occurs mainly in moribund patients.

Causes

Myoclonus may be:
- physiological, e.g. associated with sleep or a startle reaction
- essential
- secondary to:
  ▷ hypoxia
  ▷ cerebral oedema
  ▷ neurological disorders, e.g. epilepsy, neurodegenerative, post-hypoxic, post-stroke, spinal injury, trauma, tumour
  ▷ biochemical disorders, e.g. hypoglycaemia, hyponatraemia
  ▷ renal and hepatic impairment
  ▷ drug toxicity, e.g. antimuscarinics, gabapentin, opioids
  ▷ drug withdrawal, e.g. benzodiazepines, barbiturates, anti-epileptics, alcohol.

Myoclonus may be exacerbated by dopamine antagonists, e.g. antipsychotics, metoclopramide.

Management

Treat the underlying cause if possible:
- drug-related, e.g. opioids, gabapentin or pregabalin: consider dose reduction or switching to an alternative
- metabolic disturbance, e.g. hyponatraemia, uraemia.

Otherwise, a benzodiazepine should be used, e.g.:
- clonazepam 0.5mg PO at bedtime or
- midazolam 2.5–5mg SC p.r.n. or CSCI 10–20mg/24h.

Adjust the dose upwards if several p.r.n. doses are needed.

MUSCLE CRAMP

Cramp is a painful involuntary muscle spasm lasting from a few seconds to many hours or days.[25] However, some authorities refer to pain lasting >10min as painful muscle stiffness.

Cramp is a universal experience. It occurs most commonly in a single muscle in the calf and foot, but may also involve arm muscles. Cramp originates from spontaneous discharges of the motor nerves rather than from within the muscle itself. Clinical features include:
- rapid onset of acute pain with a variable rate of improvement
- visible, palpable contraction generally in one muscle or part of a muscle
- triggered by trivial movements or forceful contractions
- eased by stretching the muscle
- residual soreness.

Careful evaluation will help to:
- distinguish cramp from local or generalized muscle pain
- identify sensory loss (suggests an underlying neuropathy)

- identify the presence or absence of weakness, muscle wasting, fasciculation (suggests a lower motor neurone disorder), hyperreflexia and spasticity (suggest an upper motor neurone disorder).

Investigations will depend on the likely cause(s).

Causes

There are many causes of cramp (Box J) but, in many cases, the cause may not be obvious. Sometimes, it relates to a myofascial trigger point.

Box J Causes of cramp

Idiopathic	**Endocrine**
Old age (nocturnal leg cramps)	Hypo-adrenalism
	Hypothyroidism
Acute extracellular volume depletion	
Diuretics	**Metabolic**
Excessive sweating	Cirrhosis
GI fluid loss (diarrhoea, vomiting)	Hypomagnesaemia
Haemodialysis	Renal impairment
Lower motor neurone disorders	**Miscellaneous**
MND/ALS	Autoimmune disease
Neuropathy	Hereditary disorders
Drugs, e.g.	
ACE inhibitors	
β_2-agonists	

Management

Correct the correctable

When possible, treatment should be directed to the underlying cause. If feasible, the dose of causal drugs should be reduced or stopped.

Non-drug treatment

Cramp cannot be induced or sustained in a stretched muscle. Stretching movements (both active and passive) are an important non-drug measure. Exercise ± stretching exercises three times a day, particularly before going to bed, often reduces the frequency and severity of nocturnal calf and foot cramps. In frail patients, this may need to be done by a physiotherapist, nurse or relative.

Forced dorsiflexion of the foot for 5–10sec repeated for up to 5min stretches both calf and foot muscles. It is an uncomfortable procedure but the nocturnal benefit may outweigh the short-term discomfort.[26]

Massage and relaxation therapy are particularly important for cramp associated with myofascial trigger points.

Drug treatment

Local

Trigger points can often be made less sensitive by injection with a local anaesthetic, e.g. lidocaine 1% or bupivacaine 0.5%. If the trigger point is secondary to muscle trauma, injection of a depot preparation of a corticosteroid (methylprednisolone or triamcinolone) may help to disrupt the trigger.

Systemic

See Skeletal muscle relaxants, p.372.

REFERENCES

1   Jaiswal R *et al.* (2014) A comprehensive review of palliative care in patients with cancer. *International Reviews of Psychiatry.* **26:** 87–101.

2   Wilson KG *et al.* (2007) Depression and anxiety disorders in palliative cancer care. *Journal of Pain and Symptom Management.* **33:** 118–129.

3   Bandelow B *et al.* (2007) Meta-analysis of randomized controlled comparisons of psychopharmacological and psychological treatments for anxiety disorders. *World Journal of Biological Psychiatry.* **8:** 175–187.

4   American Psychiatric Association (2013) *Diagnostic and Statistical Manual of Mental Disorders 5th Edition.* American Psychiatric Publishing, Arlington, USA.

5   Smoller J *et al.* (1996) Panic anxiety, dyspnea, and respiratory disease. Theoretical and clinical considerations. *American Journal of Respiratory and Critical Care Medicine.* **54:** 6–17.

6   McIntosh A *et al.* (2004) *Clinical Guidelines and Evidence Review for Panic Disorder and Generalised Anxiety Disorder.* University of Sheffield and National Collaborating Centre for Primary Care, London. pp.1–421.

7   Robinson S *et al.* (2016) A review of the construct of demoralization: History, definitions and future directions for palliative care. *American Journal of Hospice and Palliative Medicine.* **33:** 93–101.

8   Lawrie I *et al.* (2004) How do palliative medicine physicians assess and manage depression. *Palliative Medicine.* **18:** 234–238.

9   Lloyd-Williams M *et al.* (2003) Which depression screening tools should be used in palliative care? *Palliative Medicine.* **17:** 40–43.

10   Miller KE *et al.* (2006) Antidepressant medication use in palliative care. *American Journal of Hospice and Palliative Care.* **23:** 127–133.

11   Breitbart W and Alici Y (2012) Evidence-based treatment of delirium in patients with cancer. *Journal of Clinical Oncology.* **30:** 1206–1214.

12   Leonard MM *et al.* (2014) Practical assessment of delirium in palliative care. *Journal of Pain and Symptom Management.* **48:** 176–190.

13   Royal College of Nursing and Alzheimer's Society This is me tool. www.alzheimers.org.uk

14   Husebo BS *et al.* (2011) Efficacy of treating pain to reduce behavioural disturbances in residents of nursing homes with dementia: cluster randomised clinical trial. *British Medical Journal.* **343:** d4065.

15 Fossey J et al. (2006) Effect of enhanced psychosocial care on antipsychotic use in nursing home residents with severe dementia: cluster randomised trial. *British Medical Journal.* **332:** 756–761.

16 Rabins PV et al. (2014) Guideline watch: practice guideline for the treatment of patients with alzheimer's disease and other dementias. *American Psychiatric Association.* www.psychiatryonline.org

17 Cocito L et al. (2001) Altered mental state and nonconvulsive status epilepticus in patients with cancer. *Archives of Neurology.* **58:** 1310.

18 NICE (2012) The epilepsies: the diagnosis and management of the epilepsies in adults and children in primary and secondary care. *Clinical Guideline* CG137. www.nice.org.uk

19 Prasad M et al. (2014) Anticonvulsant therapy for status epilepticus. *Cochrane Database of Systematic Reviews.* **9:** CD003723. www.thecochranelibrary.com

20 Glantz MJ et al. (2000) Practice parameter: anticonvulsant prophylaxis in patients with newly diagnosed brain tumors. Report of the Quality Standards Subcommittee of the American Academy of Neurology. *Neurology.* **54:** 1886–1893.

21 Miller LC and Drislane FW (2007) Treatment strategies after a single seizure: rationale for immediate versus deferred treatment. *CNS Drugs.* **21:** 89–99.

22 Walker M (2005) Status epilepticus: an evidence based guide. *British Medical Journal.* **331:** 673–677.

23 Lorenzl S et al. (2008) Nonconvulsive status epilepticus in terminally ill patients-a diagnostic and therapeutic challenge. *Journal of Pain and Symptom Management.* **36:** 200–205.

24 Lorenzl S et al. (2010) Nonconvulsive status epilepticus in palliative care patients. *Journal of Pain and Symptom Management.* **40:** 460–465.

25 Miller TM and Layzer RB (2005) Muscle cramps. *Muscle Nerve.* **32:** 431–442.

26 Coppin RJ et al. (2005) Managing nocturnal leg cramps–calf-stretching exercises and cessation of quinine treatment: a factorial randomised controlled trial. *British Journal of General Practice.* **55:** 186–191.

FURTHER READING

Khasraw M and Posner JB (2014) Neurological complications of systemic cancer. *Lancet Neurology.* **9:** 1214–27.

Van der Sheen et al. (2014) White paper defining optimal palliative care in older people with dementia: A Delphi study and recommendations from the European Association for Palliative Care. *Palliative Medicine.* **28:** 3197–3209.

12. SYMPTOM MANAGEMENT: OTHER

FATIGUE

Fatigue is a common symptom in patients with advanced illness, particularly in those with cancer, which is the focus of this section.

Fatigue is defined as a distressing persistent subjective sense of physical, emotional, and/or cognitive tiredness or exhaustion relating to cancer or cancer treatment which is not proportional to recent activity and which significantly interferes with usual functioning.[1]

Causes

The pathophysiology of fatigue is not well understood, but it is associated with:[2]
- activation of the immune system and inflammation
- altered metabolic and mitochondrial function
- hypothalamic-pituitary-adrenal (HPA) axis dysfunction
- altered neuroendocrine function.

These also contribute towards sleep disturbance, mood disturbance, cognitive impairment and cachexia-anorexia (p.108), which further impact on physical function and activity.

Influencing factors include:
- stage of disease
- type of cancer treatment
- comorbidities
- drugs, e.g. sedatives, hormone therapy
- genetic variation, impacting on, e.g. regulation of the immune response.

Multiple contributing factors are commonly present (Box A).

Box A Contributing factors to fatigue in advanced cancer

Cancer
Cachexia-anorexia
Extensive disease
Pain and other symptoms

Treatment
Chemotherapy
Hormone therapy
Immunotherapy
Radiotherapy
Sedative drugs
Surgery

Psychological
Anxiety
Depression
Distress
Insomnia

Endocrine
Hypo-adrenalism
Hypogonadism
Hypothyroidism

Metabolic
Anaemia
Chronic renal failure
Dehydration
Hypercalcaemia
Hypokalaemia
Hypomagnesaemia
Malnutrition

Concurrent disorder
AIDS
Chronic heart failure
Infection

Debility
Physical deconditioning

Evaluation

It is important to ask about fatigue, and to consider if there are potentially reversible contributing factors.

Check Hb and electrolytes routinely in fatigued ambulant patients.

Management

Reducing fatigue to a major degree is generally *not* possible in advanced disease.

Correct the correctable

When possible and appropriate, consider correcting potentially reversible contributing factors (Box A). Ensure adequate control of pain and other symptoms.[3]

If feasible, reduce the dose of sedative drugs.

Non drug management

Patient education

This involves a range of approaches, including:[4]
- listen to the patient's concerns
- explain that activity/exercise is generally beneficial; even if they exhaust themselves attending a special event or undertake a desired activity, this will not harm them

---

- 'pacing' (essential activity followed by a rest) can be helpful
- encourage good sleep hygiene, e.g.:
  ▷ avoid stimulants (e.g. caffeine, alcohol) in evenings
  ▷ avoid lying in bed at other times other than sleep
  ▷ limit day time naps to <1h
- offer practical help to aid adjustment to changing circumstances.

Exercise

Aerobic exercise such as walking and cycling is beneficial for patients with cancer-related fatigue. Exercise also reduces emotional distress and improves functional capacity and quality of life.[5]

A target of 3–5h per week of moderate activity is recommended. Patients should select a type of exercise they enjoy and be encouraged to develop an implementation strategy to ensure they undertake the activity regularly. It may be necessary to start with lighter activity and shorter periods of time and gradually build in intensity and duration.

Blood transfusion

Blood transfusion can improve fatigue and breathlessness in patients with advanced cancer, but the effect lasts only about 2 weeks. Repeat transfusions should not be offered if there is no benefit.[6]

It is important to avoid transfusions in patients who are not likely to benefit, e.g. those close to death.

Drug management

Although various drugs have been used to treat cancer-related fatigue, evidence does *not* support routine use.[7] Some may be considered in specific circumstances:
- antidepressants: for patients with depression, particularly with sleep disturbance
- corticosteroids: beneficial in the short-term (≤2 weeks); long-term data lacking
- psychostimulants: methylphenidate or modafinil may have a limited role in patients with:
  ▷ depression and a limited prognosis (<2–4 weeks)
  ▷ opioid-induced somnolence (try switching to an alternative opioid first)
  ▷ severe fatigue (when other measures insufficient, give an initial 2 week trial)
- erythropoietin: safety concerns, undesirable effects and cost restrict its use to specific instances of cancer treatment-related anaemia (see SPC).

OEDEMA

Oedema (swelling caused by excess fluid in the interstitial space of tissues) is a common feature of advanced disease. It reflects an imbalance between capillary filtration into and lymphatic drainage out of the interstitial space.

There are multiple causes which may co-exist (Box B). The underlying mechanisms include:

- increased filtration from raised hydrostatic pressure in the capillary or venous system (e.g. venous incompetence), low plasma protein concentration or local inflammation
- reduced lymphatic drainage either from damage to lymph vessels or lymph nodes or from the lymphatics being overloaded
- immobility: muscle activity is essential to maintain both venous and lymph return from dependent limbs.

Box B Causes of oedema in advanced disease

General

Drugs
- salt and water retention, e.g. NSAIDs, corticosteroids
- vasodilation, e.g. nifedipine
- mechanism uncertain, e.g. gabapentin and pregabalin

Hypo-albuminaemia

Malignant ascites

Anaemia

CHF

End-stage renal failure

Local

Venous incompetence

Venous obstruction
- extrinsic venous compression by cancer
- DVT
- IVCO
- SVCO (see p.239)

Lymphovenous stasis
- immobility and dependency
- paralysis, e.g. hemiplegia,
- paraplegia

Lymphatic obliteration/obstruction
- primary/congenital
- secondary, e.g. cancer, cancer treatment, filariasis, etc.

Leg oedema can occur in ascites, particularly when associated with secondary hyperaldosteronism. Drainage of the ascites or the use of spironolactone (an aldosterone antagonist) can result in reduced oedema.

Complications include pain and cellulitis (see p.222), and fluid leakage. Ulceration may occur when there is associated venous or arterial disease, or as a result of maceration of the tissues from fluid leakage ('lymphorrhoea').

If the clinical history and features do not indicate a likely cause, possible investigations include:
- blood tests:
  - ▷ full blood count
  - ▷ plasma albumin
  - ▷ plasma electrolytes and creatinine
  - ▷ plasma BNP (to exclude CHF)

- imaging:
  ▷ chest radiograph (to exclude, e.g. CHF, SVCO).
  ▷ ultrasound to determine venous function
  ▷ CT or MRI to determine disease status, and whether there is lymphadenopathy.

As always, management will depend on the cause.

LYMPHOEDEMA

Oedema resulting from lymphatic obliteration/obstruction is called lymphoedema, and is either primary (congenital) or secondary. Secondary lymphoedema in cancer is associated with:

- axillary or groin surgery
- postoperative infection
- radiotherapy
- lymph node metastases.

Lymphoedema in cancer can occur in any part of the body but generally affects one or more limbs ± the adjacent trunk. If left untreated, lymphoedema may become a gross and debilitating condition. Trauma and acute inflammation cause a rapid increase in swelling.

Compared with non-obstructive oedemas, lymphoedema is protein-rich, and is associated with protein-induced chronic inflammation and fibrosis.

Patients with chronic oedema (by definition >3 months) may develop many of the features of obstructive lymphoedema as a result of lymphatic overload ('lymphatic failure'). The focus in this chapter is on obstructive lymphoedema.

Evaluation

Symptoms include:
- tightness
- heaviness
- a bursting feeling if there is an acute exacerbation
- pain caused by:
  ▷ shoulder strain (because of the weight of the lymphoedematous arm)
  ▷ inflammation
  ▷ brachial or lumbosacral plexopathy (caused by the associated cancer)
- impaired function/mobility
- psychosocial distress:
  ▷ altered body image
  ▷ problems in obtaining well-fitting clothes or shoes.

Psychosocial distress is not always apparent; specific enquiry may be needed.

Some of the distinguishing features of lymphoedema (and chronic oedema) include:
- persistent swelling of part or all of the limb which over time becomes non-pitting as a result of interstitial fibrosis and which does not decrease with elevation overnight

- increased tissue turgor
- Stemmer's sign (the inability to pick up a fold of skin at the base of the second toe); *the absence of this sign does not necessarily exclude more proximal lymphoedema*
- distorted limb shape
- lymphangiectasis (dilated skin lymphatics which look like blisters)
- deep skin creases associated with cutaneous fibrosis
- hyperkeratosis (a build-up of surface keratin resulting in a warty scaly skin)
- papillomatosis (a cobblestone effect caused by dilated skin lymphatics surrounded by fibrosis)
- cellulitis
- fluid leakage ('lymphorrhoea').

When the trunk is involved:
- the subcutis feels thickened on palpation
- when a fold of skin is pinched up simultaneously on both sides of the trunk, the skin is more difficult to grip on the affected side
- underwear leaves deeper markings on the affected side
- in unilateral leg lymphoedema, the ipsilateral buttock is bigger when examined with the patient standing
- in females, there may be genital wetness from leaking lymphangiectasis.

Radiotherapy also causes subcutaneous thickening but it is qualitatively different from that in lymphoedema, i.e. it is firmer and completely non-pitting.

Explanation

When associated with incurable cancer, patients should be told that lymphoedema cannot be cured, and that the aim of treatment is to make things more comfortable.

In most cases, discomfort can be reduced by measures which reduce tension in the swollen tissues, and the prevention of further deterioration as a result of immobility and cellulitis. Thus, patients need to be educated about:
- the importance of daily skin care to improve and maintain skin integrity, and thus to minimize the likelihood of infection
- the reasons why they are susceptible to infection, e.g. skin crevices harbour bacteria, stagnant protein-rich fluid, reduced immunity
- the consequences of infection, i.e. increased swelling, more fibrosis, decreased response to limb reduction treatment
- reducing the risk of infection by protecting hands when gardening, cleaning cuts, treating fungal infections and ingrowing toenails
- seeking prompt treatment if symptoms or signs suggest infection
- the importance of limb movement and exercise
- the need for an external compression garment or multilayered bandaging.

Management

When possible, advice should be obtained from a Lymphoedema Clinic or a health professional with a special interest in lymphoedema.

Note: in advanced cancer, it is generally *not* possible to reduce the size of a lymphoedematous limb. Emphasis should be placed on preventing deterioration and easing discomfort (Box C).

Box C Palliative lymphoedema management

Prevent the preventable
Skin care

Correct the correctable
Chemotherapy if appropriate

Non-drug treatment
Positioning
Containment
Exercise
Massage

Drug treatment
Analgesics
Corticosteroids } when indicated
Diuretics } (see text)

Management of complications
Cellulitis (see p.222)
Fluid leakage
Ulceration

Prevent the preventable

Skin care

Wash and apply an emollient (moisturizer) daily. This is often best done at bedtime. Patients with flaky dry skin may well benefit initially from treatment with 50/50 liquid paraffin in white soft paraffin. Give advice about avoiding trauma, thereby reducing the likelihood of infection (Box D). Cellulitis needs prompt treatment (see p.222).

Correct the correctable

Palliative chemotherapy should be considered for potentially responsive cancers, e.g. breast, lymphoma.

Non-drug treatment

Positioning

Support a heavy limb when resting. Elevation reduces venous hypertension and enhances drainage of the venous and lymphatic systems. Pillows or specially made foam supports can be used. Maximum benefit for the arm is achieved by elevation

---

Box D Written information for patients about skin care

General information

Keep the skin supple by daily applying a moisturizer.

Swollen arm: protect the hand and arm with a glove and long sleeve when cooking, washing up or gardening; wear a thimble when sewing.

Swollen leg: wear protective footwear at all times; do not walk in bare feet.

Avoid excessive heat (e.g. very hot showers/baths, saunas, sunbeds) and sunburn on the affected area because these can increase the swelling.

Dry well between digits after washing to protect from fungal infections.

Treat fungal infection with terbinafine 1% cream once daily for 2 weeks.

If shaving within the affected area, use an electric razor to avoid cuts.

Take care when cutting toe or finger nails; use clippers rather than scissors; do not push back nail cuticles.

Treat cuts or grazes promptly by washing and applying an antiseptic; cover with a dressing.

See your GP immediately if the limb becomes hot or more swollen.

Other important points about the swollen limb:
• do not allow your blood pressure to be taken on it
• do not have needles stuck into it (blood tests, injections, acupuncture).

Summer advice

Avoid insect bites; use insect repellent cream/spray; treat bites with an antiseptic and/or an antihistamine.

Protect the swollen limb from the sun:
• sit in the shade when possible
• use a high-factor sun block, e.g. 25–30.

Equipment to take on holiday:
• emollient
• high-factor sun block
• insect repellent cream/spray
• antihistamine tablets
• antiseptic solution.

If you have had recurrent infections, take an antibacterial with you when you go on holiday in case of need.

---

to the level of the heart. With leg elevation, the patient's back also needs to be well supported to prevent back pain, possibly by using a reclining chair. Note:
• arms should not be raised above 90° because further elevation reduces the space between the clavicle and the first rib, and may obstruct venous return

- in ambulant patients with arm oedema, avoid using a sling if possible because it tends to cause pooling of fluid at the elbow and joint stiffness. If a sling is required when standing, e.g. gross oedema ± weakness from brachial plexopathy, use a broad arm sling; *not* a collar and cuff which does not provide enough support and acts as a tourniquet.

Compression/containment

If possible, a compression garment should be worn all day and removed at night; this helps prevent (or 'contain') further swelling. Modern garments are lightweight, extremely strong and machine washable and last several months. Compression garments do not fit comfortably on awkwardly shaped limbs, and soft padding with light support bandaging may need to be used instead. Likewise, if a compression garment causes pain or if the skin condition is poor.

Compression garments should fit snugly around the limb to prevent:
- a tourniquet effect if too tight, particularly when there are deep skin folds
- a collection of fluid if too loose.

In patients with swelling of the fingers, a compression glove should be worn. Leotard or bodice-style garments are available for patients with lymphoedema affecting part of the torso, but these are generally not ideal for patients with advanced cancer. Some women benefit from custom-made bras.

In advanced pelvic malignancy with bilateral leg swelling, genital and trunk oedema, compression of the legs may lead to increased truncal and genital swelling. Compression garments can be used to provide support to the genitalia, e.g. support tights, maternity garments (panty girdles), scrotal support, cycling shorts.

Exercise

Patients must wear a compression garment or bandaging during exercise; this enhances the effect of muscle contraction on lymph flow.

Encourage normal activity. However, vigorous activity should be avoided because it tends to damage the superficial fine vasculature, exacerbating lymphatic overload.

Yawning, stretching and abdominal breathing all alter intra-thoracic pressure and help to empty the thoracic and abdominal lymphatics. Walking and other limb movements help to empty the peripheral lymphatics. However, static activity, e.g. carrying a heavy object for more than a few metres, should be discouraged because it reduces both venous and lymphatic return.

A complex exercise regimen is inappropriate. In advanced cancer, exercise will mostly maintain rather than improve function. Specific exercises should be tailored to the patient's abilities and general condition:
- joints are put through a full range of movements to maintain, and possibly improve, function
- limb muscles are used to improve lymph drainage
- fibrosis may be disrupted.

To enable patients to continue to function as normally as possible with severely swollen limbs, various appliances may be helpful:

- aids for walking and dressing for those with swollen legs
- special cutlery, tin openers, scissors, etc. for those with swollen hands and arms.

If active exercises are impossible, passive exercises should be carried out at least b.d. Passive movements of a swollen limb (including hand and fingers or feet and toes) in a severely ill, bedbound patient can reduce stiffness and discomfort.

Lymphatic drainage

Lymphatic drainage (a specific type of massage with associated deep breathing) can be an important component of lymphoedema management. Superficial skin and deeper massage both help to move lymph from the initial (non-contractile) lymphatics into the deeper muscular (contractile) collecting lymphatics.

Massage is the only way of clearing oedema from the trunk. Clearing the trunk increases drainage from the limb. Areas affected by cutaneous cancer should not be massaged.

Specialized forms of massage used in Lymphoedema Clinics are generally inappropriate in patients with a short prognosis; although they may help in advanced disease for patients with midline oedema (i.e. affecting the head and neck, trunk and/or genitals). However, in most cases, the patient, a relative, close friend or carer should be taught a more straightforward form of massage ('simple lymphatic drainage').

Drug treatment

Analgesics

Optimizing non-drug measures, e.g. with good fitting garments/bandaging and supporting a limb in a comfortable position often obviates the need for analgesics. However, if needed, paracetamol and opioids are preferable because of a reported association between skin infections, NSAIDs and necrotizing fasciitis.

Corticosteroids

If lymphoedema is associated with cancer infiltrating regional lymph nodes, a trial of dexamethasone 8–12mg once daily for 1 week should be considered. By reducing peritumour inflammation, lymphatic obstruction may be reduced. If the swelling improves, dexamethasone 2–4mg once daily can be continued indefinitely. Occasionally, in breast and prostate cancer or lymphoma, corticosteroids have a more specific anticancer effect.

Diuretics

A trial of diuretic therapy may be worthwhile. However, diuretics are generally *not* of benefit unless:

- the swelling has developed or increased since the prescription of an NSAID or a corticosteroid
- there is a cardiac or venous component.

In these circumstances, prescribe furosemide 20–40mg once daily for 1 week initially; the dose is then adjusted according to response. The addition of spironolactone 50–100mg once daily may bring additional benefit but the plasma potassium concentration should be monitored.

Management of complications

Fluid leakage ('lymphorrhoea')

Leakage of lymph through macerated/broken skin can soak through dressings and clothes, and pool in shoes. It mostly occurs when the skin is thin and fragile. It may also occur in acute oedema when normal skin is rapidly stretched and literally springs a leak. Treatment comprises:
- oil-based emollient (moisturizer) around the leak, e.g. petroleum jelly
- elevation of the limb to reduce the hydrostatic pressure
  ▷ arm to shoulder level
  ▷ leg on a foot-rest
- application of supportive or short-stretch bandaging by someone trained in their use, *or*
- absorbent pads to reduce the moisture in contact with the skin.
- application of a small ostomy bag to collect fluid if compression is inadequate
- if necessary, seek specialist advice.

Cellulitis

See Quick Clinical Guide, p.222.

QUICK CLINICAL GUIDE: CELLULITIS IN LYMPHOEDEMA

Cellulitis is often associated with septicaemia (e.g. fever, flu-like symptoms, hypotension, tachycardia, delirium, nausea and vomiting). It may be difficult to identify the pathogen but, in lymphoedema, *group A Streptococcus* is the most common.

Evaluation

1 Clinical features
   - mild: pain, increased swelling, erythema (well-defined or blotchy)
   - severe: pain, increased swelling, extensive erythema with well-defined margins, blistering and weeping skin; there may be features of septicaemia, and when the leg is affected, difficulty in walking.

2 Diagnosis is based on pattern recognition and clinical judgement. Elicit:
   - present history: date of onset, precipitating factor (e.g. insect bite or trauma), treatment received to date
   - past history: details of past cellulitis, precipitating factors, antibacterials taken
   - examination: include sites of lymphatic drainage to and from inflamed area.

3 Establish a baseline
   - extent and severity of rash: if well demarcated outline with pen and date
   - level of systemic upset: temperature, pulse, BP, CRP, WBC
   - swab cuts or breaks in skin for microbiology before starting antibacterials.

4 Arrange admission to hospital for patients:
   - with septicaemia (e.g. low BP, tachycardia, high temperature, vomiting)
   - failing to respond to antibacterials (see ladder below).

Antibacterials

5 To prevent increased swelling and accelerated fibrosis, cellulitis should be treated promptly with antibacterials. Continue antibacterials until the inflammation has been completely resolved for 2 weeks; this may take 1–2 months.

6 The advice of a microbiologist should be obtained in unusual circumstances, e.g. cellulitis developing shortly after an animal bite, and when the inflammation fails to respond to the recommended antibacterials.

7 Standard treatment at home (PO)

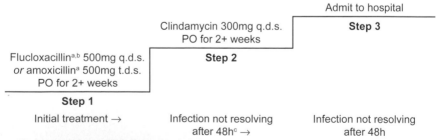

a. if a history of penicillin allergy, erythromycin 500mg q.d.s. or clarithromycin 500mg b.d. (but also see point 11 below)
b. if features suggest *Staph. aureus* infection (e.g. folliculitis, pus, crusted dermatitis), flucloxacillin should definitely be used
c. if despite 48h of a Step 1 antibacterial there are continuing or deteriorating systemic signs (± deteriorating local signs), admit to hospital; otherwise change to Step 2 antibacterial.

8 Standard treatment in hospital (IV): follow local guidelines. The following reflect the recommendations of the British Lymphology Society and Lymphoedema Support Network. Switch to PO flucloxacillin, amoxicillin or clindamycin when no fever for 48h, inflammation settling and CRP falling (see 7 above).

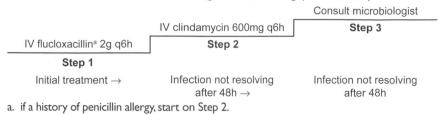

	IV clindamycin 600mg q6h	Consult microbiologist
		Step 3
IV flucloxacillin[a] 2g q6h	**Step 2**	
Step 1		
Initial treatment →	Infection not resolving after 48h →	Infection not resolving after 48h

a. if a history of penicillin allergy, start on Step 2.

9 For anogenital cellulitis, first line treatment is amoxicillin 2g IV q8h plus gentamicin 5mg/kg IV once daily; the dose of the latter to be adjusted according to renal function and gentamicin plasma concentration.

10 If ≥2 episodes of cellulitis/year, review skin condition and skin care regimen, and consider further steps to reduce limb swelling. Start antibacterial prophylaxis with:

- phenoxymethylpenicillin 250mg b.d. (500mg b.d. if BMI ≥33) for 2 years; halve the dose after 1 year if no recurrence
- if allergic to penicillins, prescribe erythromycin 250mg b.d.; if not tolerated use clarithromycin 250mg once daily (but see 11 below)
- if cellulitis develops despite the above antibacterials, consider other once daily alternatives, e.g. clindamycin 150mg, cefalexin 125mg or doxycycline 50mg; seek advice from a microbiologist and local specialist lymphoedema service
- if cellulitis develops after discontinuation of antibacterials after 2 years, treat the acute episode, and then commence life-long prophylaxis
- if recurrent anogenital cellulitis, prescribe trimethoprim 100mg at bedtime.

11 Check for important drug interactions with macrolides (clarithromycin, erythromycin); certain combinations are contra-indicated (e.g. domperidone, statins) or require close monitoring ± dose adjustment. Alternative antibacterials: cefalexin 500mg t.d.s. (but not if a history of severe penicillin allergy) or doxycycline 200mg once daily stat, then 100mg once daily. For prophylaxis, prescribe cefalexin 125mg or doxycycline 50mg once daily. Some antibacterials also interact with coumarins, e.g. warfarin.

General

12 Remember:

- if severe, bed rest and elevation of the affected limb on pillows are essential
- cellulitis is painful; analgesics should be prescribed regularly and p.r.n. Avoid NSAIDs because there is an increased risk of necrotizing fasciitis
- compression garments should not be worn until limb is comfortable
- daily skin hygiene should be continued; washing and gentle drying
- emollients should not be used in the affected area if the skin is broken.

13 Patients should be educated about cellulitis:
- why susceptible (skin crevices harbour bacteria, reduced immunity)
- causes increased swelling, more fibrosis, decreased response to compression
- daily skin care to improve and maintain skin integrity
- reduce risk, e.g. protect hands when gardening, clean cuts, treat fungal infections (terbinafine cream once daily for 2 weeks) and ingrowing toenails
- obtain prompt medical attention if cellulitis occurs.

14 When away from home, take a 2-week supply of PO flucloxacillin 500mg q.d.s. (or amoxicillin 500mg t.d.s.) for emergency use. If allergic to penicillins, erythromycin 500mg q.d.s. or clarithromycin 500mg b.d. (also see point 11 above).

FUNGATING LESIONS

A proliferative or cavitating primary or secondary cancer in the skin can lead to ulceration and fungation. This may be associated with:

- stinging, soreness, pain
- pruritus, particularly in breast cancer
- exudate
- malodour (exacerbating anorexia and nausea)
- bleeding
- infection.

A fungating cancer is distressing to the patient and may be repulsive to the carers, family and friends. Alteration of body image and malodour are distressing concomitants, and may result in social alienation and despair. Open discussion with the patient and the family is generally helpful.

Management

Discuss possibilities of disease-modifying treatments with oncologists or surgeons, e.g. radiotherapy, chemotherapy, hormone therapy, debulking surgery.

Infection

- *superficial:* proprietary metronidazole gel 0.75%; a cheaper alternative is metronidazole 200mg tablet crushed and applied to the ulcerated area mixed in lubricating gel
- *deep:* metronidazole 400mg PO q8h for 5 days
- broader spectrum antibacterials (e.g. co-amoxiclav 625mg PO t.d.s.) should be considered when there is cellulitis, systemic upset, or a lack of response to metronidazole alone.

Malodour

Controlling malodour, caused partly by tumour necrosis and partly by deep anaerobic infection, is often a major challenge. Treatment options include:

- surface cleansing (with warm water) once or twice daily
- debridement
- metronidazole: topical or systemic (see Infection above)
- live yoghurt or manuka honey topically
- counteract malodour with strong pleasant odours in the patient's living area or applied to the outer surface of the dressing, e.g. camphor, lavender.

Note: the benefit of charcoal-activated odour-absorbing dressings is questionable. Fresh air through an open window is often better than commercial air-fresheners; air filter systems are generally impractical.

Bleeding

- gentle pressure (firm pressure over a friable tumour may exacerbate bleeding)
- stop drugs which exacerbate bleeding, e.g. LMWH, low-dose aspirin prophylaxis

- review NSAID medication: consider switching to paracetamol or to celecoxib (does not exacerbate bleeding)
- PO haemostatic agents, e.g. tranexamic acid 1g q.d.s. for 1 week, then review
- topical measures, e.g. gauze soaked with tranexamic acid 500mg/5ml; sucralfate paste (crush two 1g tablets and mix in 5mL of lubricating gel, e.g. KY jelly®).

Pain

- systemic analgesics (see p.90)
- topical morphine may be helpful but not always feasible because of the extent of the ulceration
- an acute increase in pain may be caused by infection: consider antibacterials.

Associated pruritus is probably caused by inflammatory substances (e.g. PGs) and may respond to an NSAID.

Exudate

- absorbent dressing, changed as often as necessary to contain the exudate.

PRESSURE ULCERS

Pressure ulcers ('bedsores') are caused by ischaemia when skin is exposed to sustained pressure.[8,9] Pressure for periods as short as 1–2h may produce irreversible cellular changes leading to cell death. This occurs particularly over bony prominences, e.g. sacrum, greater trochanters, heels.

Many other factors make tissue ischaemia more likely (Box E). Despite best care, some patients with advanced disease will inevitably develop pressure ulcers.

Box E Risk factors for pressure ulcers	
Age >70 years	Immobility
Anaemia	Incontinence
Cachexia and weight loss	Nutrition deficiencies
Chemotherapy	Sensory impairment
Cognitive impairment	Skin fragility

Drugs:
    corticosteroids (high dose)
    NSAIDs	

Evaluation

Document the surface area of the ulcer using a transparency tracing or photograph, and an estimate of the depth.

Grade severity:

- *stage 1: non-blanching erythema*; intact skin. The area may be painful, firm, soft, warmer or cooler compared with adjacent normal skin
- *stage 2: partial thickness skin loss*; a shallow open ulcer with a pink-red wound bed without slough; may also present as a blister
- *stage 3: full thickness skin loss*; subcutaneous fat may be visible but bone, tendon or muscle not exposed. Slough may be present but does not obscure the depth of tissue loss
- *stage 4: full thickness tissue loss;* with exposed bone, tendon or muscle. Slough or eschar may be present on some parts of the wound bed; undermining and tunnelling common.[10]

Prevention

Use a validated risk scale (e.g. Braden) and check risk sites regularly.

Use a high-specification foam mattress for at-risk patients, and a high-specification foam or equivalent pressure redistributing cushion for patients who use a wheelchair or who sit for long periods.

Consider using a barrier preparation to prevent skin damage in patients at risk of skin maceration because of incontinence or excessive local moisture. Skin massage/rubbing is contra-indicated because it increases risk.

Because of limited nutritional intake, it is generally *not* possible to achieve a normal plasma albumin concentration and haemoglobin.

Encourage patients to change position at least every 4–6h, ideally more often. If unable to reposition themselves, provide assistance.

In the last few days of life, repositioning can be limited, particularly if movement causes significant distress (e.g. pain, breathlessness, agitation) and if the patient is unconscious.

Management

Patients with a prognosis of more than a few weeks may benefit from advice from a tissue viability nurse.

Most NHS Trusts in the UK have their own wound management guidelines. These will dictate the type of dressings to be used. A dressing which promotes a warm moist environment helps to promote ulcer healing.

Only consider systemic antibacterials if there is:

- spreading cellulitis *or*
- underlying osteomyelitis *or*
- clinical evidence of systemic sepsis.

Discuss the choice of antibacterials with a microbiologist.

PRURITUS

Pruritus (itch) is a dominant symptom of skin disease and also occurs in many systemic diseases (Box F).

Box F Systemic disease associated with pruritus

Endocrine
Carcinoid syndrome
Diabetes mellitus (associated with genital candidosis)
Hyperparathyroidism (secondary to chronic renal failure)[a]
Hyperthyroidism
Hypothyroidism

Haematological
Leukaemia
Lymphoma
Mastocytosis
Multiple myeloma
Polycythaemia rubra vera

Hepatic
Cholestasis
Hepatitis
Primary biliary cirrhosis

Renal
Chronic renal failure

Other
AIDS
Cancer
Multiple sclerosis

---

a. correction of hypercalcaemia leads to rapid relief; in other circumstances, hypercalcaemia is *not* associated with pruritus.

Although pruritus is limited to skin, conjunctivae or a mucous membrane (including the upper respiratory tract), the cause is not always peripheral (Box G).

Box G A neuro-anatomical classification of pruritus

Peripheral causes
Cutaneous ('pruritoceptive'), e.g.
    cutaneous mastocytosis (rare)
    drug (± rash)
    insect bite reactions
    skin diseases
    stinging nettle rash
    urticaria (most)
Neuropathic, e.g.
    post-herpetic neuralgia

Mixed peripheral and central causes
Uraemia

Central causes
Neuropathic, e.g.
    brain abscess
    brain injury
    brain tumour
    multiple sclerosis
Neurogenic, e.g.
    cholestasis
    opioid
    paraneoplastic
Psychogenic

Pruritus of cutaneous origin shares a common neural pathway with pain, but the afferent C-fibres are functionally distinct; some are stimulated by histamine and some by various other pruritogens, e.g. serotonin/5HT, substance P.[11] *This explains why some types of pruritus do not respond, or respond only poorly, to H_1 antihistamines.*

There is a wide range of causal factors; these are dependent on the underlying condition (Box H).[12]

Box H Causal factors in pruritus

Cholestasis
Autotaxin ↑
Endogenous opioids ↑
Serotonin release ↑

Old age
Dry skin
Mast cell degranulation ↑
Skin sensitivity to histamine ↑

Paraneoplastic
Histamine release from basophils
Immune response
Serotonin release ↑

Renal failure
μ- and κ-opioid receptor imbalance
Cytokines
Mast cell proliferation
Peripheral neuropathy
Skin divalent ions (Ca^{2+}, Mg^{2+}) ↑
Skin vitamin A ↑
Substance P release ↑

All drugs have the potential to cause an allergic reaction which can cause pruritus, with or without a rash. The mechanism involves the release of histamine from mast cells. The pruritus responds to H_1 antihistamines (and stopping the offending drug).

Note: there appear to be similarities between neuropathic pain, pruritus and cough. The common theme being peripheral and central sensitization of the sensory nervous system. This may explain why anti-epileptics and antidepressants have been reported as effective treatments for these very different symptoms.

Management

Correct the correctable

- dry skin (very common in old age and advanced disease):
  - ▷ avoid soap; use moisturizing soap substitutes, e.g. aqueous cream BP, Dermol® cream
  - ▷ apply bland emollient b.d–t.d.s., e.g. Diprobase® cream
- review medication: if a drug (e.g. an antibacterial) is a likely cause, it should be stopped and an alternative prescribed if necessary
- atopic dermatitis: topical corticosteroid and an emollient
- contact dermatitis: topical corticosteroid, identify causal substance, avoid further contact

- scabies: topical permethrin or malathion
- cholestatic pruritus secondary to obstruction of the common bile duct resolves if the jaundice is relieved by inserting an intraductal stent.

Non-drug treatment

- discourage scratching: file finger nails, allow gentle rubbing
- avoid prolonged hot baths
- dry the skin by patting gently with a soft towel or use a hair dryer *on a cool setting*
- avoid overheating and sweating, particularly in bed at night
- increase air humidity in the bedroom to avoid skin drying.

Drug treatment

Non-specific management

- *topical antipruritic*: levomenthol (menthol) cream BP 0.5–2% may be helpful if pruritus is localized or more intense in a limited area
- *antihistamine*: consider a trial either at bedtime or round the clock:
  ▷ a sedative H_1-receptor antagonist, e.g. chlorphenamine 4mg t.d.s.–12mg q.d.s. *or*
  ▷ a phenothiazine and H_1-receptor antagonist, e.g. promethazine 25–50mg b.d. *or*
  ▷ a TCA and H_1- and H_2-receptor antagonist, doxepin 10–75mg PO at bedtime.

The topical use of antihistamine creams should be limited to a few days in situations where histamine is involved, e.g. an acute drug rash.

Specific management

The following recommendations are presented as a step-by-step approach to drug treatment. However, the order chosen may vary depending on local preferences and availability.

Cholestasis

If stenting of the common bile duct is not possible, consider:
- sertraline 50–100mg once daily *or*
- rifampicin 150–600mg once daily (reports of severe hepatotoxicity)[13] *or*
- danazol 200mg once daily–t.d.s. (risk of hepatotoxicity and worsening cholestasis); if successful, titrate progressively downwards after 2–3 weeks (e.g. to once daily on 3 days/week) *or*
- naltrexone 12.5–250mg once daily (*unsuitable for patients needing opioids for pain relief*).[12,14]

Uraemia

- UVB phototherapy *or*
- doxepin 10mg b.d. *or*
- gabapentin 100–400mg once daily *or*
- sertraline 50mg once daily *or*
- naltrexone may be beneficial in severe uraemic itch (*unsuitable for patients needing opioids for pain relief*).[12]

Systemic opioids:

- H$_1$-receptor antagonist (benefits the minority in whom the pruritus is caused by cutaneous histamine release, see p.329) *or*
- switch opioid, e.g. morphine to oxycodone *or*
- ondansetron 8mg b.d.[12]

Hodgkin's lymphoma

- radiotherapy/chemotherapy *or*
- prednisolone 30–60mg once daily or dexamethasone 4–8mg once daily *or*
- cimetidine 800mg/24h (or alternative H$_2$-receptor antagonist) *or*
- carbamazepine 200mg b.d.[12]

Paraneoplastic/idiopathic itch

- sertraline 50–100mg once daily *or*
- mirtazapine 15–30mg at bedtime *or*
- when all else fails, thalidomide (cost prohibitive; may cause severe neuropathy when used long-term).[12]

REFERENCES

1 National Comprehensive Care Network (2014) Cancer related fatigue. In: *Clinical practice guidelines in oncology.* www.nccn.org

2 Saligan LN *et al.* (2015) The biology of cancer-related fatigue: a review of the literature. *Supportive Care in Cancer.* **23:** 2461–2478.

3 de Raaf PJ *et al.* (2013) Systematic monitoring and treatment of physical symptoms to alleviate fatigue in patients with advanced cancer: a randomized controlled trial. *Journal of Clinical Oncology.* **31:** 716–723.

4 Du S *et al.* (2015) Patient education programs for cancer-related fatigue: a systematic review. *Patient Education and Counseling.* **98:** 1308–1319.

5 Cramp F and Byron-Daniel J (2012) Exercise for the management of cancer-related fatigue in adults. *Cochrane Database of Systematic Reviews.* **11:** CD006145. www.thecochranelibrary.com

6 Preston NJ *et al.* (2012) Blood transfusions for anaemia in patients with advanced cancer. *Cochrane Database of Systematic Reviews.* **2:** CD009007. www.thecochranelibrary.com

7 Mucke M *et al.* (2015) Pharmacological treatments for fatigue associated with palliative care. *Cochrane Database of Systematic Reviews.* **5:** CD006788. www.thecochranelibrary.com

8 NICE (2014) Pressure ulcers: prevention and management of pressure ulcers. *Clinical Guideline* CG179. www.nice.org.uk

9 Haesler E (2014) *Prevention and treatment of pressure ulcers: quick reference guide.* National Pressure Ulcer Advisory Panel, European Pressure Ulcer Advisory Panel and Pan Pacific Pressure Injury Alliance. Cambridge Media: Osbourne Park, Western Australia.

10 European and US National Pressure Ulcer Advisory Panels (2014) *International Ulcer Guidelines.* www.epuap.org/guidelines/0/

11 Namer B *et al.* (2008) Separate peripheral pathways for pruritus in man. *Journal of Neurophysiology.* **100:** 2062–2069.

12 Zylicz Z *et al.* (2004) *Pruritus in advanced disease.* Oxford University Press, Oxford.

13 Howard P *et al.* (2015) Rifampin (INN Rifampicin). *Journal of Pain and Symptom Management.* **50:** 891–895.

14 Hegade VS *et al.* (2015) Drug treatment of pruritus in liver diseases. *Clinical Medicine.* **4:** 351–357.

FURTHER READING

Campos MPO et al. (2011) Cancer-related fatigue: a practical review. Annals of oncology. **22**: 1273–1279.
Ruddy KJ et al. (2014) Laying to rest psychostimulants for cancer-related fatigue? Journal of Clinical Oncology. **32**: 1865–1867.
Ryan JL et al. (2007) Mechanisms of cancer-related fatigue. The Oncologist. **12**: 22–34.

British Lymphology Society (2015) Consensus document on the management of cellulitis in lymphodema. www.thebls.com
Lymphoedema Framework (2006) Best Practice for the Management of Lymphoedema. International Consensus. London, MEP Ltd. www.woundsinternational.com/media/issues/210/files/content_175.pdf

13. EMERGENCIES

A palliative care emergency may be defined as a sudden change in a patient's condition where delay in management could result in an adverse outcome, e.g. distressing symptoms, disability or death.

Most patients receiving palliative care have a life-limiting condition but life expectancy may range from a few hours to many months, and sometimes several years. It is essential to know where each patient is in their disease trajectory before initiating investigations and treatment which cannot restore health, improve function or increase comfort, but merely serve to prolong dying.

The skill of managing emergencies in palliative care lies not only in knowing how to treat the emergency but also in deciding to what extent it is appropriate to do so. Key issues to consider are:
- the patient's recent performance status, extent of the underlying disease and prognosis (the rate at which the first two are changing provides a guide to the latter)
- the overall outcome if the emergency is treated or left untreated
- the likely effectiveness and burdens of any treatment
- the patient's wishes.

Whatever decisions are made about managing an emergency, comfort measures should always be provided to relieve distressing symptoms.

CHOKING

Choking is the sudden inability to breathe because of an acute obstruction of the pharynx, larynx or trachea. It typically occurs when food is not chewed properly and enters the upper airway. Risk factors include:
- talking or laughing while eating
- poorly fitting dentures
- impaired swallowing as a result of sedative drugs or alcohol

- neurological impairment, e.g.:
  ▷ Parkinson's disease
  ▷ pseudobulbar palsy (dysfunction of the lower cranial nerves), e.g. caused by MND/ALS, base of skull metastases, head and neck cancers
  ▷ brain tumour (primary or secondary)
  ▷ post-stroke.

Clinical features
- typically occurs while eating
- coughing or gagging
- panic
- sudden inability to talk
- hand signals, e.g. clutching or pointing to the throat
- wheezing
- cyanosis
- loss of consciousness → death.

Management
Determine if it is a partial (mild) or complete (severe) airway obstruction by asking 'Are you choking?' and proceed accordingly:

Partial
- able to speak, breathe, cough forcefully, not cyanosed
- encourage coughing to clear obstruction but do nothing else.

Complete
- unable to speak, breathe or cough, cyanosed
- give up to 5 back blows:
  ▷ stand to side and slightly behind person
  ▷ support chest with one hand and lean the person well forward to facilitate clearance of the obstructing object out of the mouth
  ▷ with the heel of your other hand give a sharp blow between the shoulder blades
  ▷ check after each blow for success; if 5 blows fail, proceed to abdominal thrusts
- give up to 5 abdominal thrusts (Heimlich manoeuvre):
  ▷ stand behind the person and lean them forward
  ▷ make a fist with one hand; put your arms around the person and grasp your fist with your other hand in the midline, halfway between the lower sternum and the umbilicus
  ▷ make a quick, hard movement inward and upward
  ▷ check after each thrust for success; if 5 thrusts fail, return to back blows
- continue alternating back blows and abdominal thrusts until:
  ▷ the obstruction is cleared
  ▷ the person can breathe and cough forcefully

- if the person loses consciousness and if appropriate, e.g. the person was not already close to death before choking:
  ▷ call for an ambulance/cardiac arrest team
  ▷ begin CPR.

A severe episode of aspiration can be a terminal event. Thus, particularly in patients with neurological impairment, and at high-risk of aspiration, it is good practice to have emergency drugs available at home for use to alleviate the inevitable distress:

- morphine 5–10mg SC/IV
- midazolam 5–10mg SC/IV
- hyoscine *butylbromide* 20mg *or* glycopyrronium 200microgram SC/IV.

As part of the *Breathing Space Programme* of the MND Association, a special box is available for MND/ALS patients via their GP to enable such medication to be kept at home in an obvious place.

An information sheet about the programme and an application form for the box can be obtained by GPs from the MND Association (www.mndassociation.org/index.html).

HYPOGLYCAEMIA

Hypoglycaemia is a blood glucose concentration lower than physiologically normal. It can be described as 'mild' if self-treated and 'severe' if assistance by another person is needed (Box A).[1]

In patients with long-standing diabetes, adrenergic warning symptoms may be absent because of autonomic neuropathy. Instead, patients present with neuroglycopenic features. Some become irritable and aggressive, and others slip rapidly into hypoglycaemic coma.

Box A Features of hypoglycaemia		
Adrenergic	**Neuroglycopenic**	
Hunger	Pallor	Mutism
Tremor	Mental detachment	Drowsiness
Sweating	Clumsiness	Seizures
Tachycardia	Mannerisms	Transient hemiplegia (rare)
	Personality change	Coma
	Confusion	

Causes

Causes of hypoglycaemia can be divided into two types:

- *fasting hypoglycaemia*: mostly caused by too much insulin or sulphonylurea in a known diabetic (Box B)
- *post-prandial hypoglycaemia*: may be caused by 'dumping syndrome' following gastric surgery, or reactive hypoglycaemia particularly after ingestion of alcohol.

Box B Causes of fasting hypoglycaemia[2]

Drugs
Drugs used to treat diabetes
   insulin
   meglitinides
   sulphonylureas
Other drugs
   alcohol
   aminoglutethimide
   pentamidine
   quinine

Organ damage
Hepatic failure
Pancreatitis

Endocrine
Addison's disease
Pituitary insufficiency

Cancer
Auto-immune (e.g. insulin receptor antibodies
   in Hodgkin's disease)
Ectopic production of insulin-like hormone
Insulin production (Islet cell tumour)

Management

A blood glucose <4mmol/L should be treated (Box C). For patients at risk, it is helpful to have a 'hypo box' containing everything necessary for treating hypoglycaemia, and keep it in a prominent place.[1,3]

Malnourished patients with reduced hepatic glycogen stores have a reduced capacity to counteract hypoglycaemia, and glucagon treatment in these patients is likely to be less effective.[2]

MEDICINAL OPIOID OVERDOSE

Causes of medicinal opioid overdose include:
- drug accumulation because of:
  - ▷ use of an opioid with a long halflife, e.g. methadone
  - ▷ reduced elimination because of renal impairment, e.g. morphine
- drug interaction, e.g. fentanyl and clarithromycin
- excessive dosing, e.g. opioid poorly-responsive pain, prescribing/administration error.

In situations where a patient has free access to their opioid, consider the possibility of a deliberate overdose.

Clinical features

- pinpoint pupils
- unconsciousness
- respiratory depression (<8 breaths/min ± cyanosis).

Box C Treatment of hypoglycaemia[4,5]

Conscious patient
1. Give *quick-acting* carbohydrate 15–20g PO:
   - 200mL of pure fruit juice
   - 100mL of Lucozade® (*not* diet version); this is preferable in renal patients
   - 150mL of Coca-Cola® (*not* diet version) *or* other non-diet fizzy drink
   - 5–6 Dextrosol® glucose tablets (or 4 Glucotabs®)
   - 3–4 heaped teaspoons *or* 4–5 lumps of sugar dissolved in water.
2. If the patient is not able to take tablets or drink but can still swallow, give 2 tubes of GlucoGel® or Dextrogel® squeezed into the mouth between the teeth and gums.
3. If the patient has a PEG, stop the feed and administer down the tube 30mL of undiluted Ribena® (*or* Lucozade® *or* Coca-Cola® as in point 1).
4. Repeat fingerstick test after 5min; if blood glucose <4mmol/L, *repeat above steps up to 3 times.*
5. Then, if blood glucose still remains <4mmol/L:
   - *if well-nourished*, give glucagon 1mg IM (can be given SC but will act more slowly)
   - *if malnourished or cachectic*, give glucose 10% 100mL IV.
6. When the blood glucose is >4mmol/L and the patient has recovered, give a *long-acting* carbohydrate of the patient's choice, e.g.:
   - two biscuits
   - one slice of bread/toast
   - 200–300mL glass of milk (not soya)
   - normal meal if due (must contain carbohydrate)/restart PEG feed.

   Note: patients given glucagon require a larger portion of *long-acting* carbohydrate to replenish glycogen stores.
7. If the patient is aggressive, give IV glucose (as below).

Unconscious patient ± seizures
- ensure airway is clear and give high-flow oxygen via a mask, check breathing and circulation, and obtain IV access. Give 20% glucose 75mL IV *or* 10% glucose 150mL IV over 10–15min.
- repeat fingerstick test 10min later: repeat glucose infusion if blood glucose <4mmol/L
- once conscious, give *quick-acting* carbohydrate drink (see points 1–3), followed by a starchy snack (see point 6)
- consider 10% glucose 100mL/h IV until the hypoglycaemic drug has been metabolized and blood glucose levels are stable.

Further measures
Review diabetes management:
- reduce insulin dose?
- stop oral hypoglycaemics?

Management

Discontinue opioid (stop CSCI/CIVI, remove TD patch):
- maintain airway
- administer oxygen to maintain SaO_2 >95%
- determine and monitor level of consciousness
- exclude hypoglycaemia (blood glucose fingerstick test)
- obtain IV access
- administer naloxone.

Naloxone is a pure antagonist which has a high affinity for opioid receptors but no intrinsic activity. It reversibly blocks access to the opioid receptor and, if given after an opioid agonist, displaces the latter because of its higher receptor affinity.

Naloxone is best given IV but, if not practical, may be given IM or SC.

Lower dose regimens must be used in patients receiving opioids for the relief of pain.[6,7] Higher dose regimens, e.g. naloxone 400microgram, will cause total antagonism leading to severe pain, and, if physically opioid-dependent, hyperalgesia and marked agitation, together with an acute withdrawal syndrome.[8] Thus, it is important to titrate the dose against respiratory function and *not* the level of consciousness.

If respiratory rate ≥8 breaths/min, and the patient easily rousable and not cyanosed, adopt a policy of 'wait and see'; consider omitting or reducing the next regular opioid dose, and subsequently continuing at a reduced dose.

If respiratory rate <8 breaths/min, and the patient comatose/unconscious and/or cyanosed:
- give naloxone 100–200microgram IV stat (e.g. 1/4–1/2 of a 400microgram/mL ampoule)
- if necessary, give 100microgram IV every 2min, until respiratory function is satisfactory.

An initial dose of 100microgram is preferable, with some guidelines recommending even smaller doses, e.g. 20–80microgram IV every 2min.[7] Diluting a 1mL ampoule containing naloxone 400microgram/mL to 10mL with 0.9% saline for injection facilitates this (20microgram = 0.5mL).

If the overdose is associated with a long-acting opioid, e.g. m/r formulation or methadone, the duration of action of the opioid will exceed that of naloxone (15–90min). Thus, even if there is an initial response to naloxone, further IV doses are likely to be needed, and it may be necessary to continue treatment with a closely monitored IVI of naloxone for up to 24h, and sometimes longer.

Wait until there has been a sustained improvement in consciousness before restarting a lower dose of opioid. It may be preferable to switch the type of opioid, e.g. to fentanyl in renal impairment; seek specialist advice.

After the administration of naloxone, if there is unexpected breathlessness and persistent hypoxaemia despite oxygen, the possibility of pulmonary oedema should be considered. Delayed-onset pulmonary oedema (48h after overdose) may also occur, associated with acute cardiomyopathy, and possibly the result of hypoxaemic cardiac muscle damage.[9] Treat as necessary with oxygen, IV furosemide, IVI nitrates, and ventilation. The pulmonary oedema generally responds to these measures and resolves within 24–48h.

Because buprenorphine has very strong receptor affinity (reflected in its high relative potency with morphine), naloxone in standard doses does *not* reverse the effects of buprenorphine and higher doses must be used, e.g. IV naloxone *2mg* stat over 90sec.

SUPERIOR VENA CAVAL OBSTRUCTION

Superior vena caval obstruction (SVCO) results from compression or occlusion of the SVC. Cancer-related SVCO (90% of cases) is generally caused by extrinsic compression of the SVC by:
* intra-thoracic primary cancer, e.g. lung cancer (80% of all cases), mesothelioma
* mediastinal lymphadenopathy, e.g. metastatic cancer, lymphoma.[10]

Most cases are subacute in onset, but can be more abrupt if a thrombosis develops (Box D).

Benign SVCO (10% of cases) is generally caused by intrinsic occlusion of the SVC by thrombus associated with indwelling venous devices, e.g.:
* central venous catheters
* cardiac devices.

Uncommon causes include post-radiotherapy fibrosis, goitre, lung tuberculosis.

Box D Clinical features of SVCO

Common symptoms
Breathlessness (50%)
Neck and facial swelling (40%)
Trunk and arm swelling (40%)
A sensation of choking
A feeling of fullness in the head
Headache

Other potential symptoms
Chest pain
Cough
Dysphagia
Cognitive dysfunction
Hallucinations
Seizures

Physical signs
Thoracic vein distension (65%)
Neck vein distension (55%)
Facial oedema (55%)
Tachypnoea (40%)
Plethora of face (15%)
Cyanosis (15%)
Arm oedema (10%)

If severe
Laryngeal stridor
Coma
Death

Management

Management is guided by liaison with oncology and radiology services, and varies according to the severity of symptoms and whether suspected or known cancer.[11,12]

Cancer-related SVCO with mild symptoms

SVCO rarely presents as an emergency because most patients develop good compensatory collateral circulation.

When SVCO is the first presentation of suspected cancer:

- investigate with appropriate imaging, e.g. CT
- biopsy mass/lymph nodes; a histological diagnosis will guide treatment with radiotherapy, chemotherapy and/or stenting
- unless there are severe symptoms, do not give high-dose corticosteroids until biopsy taken (may hinder histological diagnosis).

When SVCO occurs in someone with known cancer:

- if radio- or chemo-sensitive, e.g. lymphoma or germ cell tumour, treat accordingly
- if not sensitive, or further treatment is not an option, consider high-dose corticosteroids, e.g. dexamethasone 16mg once daily/8mg b.d. PO/IV, and insertion of a self-expanding metal stent into the SVC.

Stent insertion provides more rapid symptom relief in a greater proportion of patients than radiotherapy or chemotherapy.[11] After stenting, >90% of patients die without recurrence of the obstruction.[13]

Undesirable events are uncommon, e.g. stent misplacement, stent migration, pulmonary oedema, cardiac events, haemorrhage.

When stenting, if there is associated thrombosis, thrombectomy or thrombolytic treatment (e.g. streptokinase) may be necessary.[14] Long-term anticoagulation or anti-platelet therapy may be advisable in those who required thrombolysis.

Cancer-related SVCO with severe symptoms

Emergency treatment comprises:

- oxygen to correct hypoxaemia
- high-dose corticosteroids, e.g. dexamethasone 16mg once daily/8mg b.d. PO/IV to reduce peritumour oedema and extrinsic compression
- insertion of a self-expanding metal stent into SVC (see above).

If the patient is close to death, or has had previous SVC stents inserted and further stent insertion is not possible, provide sedation to relieve distress (see Overwhelming distress, p.253).

Management of benign SVC obstruction

Treat the underlying cause, e.g. removal of the central venous catheter, anticoagulation. There is no role for corticosteroids or diuretics.

SPINAL CORD COMPRESSION

Malignant spinal cord compression (MSCC) is a medical emergency because the outcome with paraplegia is worse than with paraparesis. The aim is to make the diagnosis and start treatment *before* the compression has irreversibly impaired nerve function, i.e. preventing the preventable.

MSCC is defined as compression of the dural sac and its contents (spinal cord and/ or cauda equina) by an extradural tumour mass. It occurs in 3–5% of patients with advanced cancer, with cancers of the breast, bronchus and prostate accounting for >60% of cases.[15] Most cases are caused by:

- vertebral collapse (85%)
- extravertebral tumour extending through an intervertebral foramen into the epidural space, e.g. lymphoma (10%).

Spinal levels of MSCC:

- thoracic (70%)
- lumbosacral (15–30%)
- compression at more than one level (30–50%).[16]

Below the level of L2 vertebra, compression is of the cauda equina i.e. peripheral nerves and *not* spinal cord.

Clinical features

See Table 1.

Table 1 Clinical features of MSCC

Feature	Incidence	Comment
Back pain	>90%	Often present for 2–3 months before diagnosis
Limb weakness	>75%	2/3 of these are unable to walk at diagnosis
Sensory level	>50%	Not a feature of cauda equina compression
Bladder and anal sphincter dysfunction	>40%	Particularly bladder: hesitancy, frequency, (late) painless retention

Pain may be caused by:

- vertebral metastasis
- nerve root compression ⎫ often exacerbated by straight-leg raising,
- cord compression ⎬ coughing, sneezing or straining
- muscle spasm.

Examination

Depending of duration of symptoms and level(s) of compression, neural signs of MSCC may include:

- in acute onset, flaccid paralysis/paraparesis

- progressing over time to:
  ▷ spasticity (increased tone, clonus and hyperreflexia in limbs below level of MSCC)
  ▷ plantar reflexes upgoing (but not if cauda equina compression)
  ▷ sensory loss with well-defined dermatomal level
  ▷ palpable bladder (urinary retention).

Signs of cauda equina compression may be asymmetric and include:
- paraparesis/flaccid paralysis with hyporeflexia and hypotonia of lower limbs
- sensory loss in a nerve root distribution; may be confined to sacrum or perineum (patient may be unaware of this until examined)
- reduced anal tone on rectal examination.

Note: cauda equina compression can present without weakness of the legs and can be easily missed.

Evaluation

Unless the patient is too ill and close to death, arrange urgent investigations:
- MRI of the whole spine is the investigation of choice
- CT may be helpful if MRI is not available.

If neither MRI nor CT are feasible, a plain radiograph of the spine will show vertebral metastasis and/or collapse at the appropriate level in 80%.

Management

Treat as an emergency unless the patient is in the last few hours or days of life. All patients must be given corticosteroids (see below). Most will receive radiotherapy; decompressive surgery is reserved for a carefully selected minority. Occasionally, chemotherapy is used as first line treatment for those with chemosensitive tumours e.g. germ cell tumour.
- liaise with MSCC co-ordinator (where available) or oncologist ± neurosurgeon or spinal surgeon to plan treatment, taking into account cancer type, prognosis and functional status of patient
- consider nursing in neutral spinal alignment (including 'log-rolling') until spinal instability is excluded on imaging, particularly if there is severe movement-related back pain or neurological symptoms
- provide pain relief.[17,18]

Corticosteroids:
- dexamethasone 16mg PO stat
- continue with 16mg PO each morning for a further 3–4 days
- maintain on 8mg PO each morning until the completion of radiotherapy or surgery
- taper (and discontinue) over 2 weeks after the completion of radiotherapy.[19]

If there is neurological deterioration during the dose reduction, the dose should be increased again to the previous satisfactory dose, and maintained at that level for a further 2 weeks before attempting to taper the dose again.

Radiotherapy

Usual primary treatment for patients who are able to walk and who do not meet criteria for surgery:

- generally delivered as fractionated therapy, e.g. 20Gy in 5 daily fractions
- for patients with a poor prognosis, established paraplegia and severe pain, a single fraction of 8Gy may be given for analgesia.

In patients who were paraparetic and paraplegic before treatment, recovery of ambulation was <40% and 13% respectively.

Surgery

Discuss with neurosurgeon or spinal surgeon if fit enough for surgery, has a prognosis of >3 months and one or more of following features present:

- paraplegia <48h with a single level of compression
- radiotherapy unlikely to be or has not been effective because patient has
  ▷ an unstable spine
  ▷ compression from intraspinal bony fragments or a collapsed vertebra
  ▷ deteriorating neurological function (particularly if occurs despite dexamethasone and radiotherapy)
  ▷ pain despite previous radiotherapy/maximum radiotherapy already received.[18,20]

Radiotherapy should also be considered after surgery.

Prognosis

Patients with paraparesis do better than those who are totally paraplegic. Loss of sphincter function is a bad prognostic sign. If the cord compression is of rapid onset (1–2 days), the most likely cause is infarction of the spinal cord as a consequence of spinal artery thrombosis secondary to compression/distortion by malignant disease. This does not respond to treatment.

For patients who do not recover mobility after treatment, median survival is 1–3 months. For those able to walk, median survival is 5–8 months.[21,22] Some patients, notably those with lymphoma or myeloma, survive 1–2 years, occasionally longer.[23]

Ongoing care

A multi-professional assessment for rehabilitation potential should be undertaken, and particular attention paid to:

- risk of autonomic dysreflexia, a life-threatening complication of paraplegia (Box E)
- bladder management – an indwelling urinary catheter may be required initially but this should be reviewed depending on response to treatment
- bowel management – a neurological bowel management plan may be required
- discharge planning.

Box E Autonomic dysreflexia[24]

Occurs mostly with complete spinal cord transections above T7, but also reported as low as T10 and with incomplete transections.

Patients at risk of autonomic dysreflexia should be educated about ways to avoid it (particularly the importance of good bladder/bowel management) and how to identify and manage an episode.

Most commonly caused by a distended bladder or rectum (or another nociceptive stimulus *below* the level of the lesion) causing sympathetic autonomic overactivity resulting in vasoconstriction and hypertension.

This stimulates parasympathetic overactivity *above* the lesion via the carotid and aortic baroceptors resulting in vasodilation and bradycardia.

As a general rule, headache in someone with paraplegia/tetraplegia should lead to action.

Clinical features

Sudden uncontrolled rise in blood pressure:
- systolic pressures reaching up to 300mmHg (typically 180–200mmHg)
- diastolic pressures reaching up to 220mmHg (typically 100–150mmHg)
- pounding headache.

Other features may include:
- feelings of anxiety
- blurred vision
- nasal congestion
- breathlessness
- bradycardia (relative to usual resting heart rate)
- profuse sweating above the level of the spinal injury
- *blotchy skin rash or flushed above the level of the spinal injury* (due to parasympathetic activity)
- *cold with goose pimples below the level of injury* (due to the sympathetic activity).

Management

Confirm diagnosis (blood pressure >180/100 *or* 20–40mmHg higher than normal).

Provided the spine is stable, sit the patient up with legs down, and remove any tight clothing, e.g. socks and shoes.

Identify and remove the noxious stimulus, e.g.:

Box E Contd.

For patients with a catheter:

- check that the tubing is not blocked or kinked
- if blocked, remove the catheter, and re-catheterize using a lidocaine lubricant (despite loss of sensation).

For patients without a catheter:

- if bladder distended and patient unable to pass urine, insert catheter using a lidocaine lubricant.

If bladder distension excluded, gently examine the anus and rectum using a gloved finger lubricated with lidocaine jelly; remove any faeces.

If symptoms persist (and/or systolic blood pressure >150mmHg) give a vasodilator. If the patient has not used a phosphodiesterase 5 inhibitor within the last 48h:

- glyceryl trinitrate SL 300–600microgram (tablets) or 400microgram (spray); repeat every 5–10min if necessary up to a maximum of three doses.

If blood pressure remains high (or if the patient has used a phosphodiesterase 5 inhibitor), options include:

- captopril 25mg SL
- nifedipine 10mg PO (bite into and swallow the liquid contents of an immediate-release capsule).

Monitor blood pressure and heart rate every 5min. Continue to search for a cause if none yet found. A Spinal Cord Injury Centre can be contacted for further advice.

Admit to hospital those failing to respond to the above; they may require an IV hypotensive drug, e.g. hydralazine 20mg or labetolol 10mg, and management in a high-dependency unit.

HYPERCALCAEMIA

Hypercalcaemia is a raised *corrected* plasma calcium concentration (normal range 2.2–2.6mmol/L). 'Correction' for variation in the plasma albumin concentration is generally done by the laboratory.

Hypercalcaemia occurs in 10–20% of patients with cancer, most common in squamous cell cancers of the lung, head and neck, kidney and cervix uteri.

Generally, it is a paraneoplastic phenomenon, relating to the ectopic production of parathyroid hormone-related peptide, and is thus unrelated to the extent of bone metastasis.

Diagnosis is based on clinical suspicion and confirmed by blood tests. Primary hyperparathyroidism is the main differential diagnosis.

Clinical features

Hypercalcaemia can cause a range of non-specific symptoms (Box F). Severity relates more to the rate of increase in the plasma calcium concentration than to the actual concentration. Most patients who develop hypercalcaemia have disseminated disease; many die in <3 months and 80% within 1 year.[25]

Box F Symptoms of hypercalcaemia

Mild
Polyuria   } not constant
Polydipsia/thirst } features
Fatigue
Lethargy
Mental dullness
Weakness
Anorexia
Constipation
Increasing pain

Severe
Nausea   } → dehydration and
Vomiting   } cardiovascular collapse
Ileus
Delirium
Drowsiness
Coma

Management

Stop and think! Are you justified in treating a potentially fatal complication in a moribund patient?

The following criteria jointly justify the correction of hypercalcaemia:
• corrected plasma calcium concentration of >2.8mmol/L
• symptoms attributable to hypercalcaemia
• first episode or long interval since previous one
• previous good quality of life (in the patient's opinion)
• medical expectation that treatment will achieve a durable effect (based on the results of previous treatment)
• patient willing to undergo IV therapy and requisite blood tests.

IV fluids

Initial treatment is with IV 0.9% saline 2–3L/24h. This helps by correcting dehydration and by beginning to reduce the plasma calcium concentration.

Bisphosphonates

Definitive treatment is with a bisphosphonate (see p.359). Because of the risk of renal toxicity, patients must be well hydrated before their use.

HAEMORRHAGE

In advanced cancer, bleeding contributes significantly to the patient's death in about 5%. External catastrophic bleeding is less common than internal occult bleeding.

Surface bleeding

Surface bleeding may be caused by a primary cancer or metastasis, or be associated with drugs or a concurrent illness. Bleeding may present as:
* haematemesis and/or melaena
* rectal haemorrhage
* vaginal haemorrhage
* haemoptysis (see p.160)
* bleeding from a fungating wound (see p.225)
* nosebleed
* haematuria.

Other causes of bleeding

Platelet disorders

* present as petechial rash, excessive bruising (purpura) and/or bleeding from nose/gums/bladder
* causes include marrow replacement with cancer (e.g. acute myeloid leukaemia, myeloma), drugs (e.g. chemotherapy, carbamazepine, heparin), idiopathic thrombocytopenic purpura, sepsis, disseminated intravascular coagulation (DIC).

Coagulation disorders

* present as bruising and bleeding into joints or muscles
* causes include severe liver impairment, phytomenadione (vitamin K_1) deficiency, DIC.

Management

Validate the patient's and family's concern; never say, 'Don't worry', but 'You must be worried about it.'

If the patient is well enough, check:
* FBC
* prothrombin time (PT)
* activated partial thromboplastin time (APTT).

Additional investigations may be required; seek advice from a haematologist.

Correct the correctable

Can the cancer be modified?

Liaise with oncologist in case further anticancer treatment is possible. Radiotherapy can be effective for surface bleeding, e.g. skin, lungs, oesophagus, rectum, bladder, uterus, vagina.

Can other factors be modified?
- review drug chart and stop anticoagulants (e.g. LMWH, warfarin), anti-platelet drugs (e.g. aspirin, clopidogrel) and drugs which impair platelet function (e.g. SSRIs, most NSAIDs)
- treat vitamin K deficiency
- treat concurrent illness, e.g. infection (may worsen haematuria, haemoptysis).

Physical management of bleeding from accessible sites
- gauze applied with pressure for 10min soaked in the contents of an ampoule for injection of:
  ▷ tranexamic acid 500mg in 5mL (wounds/anterior epistaxis) *or*
  ▷ adrenaline (epinephrine) (1 in 1,000) 1mg in 1mL (wounds; short-term only)
- silver nitrate sticks applied to bleeding points (nose, mouth, wounds)
- haemostatic dressings, i.e. alginate (e.g. Kaltostat®, Sorbsan®)
- sucralfate paste; two 1g tablets crushed in 5mL water-soluble gel, e.g. KY jelly® (wounds).

Drugs

Systemic drugs:
- antifibrinolytic drug, e.g. tranexamic acid 1g PO q.d.s.[26]

Topical drugs for cancer bleeding from less accessible sites

Generally used only if other options/PO tranexamic acid have failed; instillations should be warm, ideally body temperature:
- *mouth (use as mouthwash, can be swallowed after use):*
  ▷ tranexamic acid solution 500mg/10mL (5%) 10mL q.d.s.; use special order mouthwash or dilute one 500mg/5mL ampoule for injection with 5mL water
  ▷ sucralfate oral suspension 2g in 10mL b.d.
- *rectum (instil as enema):*[27,28]
  ▷ tranexamic acid solution 5g/100mL (5%) 100mL once daily or b.d.; use special order mouthwash or dilute ten 500mg/5mL ampoules for injection with 50mL water
  ▷ sucralfate oral suspension 2g in 10mL b.d.
- *bladder (via urinary catheter):*[29,30]
  ▷ continuous irrigation with 0.9% saline
  ▷ tranexamic acid solution 5g/100mL (5%) 100mL once daily or b.d.; dilute ten 500mg/5mL ampoules for injection with 50mL sterile water
- *lungs*
  ▷ nebulized tranexamic acid, see p.160.

Small bleeds may be a 'herald' or a 'warning' that a severe haemorrhage is relatively imminent. Consider carefully whether this possibility should be discussed with the patient so that their wishes can be determined and treatment planned, should severe haemorrhage develop (see p.259).

Thrombocytopenia and DIC

In palliative care, bleeding from severe thrombocytopenia or DIC is very likely to be a terminal event. Although liaison with a haematologist should be considered to discuss emergency platelet transfusions, it is likely to be most appropriate to manage this in the same way as severe haemorrhage (see below).

Severe haemorrhage

Massive haemorrhage from a major artery (neck, lungs, groin) is a rare rapidly fatal complication of cancer, particularly of the neck or lung. It is more likely after surgery and/or radiotherapy. It is generally *not* expected, and death typically occurs in seconds rather than minutes.

Readily available 'crisis' medication is often recommended (e.g. midazolam), but unless *immediately* available, it is of *no use* in the event of a massive haemorrhage. *Sitting with the patient and holding their hand is the only realistic comfort measure.*[31]

In practice, it is often not possible to keep medication for emergency use by a patient's bed. Thus, the patient would be left alone during those final seconds of consciousness while midazolam was obtained and administered. Even if this was done by a second person, the patient would be dead before the medication could take effect.

However, if the patient does not die immediately, local pressure should be applied with packing. The more superficial material can be changed if it becomes saturated with blood. A green surgical towel may make the extent of blood loss less obvious and less disturbing to the patient and family.

Further management will depend on the extent of the bleeding, the stage of the cancer, the patient's performance status and their previously stated wishes.

On occasion, it may be appropriate to:
• give midazolam 5–10mg buccal/SC/IV (if the patient is distressed)
• monitor heart rate, blood pressure, oxygen saturation
• insert a large bore IV cannula (16G)
• infuse IV crystalloid fluid 1–2L
• take blood for FBC, urea and electrolytes, coagulation status (PT, APTT), blood group and cross match.

Check the pulse every 30min: if it is steady or decreases, this suggests that bleeding has stopped. If the patient survives 24h, consider a blood transfusion.

Massive haemoptysis

Although about 20% of patients with lung cancer experience haemoptysis, the incidence of fatal massive haemoptysis is only 3%.

Massive haemoptysis is most likely with squamous cell cancer lying centrally or causing cavitation.

In a patient with a poor prognosis, conventional life-saving interventions, e.g. resuscitation, interventional bronchoscopy, arterial embolization, are generally *not* appropriate (Box G).

If the patient survives, the situation will need to be reviewed with the patient and family after 1–2 days. Life-support measures may need to be considered, e.g. blood transfusion.

Box G Palliative management of massive terminal haemoptysis

Anticipation

When there is potential for life-threatening haemoptysis (suggested by increasing volume and frequency), this should prompt a team discussion with the patient and family to agree an appropriate management plan, including a 'do not attempt cardiopulmonary resuscitation' decision.

Have dark towels, dark sheets/blankets or absorptive dressings available to reduce the visual impact of large amounts of fresh blood.

If practical, have a syringe containing morphine and one containing midazolam 10mg drawn up and kept in a convenient safe place, or have ampoules readily available.

The dose of the opioid will depend on whether the patient is already receiving morphine regularly. If not, 10mg will be appropriate; otherwise use the equivalent of a q4h dose. The aim is to reduce fear, not necessarily to render the patient unconscious.

If massive haemoptysis occurs

Untreated massive haemoptysis has a mortality rate >50%. Do not leave the patient alone until the situation has resolved one way or the other.

Maintain the airway: ideally, the patient should lie bleeding side down (if known) to reduce the impact on the other lung. Otherwise allow the patient to adopt the position in which they feel most safe/comfortable.

Administer morphine and midazolam SC but IV or IM if the patient is shocked and peripherally vasoconstricted.

ACUTE SEVERE PAIN

Unrelieved pain should always be treated with urgency (see p.81). The following describes some of the situations which cause acute severe pain, even in patients taking regular analgesics.

Note: a common misconception among the general public is that death is heralded by an agonizing crescendo of pain, totally resistant to analgesics. Thus, sudden severe pain may be interpreted by a patient and their family that death is imminent, with resultant panic. Explanation of the likely cause of the pain, what can be done about it, and what can be expected over the coming days is a crucial aspect of management.

Intrahepatic haemorrhage

Occasionally with liver metastases, the patient experiences increasingly severe right upper quadrant pain. Unless associated features suggest an alternative diagnosis, e.g. perforated peptic ulcer or cholecystitis, the likely diagnosis is an intrahepatic haemorrhage causing acute distension of the hepatic capsule. When this is the case:

- give *double* the previous oral analgesic morphine requirement *or*
- if the patient has already taken an extra rescue dose of morphine with inadequate relief, *treble* the previous oral morphine dose; the presence of severe pain despite an additional dose of morphine indicates that the dose can be safely increased to this level.[32]

This is an acute phenomenon which resolves as the hepatic capsule adapts and the haematoma is resorbed. Thus, the patient should be told that, in about a week, analgesic requirements are likely to be back to pre-haemorrhage levels. Tentative dose reductions should be made after 3 days, or sooner if the patient is comfortable but complaining of drowsiness. Failure to reduce the dose may result in increased undesirable opioid effects, e.g.:

- nausea and vomiting
- drowsiness
- delirium.

Pathological fracture (acute collapse) of a vertebra

A fracture is called 'pathological' if it occurs in bone weakened by a disease process (e.g. cancer, metastases, osteoporosis, infection) or from trauma insufficient to fracture a normal bone. The commonest cause of pathological fracture in palliative care is metastatic bone disease. Vertebral collapse from osteoporosis is more common in the elderly and those receiving long-term corticosteroids.

When possible, a preventive strategy should be adopted, e.g. bisphosphonates in patients with myeloma or breast cancer (see p.359).

MSCC, suggested by radicular pain, motor weakness, sensory symptoms and bladder dysfunction, should be excluded, e.g. by MRI (see p.241).

For patients *not* taking regular analgesics, give:

- morphine 5–10mg SC/IV (preceded by metoclopramide 10mg IV over ≥3min); IV allows rapid titration of morphine, e.g. repeat 1mg boluses every 2–3min until acceptable pain relief
- an NSAID PO, e.g. ibuprofen 400mg t.d.s. or naproxen 500mg b.d.; occasionally IM diclofenac or SC ketorolac are used.

However, typically the patient is already taking an NSAID and morphine regularly for pre-existing bone pain. In this case, give:

- a *double* dose of morphine PO *or*
- an injection of morphine equal in mg to the previous regular PO dose; this will have 2–3 times the effect of the oral dose.

If these have failed to give adequate relief, it may be necessary to *treble* the previous satisfactory dose of morphine for several weeks (after which it is generally possible to reduce the dose again over several days/weeks to its pre-collapse level).

For severe incident pain on movement, use pre-emptive analgesia; if available, nitrous oxide (50% with oxygen) before and during movement can be used.

In addition, consider:

- for patients with associated nerve compression pain, dexamethasone 4–8mg once daily (see p.365)
- for patients with associated muscle spasm, diazepam, 5mg stat and 5–10mg at bedtime.

Increasingly, multidisciplinary teams comprising oncologists and orthopaedic and spinal surgeons are available to guide management of bone metastases. Specialist options include:

- palliative radiotherapy; generally beneficial but may take 4–6 weeks to achieve maximal relief
- bisphosphonates (see p.359)
- epidural analgesia with morphine and bupivacaine for severe incident pain
- percutaneous vertebroplasty (i.e. injection of bone cement containing polymethylmethacrylate into the fractured vertebral body) or balloon kyphoplasty under fluoroscopic guidance
- orthopaedic surgery, particularly with MSCC, e.g. decompression and stabilization.[17]

Depending on the primary site, surgery may be followed by radiotherapy, chemotherapy or hormone therapy. These should also be considered for patients unable to undergo surgery.

Pathological fracture of a long bone

The commonest cause of a pathological fracture in palliative care is metastatic bone disease. Where possible, a preventive strategy should be adopted, e.g.:

- local radiotherapy to a bone metastasis
- bisphosphonates in patients with myeloma or breast cancer (see p.359)
- orthopaedic surgery: prophylactic fixation or stabilization.

If a pathological fracture occurs, provide immediate analgesia (see above).

Surgery offers the most reliable and rapid means of controlling pain and of restoring function, and should be considered unless the patient is close to death. It requires the patient to be willing and generally fit enough to undergo an operation and the presence of enough bone for stable fixation. Radiotherapy can be considered after surgical stabilization.[33–35]

If surgery is planned:

- ensure sufficient regular analgesia is provided
- continue pre-fracture analgesics postoperatively and prescribe sufficient p.r.n. postoperative medication.

Humerus

In addition to analgesia, immediate care is normally conservative:

- use a loosely fitting sling to part-immobilize the limb; the sling should allow the arm to hang down freely (improves bone alignment and reduces muscle spasm)
- encourage patient to keep the arm in this position as much as possible and to sleep in a semi-erect position
- encourage patient to use their fingers as much as possible and, at least twice a day, remove arm from the sling and straighten the elbow completely to prevent joint stiffening.

Alternative measures include:

- splint arm to trunk, e.g. with Netelast® and/or Velcro® *or*
- fracture braces (humeral shaft).

If pain remains a major problem despite regular oral analgesia, consider a nerve block or epidural analgesia.

Femur

In addition to analgesia, immediate care includes:

- immobilize leg with pillows
- administer a local anaesthetic femoral nerve block before obtaining a radiograph
- use appropriate nursing techniques for turning the patient in bed, e.g. 'logrolling'

If treating conservatively, because surgery is inappropriate, consider:

- skin traction or splinting (seek specialist advice)
- epidural analgesia.

OVERWHELMING DISTRESS

Occasionally, a patient who is imminently dying becomes severely distressed, most commonly because of an agitated delirium but sometimes because of pain or breathlessness.[36]

When specific measures fail to relieve, it may be necessary to deliberately reduce the patient's awareness by giving sedatives. This is a treatment of last resort, i.e. for use when all else has failed. The aim is to relieve suffering, *not* to kill the patient (see p.26).

Sedation must always be proportionate, and progressive only if necessary. Sedation is a continuum: with p.r.n. sedation at one end and continuous deep sedation (CDS) at the other (Figure I and Box H).

Abrupt deep sedation is rarely necessary, e.g. when there is sudden massive unstoppable arterial haemorrhage (see above). In the imminently dying, it is uncommon to lighten the depth of the sedation once the patient is settled.[37]

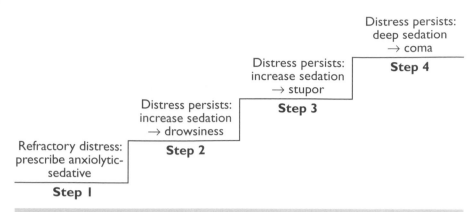

Figure 1 Proportionate progressive sedation for intolerable refractory distress in the imminently dying.

Box H Drugs for sedation in the imminently dying

For more information, see Essential PCF, p.352 and p.356.

First-line drugs

Midazolam

- start with 2.5–5mg stat and q1h p.r.n.
- if necessary, increase progressively to 10mg SC/IV stat
- maintain with CSCI/CIVI 10–60mg/24h.

Consider adding in an antipsychotic if midazolam 30mg/24h is inadequate to settle the patient.

Haloperidol

- start with 2.5–10mg SC stat and q1h p.r.n. (1–5mg SC q1h in the elderly)
- maintain with CSCI 10–15mg/24h.

Second-line drugs

Levomepromazine

Generally given only if it is intended to reduce a patient's level of consciousness:

- start with 25mg SC stat and q1h p.r.n. (12.5mg in the elderly)
- if necessary, titrate dose according to response
- maintain with 50–300mg/24h CSCI.

Although high-dose levomepromazine (≥100mg/24h) is best given by CSCI, smaller doses can be given as an SC bolus at bedtime–b.d., and p.r.n.

Some centres use smaller doses first-line, e.g. 12.5mg SC stat and q1h p.r.n. (6.25mg in the elderly).

Third-line drugs

Phenobarbital
Propofol } Specialist use only, for patients failing to respond to the above.

A small number of dying patients experience persistent overwhelming existential distress despite optimal psychosocial and spiritual support.[38] Management of this must be supervised by professionals skilled in psychological evaluation.

Psychosocial and spiritual support must continue to be offered and, if used, sedation should be undertaken in a proportionate and progressive manner. Respite sedation for a few hours each day or for 2–3 days are normally the first steps, and often are sufficient (see p.26).[37] A decision about CDS should be made only by a specialist palliative care team, and after discussion with both the patient and their family.

REFERENCES

1 Diabetes Control and Complications Trial Research Group (1993) The effect of intensive treatment of diabetes on the development and progression of long-term complications in insulin-dependent diabetes mellitus. New England Journal of Medicine. 329: 977–986.

2 Holroyde C et al. (1975) Altered glucose metabolism in metastatic carcinoma. Cancer Research. 35: 3710–3714.

3 Sinclair A et al. (2013) End of life diabetes care: A strategy document commissed by diabetes UK. Clinical care recommendations 2nd edition. www.diabetes.org.uk/end-of-life-care

4 NHS Diabetes (2010) The hospital management of hypoglycaemia in adults with diabetes mellitus. www.diabetes.nhs.uk/

5 NHS Diabetes (2011) Recognition, treatment and prevention of hypoglycaemia in the community. www.diabetes.nhs.uk/

6 NHS England (2014) Risk of distress and detah from inappropriate doses of naloxone in patients on long-term opioid/opiate treatment. Patient Safety Alert. NHS/PSA/W/2014/2016R. www.cas.dh.gov.uk

7 UK Medicines Information (2015) What naloxone doses should be used in adults to reverse urgently the effects of opioids or opiates? Medicines Q&A. 227.223. www.evidence.nhs.uk

8 Cleary J (2000) Incidence and characteristics of naloxone administration in medical oncology patients with cancer pain. Journal of Pharmaceutical Care in Pain and Symptom Control. 8: 65–73.

9 Paranthaman SK and Khan F (1976) Acute cardiomyopathy with recurrent pulmonary edema and hypotension following heroin overdosage. Chest. 69: 117–119.

10 Wilson LD et al. (2007) Clinical practice. Superior vena cava syndrome with malignant causes. New England Journal of Medicine. 356: 1862–1869.

11 Warner P and Uberoi R (2013) Superior vena cava stenting in the 21st century. Postgraduate Medical Journal. 89: 224–230.

12 Watkinson AF et al. (2008) Endovascular stenting to treat obstruction of the superior vena cava. British Medical Journal. 336: 1434–1437.

13 Rowell NP and Gleeson FV (2001) Steroids, radiotherapy, chemotherapy and stents for superior vena caval obstruction in carcinoma of the bronchus. Cochrane Database of Systematic Reviews. 4: CD001316. www.thecochranelibrary.com

14 NICE (2004) Interventional procedure overview of stent placement for vena cava obstruction. IPG79. www.nice.org.uk

15 Loblaw DA et al. (2005) Systematic review of the diagnosis and management of malignant extradural spinal cord compression: the Cancer Care Ontario Practice Guidelines Initiative's Neuro-Oncology Disease Site Group. Journal of Clinical Oncology. 23: 2028–2037.

16 Prasad D and Schiff D (2005) Malignant spinal-cord compression. *Lancet Oncology*. **6**: 15–24.
17 NICE (2008) Metastatic spinal cord compression. *Clinical Guideline* **75**. www.nice.org.uk
18 Quraishi NA and Esler C (2011) Metastatic spinal cord compression. *British Medical Journal*. **342**: d2402.
19 Klimo P, Jr and Schmidt MH (2004) Surgical management of spinal metastases. *Oncologist*. **9**: 188–196.
20 Patchell RA et al. (2005) Direct decompressive surgical resection in the treatment of spinal cord compression caused by metastatic cancer: a randomised trial. *Lancet*. **366**: 643–648.
21 Helweg-Larsen S et al. (2000) Prognostic factors in metastatic spinal cord compression: a prospective study using multivariate analysis of variables influencing survival and gait function in 153 patients. *International Journal of Radiation Oncology, Biology and Physics*. **46**: 1163–1169.
22 Maranzano E et al. (2005) Short-course versus split-course radiotherapy in metastatic spinal cord compression: results of a phase III, randomized, multicenter trial. *Journal of Clinical Oncology*. **23**: 3358–3365.
23 Conway R et al. (2007) What happens to people after malignant cord compression? Survival, function, quality of life, emotional well-being and place of care 1 month after diagnosis. *Clinical Oncology*. **19**: 56–62.
24 Milligan J et al. (2012) Autonomic dysreflexia: recognizing a common serious condition in patients with spinal cord injury. *Canadian Family Physician*. **58**: 831–835.
25 Stewart AF (2005) Clinical practice. Hypercalcemia associated with cancer. *New England Journal of Medicine*. **352**: 373–379.
26 Bennett C et al. (2014) Tranexamic acid for upper gastrointestinal bleeding. *Cochrane Database of Systematic Reviews*. **11**: CD006640. www.thecochranelibrary.com
27 Kochhar R et al. (1988) Rectal sucralfate in radiation proctitis. *Lancet*. **332**: 400.
28 McElligott E et al. (1991) Tranexamic acid and rectal bleeding. *Lancet*. **337**: 431.
29 West N (1997) Prevention and treatment of hemorrhagic cystitis. *Pharmacotherapy*. **17**: 696–706.
30 Choong SK et al. (2000) The management of intractable haematuria. *BJU International*. **86**: 951–959.
31 Harris DG et al. (2011) The use of crisis medication in the management of terminal haemorrhage due to incurable cancer: a qualitative study. *Palliative Medicine*. **25**: 691–700.
32 Hagen N et al. (1997) Cancer pain emergencies: a protocol for management. *Journal of Pain and Symptom Management*. **14**: 45–50.
33 Townsend P et al. (1995) Role of postoperative radiation therapy after stabilization of fractures caused by metastatic disease. *International Journal of Radiation Oncology, Biology and Physics*. **31**: 43–49.
34 Malviya A and Gerrand C (2012) Evidence for orthopaedic surgery in the treatment of metastatic bone disease of the extremities: a review article. *Palliative Medicine*. **26**: 788–796.
35 Eastley N et al. (2012) Skeletal metastases - the role of the orthopaedic and spinal surgeon. *Surgical Oncology*. **21**: 216–222.
36 de Graeff A and Dean M (2007) Palliative sedation therapy in the last weeks of life: a literature review and recommendations for standards. *Journal of Palliative Medicine*. **10**: 67–85.

37 Cherny NI and Radbruch L (2009) European Association for Palliative Care (EAPC) recommended framework for the use of sedation in palliative care. *Palliative Medicine*. **23**: 581–593.
38 Morita T (2004) Palliative sedation to relieve psycho-existential suffering of terminally ill cancer patients. *Journal of Pain and Symptom Management*. **28**: 445–450.

FURTHER READING

Currow D and Clark K (2006) *Emergencies in Palliative and Supportive Care*. Oxford University Press, Oxford.
Fisher R and Fay J (2014) Primary care management of palliative care emergencies. *InnovAiT: Education and inspiration for general practice*. **7**: 581-586.

14. END-OF-LIFE CARE: PLANNING AND LAST DAYS OF LIFE

INTRODUCTION

Many people live without really considering their own mortality. However, the diagnosis of a life-limiting condition, and particularly the awareness of progressive physical deterioration, will prompt many patients (and those close to them) to face their impending death. This is generally psychologically and spiritually demanding, and the extent to which a patient is able to do this, and discuss it with others, varies.

A person may accept that their life is drawing to a close but still make no specific arrangements. However, pro-active planning is now encouraged.[1-3] This encompasses:
- *Advance Care Planning (ACP)*: enables a patient with capacity to record their wishes so that, should they later lose capacity, the ACP can direct or influence decisions about care and treatment. Documentation includes:
  ▷ an informal statement of wishes and preferences
  ▷ a formal Advance Decision to Refuse Treatment (England/Wales) or Advance Decision (Scotland)
  ▷ a Lasting Power of Attorney (England and Wales) or Welfare Attorney (Scotland)
- *End-of-life care planning*: discussion about a patient's wishes and goals as they enter the last days, weeks or few months of life. It covers areas such as symptom management, nutrition and hydration, psychological and social support and co-ordination of care, and results in an individualized end-of-life (EOL) care plan.

Although terminology overlaps, the processes involved are separate. Although few people undertake ACP, many patients will work with the healthcare team to create an individualized EOL care plan.

MENTAL CAPACITY AND DECISION-MAKING

All adult patients are presumed to have mental capacity to make decisions about their care. This means that a patient can agree to or refuse any examination, investigation or treatment. Patients must be given appropriate information and support to maximize their capacity to make decisions.

When making decisions with a patient, a health professional must be satisfied that the patient has mental capacity. If in doubt, the patient's capacity should be evaluated (Box A).

Box A Mental capacity[4]

Over 16s are presumed to have mental capacity unless shown otherwise but refusal of life-sustaining treatment by a 16 or 17 year-old may be overridden by a parent or a court.

Evaluation of capacity is made in relation to a particular decision (e.g. choice of treatment) at a particular time.

Evaluation will normally involve discussion with the person's family, friends or carers, or an Independent Mental Capacity Advocate (IMCA) if one has been appointed previously.

Capacity can vary over time, so health and social care professionals should identify the time and manner most suitable to the patient to discuss treatment options. It may be necessary to call upon a psychiatrist or clinical psychologist to provide an expert opinion.

Loss of capacity may be temporary, e.g. because of a reversible condition. If a patient who lacks capacity could regain it soon (e.g. after receiving treatment) and if feasible, defer decision-making until then.

The two stage test

1. *Diagnostic*: does the patient have an impairment of the mind or brain which means they are unable to make the decision for themselves?
2. *Functional*: the patient is *unable* to:
   - understand the information relevant to the decision, including the likely consequences of making or not making the decision
   - retain that information for as long as is necessary to make and communicate the decision
   - use that information as part of the process of making the decision
   - communicate the decision by some means (nonverbal or verbal).

All evaluations of capacity should be documented in the patient's clinical records. If borderline, a decision that the patient lacks capacity should be based on probability, i.e. it is more likely that they lack capacity than retain it.

A team approach should be used to determine capacity. However, the final responsibility remains with the senior professional involved.

If uncertainty persists, the court should be asked to adjudicate.

A patient can be regarded as lacking capacity to make decisions about their care only if they fail the test for capacity.

If a patient is found to be lacking capacity, it is the responsibility of the health professional to find out if the patient has completed any form of ACP.

Making decisions when a patient lacks capacity[5]

If a patient does not have capacity to make a particular decision, then the health professional must find out if the patient has made any form of advance decision.

There are two legal means by which a patient may have made their wishes known when they still had capacity (Box B).

Box B Legal options for making future wishes known

England and Wales[6]

Advance Decision to Refuse Treatment: legally binding if valid and applicable.

Lasting Power of Attorney for Welfare: person(s) chosen by the patient to make decisions on their behalf.

Scotland[7]

Advance Directive: potentially legally binding, but not yet tested in the courts.

Welfare Power of Attorney: person(s) chosen by the patient to make decisions on their behalf.

Northern Ireland

There is *no* law permitting the appointment of legal proxies (Power of Attorney) to make healthcare decisions.

Primary legislation does *not* cover advance refusals, but likely that principles established in English Law would apply.

If there is no relevant Advance Decision/Directive and no relevant legal proxy, then the responsible doctor must make decisions for the patient's overall benefit (see below).

If there is disagreement, a second opinion should be sought. Occasionally a court order may be necessary, or a court deputy (England/Wales) or guardian/intervener (Scotland) appointed to make decisions for the patient's overall benefit.

When court proceedings are in process or in an emergency, health professionals may provide treatment necessary to prevent a serious deterioration in a patient's condition.

Advance refusal of treatment

This is a set of instructions that an adult with mental capacity can make to refuse treatment should they lose capacity in the future. It is called an Advance Decision to Refuse Treatment (ADRT) in England and Wales, and an Advance Directive in Scotland. It is sometimes called a 'living will'. An advance refusal can be written by a person over 16 in Scotland, over 18 elsewhere in the UK.

A valid and applicable ADRT is as legally binding as a contemporary refusal of treatment made by a person with capacity (Box C). Valid and applicable advance refusals are likely to be legally binding in Scotland and Northern Ireland, although this has not yet been tested in the courts.

Box C Advance Decision to Refuse Treatment[6]

An ADRT can be verbal, but for clarity people should be encouraged to produce a written one:
- there is no official format for a written ADRT *unless life-sustaining treatment is refused*
- there is no official review period for an ADRT.

Although it is recommended that people talk to their GP, consultant and/or solicitor before formulating an ADRT, this is not a legal requirement.

An ADRT can refuse:
- treatment of any kind
- clinically-assisted nutrition and hydration (these are regarded as treatment)
- life-sustaining treatment.

To refuse life-sustaining treatment, an ADRT must be written (e.g. recorded in the medical notes or written by the person) and:
- contain a specific statement that the person wishes it to apply even though treatment refusal may result in earlier death
- be signed by the person and by a witness (or on their behalf in their presence).

An ADRT *cannot*:
- make a legally-binding request for treatment
- refuse basic care, e.g. shelter, warmth, hygiene measures, the offer of oral food and fluids
- be used by a person to make a request for their life to be ended.

An ADRT is valid if:
- the patient had mental capacity when it was made (see Box A)
- it was made voluntarily, i.e. the patient was not coerced into making it
- the patient was informed as to the nature and purpose of the treatment they are refusing.

An ADRT is applicable if:
- there is a refusal of a specific treatment, e.g. CPR, chemotherapy
- the treatment in question is that specified by the ADRT
- the circumstances in which the refusal is to apply are specified and exist at the time the decision needs to be made.

An ADRT may *not* be valid or applicable if:
- there have been changes in circumstances which give reasonable grounds for believing these would have affected the person's refusal, e.g. a new treatment has been discovered for the person's illness
- since making the ADRT, the person has done anything clearly inconsistent with the ADRT remaining their fixed decision
- since making the ADRT, the person has subsequently withdrawn their decision (verbally or in writing)
- the patient has subsequently conferred power to make that decision on an attorney.[8]

It is good practice to ask the patient, family member or GP if an advance refusal exists. It is the responsibility of the healthcare team to check whether the advance refusal is valid and applicable to the decision in question. Even if not, it may still provide insight into the person's wishes and preferences.

If a health professional has a conscientious objection to complying with an advance refusal, this should be discussed with other members of the healthcare team. If necessary, care of the patient should be transferred to another health professional who is able to comply with the ADRT.

If the patient is, or is liable to be, detained under the Mental Health Act 1983, an advance refusal may not apply. Clarification should be sought from a psychiatrist.

Lasting Power of Attorney (LPA)

Different statutes cover proxy decision-making in England and Wales, and Scotland (Box D). Northern Ireland has no provisions for appointment of legal proxies.

Making decisions for a patient's overall benefit

Where there is no advance refusal or legal proxy with authority to make a decision for a patient who lacks capacity, the decision is made by the doctor responsible for the patient's care.

In England, Wales and Northern Ireland decisions which are made on behalf of mentally incapacitated patients by health professionals or welfare attorneys must be in their 'best interests'. In Scotland it must be considered whether a treatment 'benefits' the patient. 'Overall benefit' is used in GMC guidance to cover both terms.

Overall benefit is not limited to medical benefit but encompasses all of a patient's interests, including psychological and social ones (Box E). A patient may have written a statement of wishes and preferences to help doctors to understand their wishes when making a decision for their overall benefit (Box F).

When everyone appropriate has been consulted, it can be helpful to create a 'balance sheet' listing the advantages and disadvantages of the various options to aid decision-making. A decision about life-sustaining treatment must not be motivated by a desire to bring about the patient's death.

The final decision must be the least restrictive of the patient's future choices, and for their overall benefit.[5] A formal 'best interests meeting' may sometimes be helpful, e.g. if there is disagreement about an important decision such as the patient's place of care or the withdrawal of treatment.

Independent Mental Capacity Advocate

Most adults who lack capacity and who have not written an ADRT or appointed a welfare attorney, will have family, friends or carers who can and should be consulted about their views if a decision needs to be made on their behalf.

Box D Power of Attorney

England and Wales

Lasting Power of Attorney (LPA) is covered by statute law in England and Wales.[9] Over 18s who have capacity can make an LPA to appoint one or more persons as Attorney(s) to take decisions on their behalf if and when they lose capacity.

An LPA can cover decisions relating to healthcare and/or personal welfare (Personal Welfare Attorney), and/or property and financial affairs (Property and Affairs Attorney).

A Personal Welfare Attorney can refuse treatment on behalf of an incapacitated person, but can only refuse life-sustaining treatment if the LPA specifies this.

A Personal Welfare Attorney cannot demand inappropriate medical treatment.

Before relying on the authority of the Welfare Attorney, health professionals must be satisfied that:
- the patient lacks capacity to make the decision
- the LPA has been registered with the Office of the Public Guardian
- a statement has been included in the LPA specifically authorizing the Welfare Attorney to make decisions relevant to the current situation
- the decision being made by the Welfare Attorney is in the patent's best interests.

Scotland

In Scotland, the Adults with Incapacity statute applies,[7] under which over 16s may appoint someone as Welfare Attorney to take decisions on their behalf if and when they lose capacity.

The Sheriff may appoint a Welfare Guardian with similar powers.

A Welfare Attorney or Guardian cannot demand inappropriate medical treatment.

Before relying on the authority of a Welfare Attorney, health professionals must be satisfied that:
- the patient lacks capacity to make the decision
- the Attorney or Guardian has specific power to consent to treatment
- the decision being made by the Attorney will benefit the patient
- the Attorney has taken account of the patient's past and present wishes as far as they can be ascertained.

When there is disagreement between health professionals and welfare attorney or guardian, an application can be made to the Mental Welfare Commission of Scotland to appoint a 'nominated medical practitioner' to give an opinion.

This opinion is final unless appealed by either party to the Court of Sessions.

Box E Checklist for determining overall benefit[5]

Involve the person as much as possible in making the decision, even if they lack capacity to make the final decision.

Find out the person's past and present wishes, feelings and views which might be likely to influence the decision and may have been expressed:
- verbally
- in writing, e.g. a statement of wishes and preferences (Box F)
- through behaviour or habits
- through any religious, cultural or moral beliefs or values.

Consult and take into account the views of any:
- court-appointed Guardian or Welfare Attorney (when these do not have power to make this specific decision)
- other members of the healthcare team
- others previously named by the person, e.g. carers, close family and friends, as far as possible and when appropriate
- Independent Mental Capacity Advocate (IMCA, see below).

Avoid discrimination, e.g. age, appearance, condition or behaviour.

Box F Statement of wishes and preferences[10]

This is a statement recorded by the patient to convey their:
- wishes and preferences about future treatment and care, e.g.:
  ▷ personal preferences
  ▷ who they want involved in future decision making
  ▷ types of medical treatment which may or may not be wanted
  ▷ place of care
- beliefs or values that govern how they make decisions in order to guide future decision making.

Statements of wishes and preferences or documented conversations the patient has had with their family or other carers, may be recorded in the medical notes.

Such statements are not legally binding.

Acts which are illegal cannot be included, e.g. assisted suicide.

When a patient lacks mental capacity, a professional carer formulating a decision about care or treatment must take any statement of wishes and preferences into account when trying to determine the patient's best interests.

If not documented in the medical notes, relatives or other carers should be contacted to determine whether any statement of wishes or preferences exists, or for help in determining the patient's probable wishes.

In England and Wales, statute law stipulates that, when there is no appropriate third party to consult, an Independent Mental Capacity Advocate (IMCA) should be appointed for the person if decisions have to be made about:
- serious medical treatment, e.g. chemotherapy, major surgery, withholding or withdrawing clinically-assisted nutrition and hydration:
  ▷ when the likely benefits and possible burdens are finely balanced
  ▷ when a decision between choice of treatment is finely balanced
  ▷ when what is proposed is likely to have serious consequences, e.g. potentially shortening the person's life or causing prolonged severe pain (or other major distress)
- moving the person into long-term care (>28 days in a hospital or >8 weeks in a care home)
- a long-term move (>8 weeks) to a different hospital or care home
- adult protection (in England).[6]

The role of the IMCA is to obtain as much information as possible about the person's wishes, feelings, beliefs and values from associated third parties. The IMCA will then prepare a written report for the healthcare team, which must be taken into account by whoever makes the final decision.

Deprivation of Liberty Safeguards (DoLS)

Deprivation of Liberty Safeguards (DoLS) are derived from an amendment to the MCA 2005, and apply to *persons without capacity* aged over 16 in England/Wales only.[11] DoLS apply to patients in a care home, hospital or hospice, but not at home.

It is unlawful to provide care or treatment for a patient which amounts to a deprivation of their liberty. To determine if a patient without capacity is at risk of being deprived of their liberty by their care or treatment, apply the 'acid test' (Box G).

If a patient is identified as being deprived of their liberty, or at risk of such, the doctor (or care home manager) in charge of their care must consider whether it is in the patient's best interests and if there are any less restrictive ways of caring for them.

If it is considered to be in the patient's best interests and there is no less restrictive care regimen possible, then authorization must be sought to deprive the patient of their liberty (Box H).

Box G Deprivation of liberty test

To determine whether a patient without capacity is being deprived of their liberty, apply the 'acid test' by asking:
- is the patient subject to continuous supervision and control
- is the patient free to leave?

If the patient is subject to continuous supervision and control, and is not free to leave, then they have been deprived of their liberty.[12]

'Control' includes physical and/or chemical restraint.

Box G Contd.

A patient is deemed not to be 'free to leave' if measures are in place to prevent them from leaving (e.g. distraction door locks, restraint) or if staff are opposing the wishes of relatives or carers to take them home.

A patient dying in a hospice is unlikely to be considered deprived of their liberty if they consented to the admission and the treatment plan offered.

Factors likely to be taken into account when considering whether a patient dying in a hospice is being deprived of their liberty include:
- their circumstances or treatment are no longer covered by consent to the admission or initial treatment plan
- they are receiving sedatives to decrease anxiety and agitation, particularly if over a period of weeks and without advance consent
- they are undergoing chemical restraint
- they are under constant supervision because of terminal agitation
- if they are mobile but prevented from leaving the hospice grounds because they are a danger to themselves.

Box H Obtaining authorization for depriving patients without capacity of their liberty

Authorization can be obtained by:
- DoLS authorization *or*
- detention under the Mental Health Act 1983 *or*
- a court order.

A DoLS authorization may be *urgent authorization* issued by the hospital or care home and valid for 7 days or *standard authorization* up to maximum 12 months.

Standard authorization is obtained from the appropriate supervisory body:
- the Local Authority for patients in a care home
- the Clinical Commissioning Group (England) or Local Health Board (Wales) for patients in hospital.

When DoLS authorization is requested, an evaluation by a trained assessor will be carried out.

If authorization is granted, someone is appointed to represent the interests of the patient. This person is called the Relevant Person's Representative (RPR) and is normally a relative or friend of the patient.

If a patient dies while under a DoLS authorization, this is considered as a death 'in state detention' and the coroner should be notified.

The coroner will undertake an investigation and issue a death certificate (or advise when one can be issued). Practices may vary according to region and coroner (see p.387).

END-OF-LIFE CARE PLANNING

End-of-life (EOL) care planning aims to improve a patient's care and choices. It should not be left until the last moment, but done when it seems likely that the patient will die within the next year. It is estimated that at, any one time, over 30% of hospital patients are in their last year of life.[13]

Estimating prognosis is difficult. However, if a patient has an incurable progressive life-threatening condition, e.g. cancer, heart failure, COPD, or increasing frailty ± dementia, consider EOL care planning if they have:

- two or more unplanned hospital admissions in the last six months *or*
- persistent symptoms despite best treatment *or*
- poor or deteriorating performance status *or*
- organ failure secondary to the underlying illness.

A negative answer to the question, 'Would I be surprised if the patient were to die in the next 12 months?' should also prompt EOL care planning.

However, EOL care planning can be done any time by anyone, e.g. a well person prompted to do so by the death of a relative or friend.[14] EOL care planning involves discussion between a health professional and the patient, and (if the patient wishes) relatives/informal carers.

The topic should be introduced sensitively, exploring how much information the patient would like to know about their illness and prognosis. It is a voluntary process and there should be no pressure to take part. A choice not to confront future issues should be respected.

EOL discussions should identify:

- their concerns
- their understanding of their illness and prognosis
- important values including cultural, religious or spiritual preferences
- personal goals for care.

When these have been established, current treatment and care should be reviewed. Agreement with the patient should be sought on goals for further treatment, including:

- focusing on what can be done to support the patient to live well
- indicating what would no longer be of real benefit, e.g. CPR (see p.17)
- discussing whether admission to hospital would be appropriate if and when there is further physical deterioration
- preferred place of care; where the patient would like to be cared for during their final illness.

Patients' priorities differ, and the process of shared decision-making should be individualized accordingly. Discussion should be:

- documented
- reviewed regularly, in accordance with the patient's desire and ability to be involved in decision-making
- communicated to key persons involved in their care.

With their permission, patients should be placed on the GP's end-of-life register.[1] As part of this process, patients may choose to complete a document such as an Emergency Care and Treatment Plan.[15] This summarizes the patient's decisions about what care and treatment they would want should their health deteriorate rapidly and they become unable to participate in decision-making.

LAST DAYS OF LIFE

Hospital is the commonest place of death in England and Wales (Table 1), and across the developed world. This presents a particular challenge because acute hospitals do not generally provide the best environment for holistic care.

Table 1 Main place of death England and Wales 2014[a]

Hospital	Home	Care home	Other communal establishment[b]	Elsewhere[c]
48%	23%	21%	6%	2%

a. Office of National Statistics data based on some 500,000 deaths
b. includes hospices, but also hotels, common lodging houses, colleges, sheltered accommodation, and prisons
c. includes road traffic accidents and other outdoor deaths.

This is partly because the focus tends to be on improving organ function. This may lead to attempts to fix what cannot be fixed, regardless of the patient's priorities. Regrettably, it is *not* routine to ask the patient (and family) what is important to them, and the fact that someone is dying may be completely overlooked.[16]

In the UK, national guidelines have been developed to facilitate patient-focused care, based on five Key Priorities (Box 1).[2,3]

Box 1 One chance to get it right: five priorities[2]

1. The possibility (of dying in the next hours or days) is recognized and communicated clearly, decisions made and actions taken in accordance with the person's needs and wishes, and these are regularly reviewed and decisions revised accordingly.

2. Sensitive communication takes place between the healthcare team and the dying person, and those identified as important to them.

3. The dying person, and those identified as important to them, are involved in decisions about treatment and care to the extent that the dying person wants.

4. The needs of families and others identified as important to the dying person are actively explored, respected and met as far as possible.

5. An individual plan of care, which includes food and drink, symptom control and psychological, social and spiritual support, is agreed, co-ordinated and delivered with compassion.

It is crucial that what is important to dying patients and families provides the focus for care, namely:

- effective communication
- expert and compassionate care
- trust and confidence in the carers.[17]

Recognizing when a patient may be in the last days of life

The first priority requires a team decision led by the senior responsible clinician. This may be the GP or Consultant, who should be responsible for all important decisions, delegating to colleagues as and when appropriate.

Failure to recognize the dying phase can have profound implications for the patient and their loved ones. This may lead to the patient and family:

- being unaware that death is imminent
- losing trust in the healthcare team as the patient's condition clearly deteriorates without any acknowledgement
- getting conflicting messages from the healthcare team
- being more likely to die with unrelieved symptoms and less likely to be in the care setting of their choice
- having inappropriate CPR
- having their psychological, cultural and spiritual needs neglected
- having a more difficult bereavement.

Estimating prognosis for individual patients is difficult, even when death is imminent.[18] On a population level, it is statistically possible to estimate prognosis, based on disease severity and other factors; but statistics may be meaningless for an individual, and potentially harmful. However, several variables are associated with decreased survival in patients with cancer (Box J).[19]

Using such variables, attempts have been made to produce a reliable prognostic index. However, even the best of the currently available scales provide only general guidance based on probability, and are little used outside research settings.

In practice, if a patient is functionally deteriorating *in the absence of a reversible cause* or has declined treatment, the following 'rule' is commonly used in palliative care for patients with cancer to guide decision-making: if a patient is deteriorating:

- month by month, they probably have several months to live
- week by week, they probably have only weeks to live
- day by day, they probably have only days to live.

Further, *in the absence of a reversible cause* for the deterioration, the following features collectively indicate that a patient almost certainly has only days or hours to live:

- physically wasted and profoundly weak → bedbound
- drowsy for much of the day → coma
- very limited attention span → disoriented (→ agitated delirium)
- unable to take tablets or has great difficulty swallowing them
- little or no oral intake of food and fluid

Box J Factors associated with decreased survival in cancer patients[19]		
Clinical features	**Biological factors**	**Other**
Anorexia	Anaemia	Co-morbidity
Ascites	Hypercalcaemia	Metastatic disease
Breathlessness	Hypo-albuminaemia	Older age
Delirium	Hyponatraemia	Poor performance status
Dry mouth	Leucocytosis	Primary site of cancer,
Dysphagia	Lymphocytopenia	e.g. SCLC, ovary, pancreas,
Fever	Proteinuria	glioblastoma
Nausea	Raised CRP	Single status
Oedema	Raised LDH	
Pain		
Tachycardia		
Tiredness		
Weight loss		

- altered breathing pattern, e.g. Cheyne-stokes breathing, noisy rattling breathing, periods of apnoea
- signs of reduced cardiac function, e.g. mottling of skin, cold extremities, tachycardia, weak peripheral pulses.

Communicating and managing uncertainty at the end of life

Sometimes it can be difficult to know if an acute deterioration is reversible. Consequently, concluding that a patient is imminently dying may turn out to be wrong. Surprisingly, a patient's condition may stabilize or even improve, albeit temporarily. Thus, treatment at the end of life needs to be reviewed regularly in case the patient rallies unexpectedly.

Doubt should be sensitively shared with the patient and those important to them. Sometimes, further disease-modifying treatment should be considered, but care needs to be taken about how this is explained to the patient and their family so they are clear about the potential outcomes, e.g.:

'Your husband is seriously ill and could die. We are doing all we can but are worried that the treatment may not work.'

'It is important that you (and anyone else important to mother) know that while we are doing everything we can to help her get better, she is seriously ill and may not recover. If your mother gets any worse, she could deteriorate very quickly... time may be very short.'

Uncertainty should not lead to 'prognostic paralysis' which can prevent patients and their families from receiving appropriate supportive end-of-life care. If the needs of these patients can be identified at an appropriate time, discussion of the patient's wishes, anticipation of clinical problems and patient-centred planning can be done in a timely fashion rather than during a crisis. Some hospitals use the AMBER care bundle to provide a systematic approach to the care of patients in this situation.[20]

Once it has been established that the patient is, or may be, entering the last hours and days of life, and this has been sensitively communicated to the patient and those important to them (where appropriate), a lead health professional should be identified to encourage shared decision making.

Discussion should then focus on identifying the patient's goals and values (see EOL care planning above). If not already discussed, decisions will need to be made about:
- where the patient wants to be cared for during their final illness, and what support is available for them
- ceilings of care, e.g. whether treatment with antibiotics or CPR is appropriate
- hydration and nutrition (see p.18)
- symptom management and anticipatory prescribing (see below)
- stopping unnecessary drugs (see below), observations and investigations
- addressing psychological and spiritual needs.

These decisions should be documented in an individualized care plan which should:
- facilitate discussions between the healthcare team and patient/family
- ensure all aspects of EOL care planning are addressed
- provide support materials for decision-making, e.g. information leaflets for patient and family, useful contact details
- provide guidance on symptom management
- facilitate communication between all members of the healthcare team caring for the patient.

The care plan should be regularly updated and reviewed, as necessary and as the patient wishes.[1,3]

MANAGING DIABETES MELLITUS AT THE END OF LIFE

As patients approach death, food intake decreases. In those with diabetes, there is an increasing risk of hypoglycaemia (see p.235). It is thus necessary to reduce antidiabetic drugs in parallel with the reduced calorific intake.

In patients with type 2 diabetes, it is generally possible to completely stop oral hypoglycaemics. With insulin-dependent type 1 diabetes the situation is more complex because completely stopping insulin may seem like actively hastening death, and may be deeply upsetting to the patient and/or family.

Vigilance is required to ensure that symptoms of hypo- or hyperglycaemia are not confused with symptoms associated with dying.

Insulin-dependent diabetes mellitus

Reduce the dose of insulin as oral intake diminishes:
- simplify regimen:
  ▷ long-acting insulin once daily *or*
  ▷ intermediate-acting insulin b.d.

- avoid symptomatic hypo- or hyperglycaemia by keeping blood glucose levels between 6–15mmol/L
- limit fingerstick blood glucose tests to once daily before evening meal.

Generally, insulin injections are continued until the patient is imminently dying and comatose (*not* because of hypoglycaemia or diabetic keto-acidosis) and when all other life-sustaining treatments have been stopped.

The decision to stop insulin should be discussed with the patient (when they still have capacity), and with the family.

Non-insulin dependent diabetes mellitus

When the patient is no longer able to swallow:
- stop antidiabetic medication and blood glucose monitoring
- consider stopping low-dose insulin, e.g. insulin <15 units total daily dose.

However, if the patient requires a total daily dose of >15 units of insulin, manage as for insulin-dependent diabetes.[21]

MAINTAINING COMFORT AT THE END OF LIFE

Symptom relief at the end of life is generally a continuation of what is already being done. However, previously well-managed symptoms can recur or new ones develop. Because time is short, there is a greater need for urgency; tomorrow may be too late.

Even when a patient is close to death, careful evaluation is still necessary. Moribund patients may call out repeatedly. Is this because they are:
- in discomfort from, e.g. the cancer, dry mouth, joint stiffness, bedsore, distended bladder?
- distressed by unexpected disturbance? (Warn them before moving them.)
- checking that someone is with them? (Assure them by talking to them.)
- delirious?

Careful observation, examination and discussion with the nurses, other carers and family will help to determine the cause and guide management.[3,22]

Review medication

When patients are clearly approaching death:
- *simplify medication:*
  ▷ stop long-term prophylactic medication, e.g. statins, antihypertensives, warfarin
  ▷ stop laxatives, antidepressants, and NSAIDs when the patient is moribund
- *anticipate and prescribe drugs* for possible problems, e.g.:
  ▷ pain
  ▷ breathlessness
  ▷ nausea and vomiting
  ▷ agitation and delirium
  ▷ death rattle (noisy rattling breathing)

- *prescribe drugs SC/IV* as well as PO in case swallowing becomes difficult
- *review the need for clinically-assisted hydration:* discuss the risks and benefits with patient and family (see p.18) and agree whether to continue, reduce or stop (see p.276)
- *stop unnecessary procedures:* e.g. routine checking of vital signs.

Drug choice will be guided by the patient's current symptoms, previous drug requirements and local guidelines. *Prescribe drugs regularly if the patient was taking them regularly* when they could swallow and 'as needed'. Certain drugs should be routinely available to cover the most common symptoms (Table 2).

Table 2 Drugs which should routinely be available at the end of life (all given SC and q1h p.r.n.)

Symptom	Drug	Comments
Pain	Morphine	Dose depends on current morphine dose; if opioid naïve, use 2.5–5mg SC
Breathlessness	Morphine	Dose depends on current morphine dose; if opioid naïve, use 2.5–5mg SC
		Combine with midazolam 2.5–5mg SC
Nausea and vomiting	Haloperidol 1–2.5mg	See QCG Nausea & vomiting, p.123
Agitation, restlessness	Midazolam 2.5–5mg	But if delirium, combine with an antipsychotic (see below)
Delirium	Haloperidol 1.5–5mg *or* Levomepromazine 12.5–25mg ± Midazolam 2.5–5mg	If haloperidol insufficient consider the more sedative levomepromazine. Midazolam alone can exacerbate delirium
		Continuous deep sedation rarely necessary (see p.253)
Noisy rattling breathing	Hyoscine *butylbromide* 20mg	See QCG Management of death rattle (noisy rattling breathing), p.280

Prescribing all these drugs 'q1h p.r.n.' facilitates rapid dose titration. However, if after several q1h doses there is no benefit or any benefit is short-lived, it is important to consider if an alternative or an additional drug is needed.

If the patient is at home/in a care home, ensure medication is available in a 'Just-in-case' box.

Continuous subcutaneous infusion

The administration of commonly used symptom relief drugs by continuous subcutaneous infusion (CSCI) is standard practice in patients for whom swallowing has become increasingly difficult or impossible. Other indications include:

- persistent nausea and vomiting/bowel obstruction
- coma.

Ambulatory battery-powered infusion devices are generally used. The injectable formulation must be relatively non-irritant. For most drugs, this route is off-label but such use is supported by widespread clinical documentation.

Before setting up a CSCI, it is important to explain to the patient and family:

- the reason(s) for using this route
- how the infusion device works
- the advantages and possible disadvantages of CSCI (Box K).

Box K Advantages and disadvantages of CSCI

Advantages

Round-the-clock comfort because plasma drug concentrations are maintained without peaks and troughs.

Less need for repeated injections.

Generally needs to be loaded once daily.

Control of multiple symptoms with a combination of drugs.

Independence and mobility maintained because the infusion device is lightweight and can be worn in a holster.

Patient preference.

Saving nurses' time.

Disadvantages

Lack of flexibility if more than one drug is being administered.

Lack of reliable compatibility data for some mixtures.

Possible inflammation and pain at the infusion site.

Although uncommon, problems with the infusion device can lead to episodic pain (or other symptom) if the problem is not resolved quickly.

If symptoms are controlled, start the CSCI 1–2h before the effect of the previous medication will wear off. If symptoms are uncontrolled, set up the CSCI immediately with stat doses of the same drugs.

Although often administered by CSCI, several drugs with a long duration of action, e.g. dexamethasone, levomepromazine, can be given as a bolus SC or IV injection once daily or b.d. (Table 3).

Table 3 Drugs which can be given once daily or b.d. instead of by CSCI

Drug	Plasma halflife (h)	Duration of action (h)
Dexamethasone	3–4.5	36–54
Furosemide	0.5–2	6–8
Haloperidol	13–35	≤24
Levomepromazine	15–30	≤24

Appropriate bolus doses of p.r.n. medication must also be prescribed. To avoid potential problems with drug incompatibility, these are given via a separate SC needle/cannula (left *in situ* for this purpose) and flushed with compatible diluent.

Oral fluids and clinically-assisted hydration

In the last days of life, patients should be helped to drink if they wish to and are able to, even if this only amounts to frequent sips of fluid.[3]

With increasing weakness, there may be concerns about impaired swallowing and risk of aspiration. Generally, in those close to death, a formal swallow assessment by a Speech and Language Therapist is not appropriate, *but a dying patient should not be denied drinks just because a swallow assessment has not been performed.*

Explain to the patient and family that aspiration of small amounts of water is unlikely to be harmful, other than triggering cough. Demonstrate ways that would help the patient to drink as safely as possible, e.g. take small amounts at a time, sit upright, swallow twice after each sip.

The role of clinically-assisted hydration is less clear. On the one hand, fluid depletion may be beneficial as a result of:

- reduced pulmonary, salivary and GI secretions, with a consequent reduction in cough, 'death rattle' and vomiting
- reduced urinary output, and thus less incontinence and need for an indwelling urinary catheter
- less oedema and ascites with fewer associated symptoms.

On the other hand, it is argued that clinically-assisted hydration decreases the risk of symptoms such as:

- delirium, or opioid toxicity, particularly if renal failure develops
- sedation and myoclonus
- constipation, pressure sores and dry mouth.

The evidence is mixed, and a systematic review concluded that there was insufficient evidence to draw firm conclusions about either benefit or harm from clinically-assisted hydration in dying patients.[3]

Such conflicting data emphasize the need for individual evaluation and review. When there is uncertainty about the potential benefit of clinically-assisted hydration, a time-limited trial with specific goals could be undertaken, e.g. give 0.9% saline 1L/24h SC/IV for 48h, and see if the specific symptom improves.

The uncertainty of benefit should be discussed with the patient and family. However, it can be explained that parenteral fluids are unlikely to either prolong life or hasten death in this setting.[23]

Mouth care

In moribund patients the mouth should be moistened every 30min with water from a water spray, dropper or sponge stick or ice chips placed in the mouth. In addition:
- smear the lips with a greasy emollient, e.g. white soft paraffin (petroleum jelly, Vaseline®) q4h to prevent cracking
- use a room humidifier or air-conditioning when the weather is dry and hot.

Incontinence and retention of urine

In patients close to death, incontinence is generally best managed by an indwelling urinary catheter. This provides maximum comfort with minimum ongoing disturbance.

A loaded rectum may well be the cause of retention in dying patients. This may necessitate treatment with a laxative suppository, an enema, or digital evacuation of the rectum.

Pain

Generally, pain will not be troublesome at the very end if relief has previously been good and analgesia is maintained.

Most patients dying from cancer will be taking a strong opioid (e.g. morphine, oxycodone). The strong opioid will need to be given by CSCI when the patient loses the ability to swallow.

Occasionally, patients who have been taking an NSAID suffer renewed pain if the NSAID is stopped when swallowing prevents PO drug administration. Should this happen, an NSAID can be given rectally (e.g. diclofenac 50mg t.d.s. PR) or by injection (e.g. diclofenac 25–50mg SC stat & 75mg/24h CSCI).

Breathlessness

Patients often fear suffocating to death, and a positive approach to the patient, their family and colleagues about the relief of terminal breathlessness is important:
- no patient should die with distressing breathlessness
- failure to relieve terminal breathlessness is a failure to utilize drug treatment correctly.

Because of fear, inability to sleep and exhaustion, patients and their carers generally accept that drug-related drowsiness may need to be the price paid for reduced breathlessness. However, some patients become mentally brighter when anxiety is reduced by light sedation, and there is an associated improvement in their breathlessness.

In dying patients, the time for measures to correct the correctable and for introducing new non-drug treatments is past (see p.148). A combination of morphine and midazolam is generally effective in relieving distressing breathlessness.[24]

In opioid naïve patients, give:
- morphine 10mg + midazolam 10mg CSCI/24h, *and*
- morphine 2.5–5mg + midazolam 2.5–5mg SC q1h p.r.n.

For patients already taking an opioid, increase the regular and p.r.n. opioid dose by 25–33%.

When death is imminent, in the absence of respiratory distress, oxygen should *not* be used routinely even for severe hypoxaemia. Further, in most of those already receiving oxygen, it is possible to discontinue it without causing distress.[25]

Agitation and delirium

Not all agitated dying patients are delirious, but most delirious patients are agitated (see p.196). Note:
- mild delirium is not always easy to detect
- the use of a benzodiazepine alone may precipitate or exacerbate delirium
- an antipsychotic (e.g. haloperidol) is required if a patient manifests features suggestive of delirium
- if in doubt, treat an agitated dying patient with both an antipsychotic and midazolam (see p.253).

Death rattle (noisy rattling breathing)

Death rattle occurs in about 50% of dying patients. Because the patient is generally unconscious, management is often more to relieve the distress of the family and other patients.

Those around the patient can be helped to cope with the noisy respirations by:
- *exploration* of their concerns and fears relating to the rattle
- *explanation* of the cause of the rattle, and that it generally does not cause distress to a comatose person.

This alone may be sufficient to relieve any distress.

If the rattle is associated with distressing breathlessness in a semiconscious patient, supplement the recommendations below with an opioid (e.g. morphine) and an anxiolytic sedative (e.g. midazolam).

Traditionally, death rattle has been treated with a secretion-drying antimuscarinic drug (see QCG below). However, their use in undistressed unconscious patients has been questioned because there is not strong evidence of benefit but a risk of undesirable effects (see Antimuscarinics, p.349).[25–27]

Nonetheless, antimuscarinics are widely used, with up to 2/3 of patients appearing to respond.[26,27] Possible reasons for a failure to respond to antimuscarinics include:
- the underlying cause of the rattle
- the inability to dry up existing secretions in the pharynx.

Antimuscarinics will probably be most effective for rattle associated with saliva pooling in the pharynx and least effective for rattle caused by infective bronchial secretions, pulmonary oedema, or gastric reflux, which may benefit from alternative measures (see QCG).

Further, because antimuscarinics (if used) do not affect existing secretions, they are best given as soon as the rattle develops. Some also advocate gentle suctioning of the pharynx to remove existing secretions.[28]

Glycopyrronium, hyoscine *butylbromide* and hyoscine *hydrobromide* are equally effective. Hyoscine *butylbromide* is widely used because it is the cheapest and is free of CNS effects. In contrast, hyoscine *hydrobromide* acts centrally and, although anti-emesis and sedation will generally be beneficial, occasional paradoxical CNS stimulation may precipitate or exacerbate an agitated delirium.

Note: because atropine normally stimulates rather than sedates, it should *not* be used for death rattle unless an alternative is unavailable.

QUICK CLINICAL GUIDE: DEATH RATTLE (NOISY RATTLING BREATHING)

Death rattle occurs in about 50% of dying patients. It is caused by fluid collecting in the upper airway, arising from one or more sources:
- saliva (most common)
- bronchial mucosa (e.g. inflammation/infection)
- pulmonary oedema
- gastric reflux.

Rattling breathing can also occur in patients with a tracheostomy.

Non-drug treatment
- if the patient is unconscious, ease the family's distress by explaining that the rattle is not distressing to the patient
- position the patient semiprone to encourage postural drainage; but upright or semi-recumbent if the cause is pulmonary oedema or gastric reflux
- suction of the upper airway but, because it can be distressing, generally restrict use to unconscious patients.

Drug treatment

If the rattle is associated with distressing breathlessness in a semiconscious patient, supplement the recommendations below with an opioid (e.g. morphine) and an anxiolytic sedative (e.g. midazolam).

Saliva

Because they do not affect existing secretions, an antisecretory drug should be given SC as soon as the rattle begins (Table). Hyoscine *butylbromide* is widely used because it is the cheapest and is free of CNS effects.

CSCI treatment is generally started at the same time as the first or second SC dose; increase the dose if ≥ 2 p.r.n. doses/day are needed.

Table Antimuscarinic drugs for death rattle

Drug	Stat and p.r.n. SC dose	CSCI dose/24h
Hyoscine *butylbromide*	20mg	20–120mg
Hyoscine *hydrobromide*	400microgram	1,200–1,600microgram
Glycopyrronium	200microgram	600–1,200microgram

In end-stage renal failure, do *not* use hyoscine *hydrobromide* because of an increased risk of delirium. Use hyoscine *butylbromide* (dose unchanged) or glycopyrronium (dose halved) instead.

Respiratory tract infection

Generally, it is *not* appropriate to prescribe an antibacterial in an imminently dying patient. Rarely, one may be indicated if death rattle is caused by profuse purulent sputum in a semiconscious patient.

Pulmonary oedema

Consider furosemide 20–40mg SC/IM/IV q2h p.r.n. Beware precipitating urinary retention.

Gastric reflux

Consider metoclopramide 20mg SC/IV q3h p.r.n. ± ranitidine 50mg SC/IV b.d.–q.d.s.

Antimuscarinics block the prokinetic effect of metoclopramide; avoid concurrent use if possible.

PROFESSIONAL AND PERSONAL ISSUES

Palliative care places many stresses on health professionals. These include:
- breaking bad news
- coping with the failure to cure
- repeated exposure to the death of people with whom you have formed a supportive relationship
- involvement in emotional conflicts
- absorption of anger and grief expressed by patients and families
- role-blurring in multiprofessional teamwork.

These all make you think about your own mortality, your own limitations (personal and professional), and your own beliefs. Further, it becomes necessary to deal honestly with your personal emotions: anger, grief, hurt. This will require a process of transformative adaptation to enable you to keep caring for patients and yourself.[29]

Various factors and strategies can help to develop resilience, preserve emotional and physical health, and hopefully avoid burnout.

Relating to self:
- a good work–life balance
- good self-esteem
- flexibility
- humour
- humility
- setting realistic goals.

Relating to teams:
- mutual respect and support
- good communication with each other
- sharing decision-making and responsibility.

Good healthcare teams will aim to develop these aspects in individual members, and thus improve the functioning of the team.

Often, informal structures are sufficient to deal with conflict. Sometimes more structured support in the form of individual or group supervision is helpful, facilitated by someone outside the team, e.g. a psychologist, counsellor or chaplain. Occasionally more in-depth psychological help may be needed.

Nonetheless, for those working in end-of-life care, the rewards generally far outweigh the challenges:
- achieving symptom relief and/or resolving other complex issues
- facilitating psychological adjustment
- belonging to a supportive team
- working holistically and thoroughly
- being inspired by patients, relatives, and colleagues
- personal development from being constantly challenged
- doing something obviously worthwhile.

However, there will be times when even the most resilient person will be stretched by a particular set of challenging circumstances at work, at home, or both. Having the humility to recognize your vulnerability, and having supportive colleagues concerned about your wellbeing are key to sustaining commitment in end-of-life care.

Just being there

For patients and families, being told 'there's nothing more we can do for you', leads to a sense of loneliness, hopelessness and despair. The same is true of health professionals.

Indeed, there are times when a doctor or nurse feels they have nothing more to offer. At such times we have to rely on who we are as individuals, and the value which *just being there* brings (Figures 1–4).

When there is nothing to offer except ourselves, a belief that life has meaning and purpose is personally sustaining. However, to speak glibly of this to a patient who is in despair is cruel. At such times, actions speak louder than words.

Having the strength to *just be there* with a dying patient, without particular words or actions, demonstrates a shared humanity which goes beyond patient/professional roles. This can sustain both the patient and the health professional.

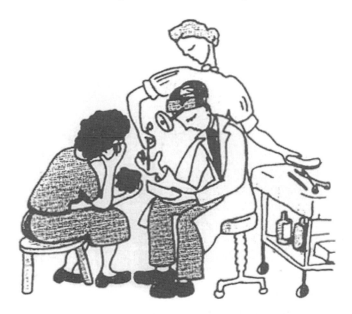

Figure 1 This shows the doctor, armed with his competence and his instruments and protected by the multiprofessional team. Reproduced with permission.[30]

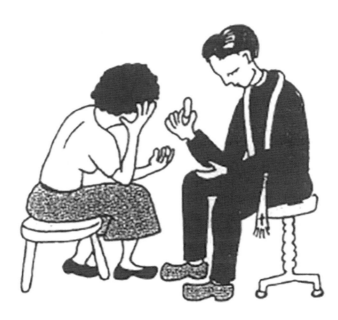

Figure 2 A priest performing his sacramental ministry. Here we see him wearing his stole and clerical collar protected by having a role to play and a ritual to perform. Reproduced with permission.[30]

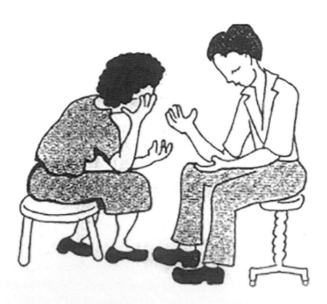

Figure 3 A patient meeting with either doctor or clergyman when he has exhausted the physical aspects of his ministry. He is left with his hands empty, but with his resources of counselling still available. Reproduced with permission.[30]

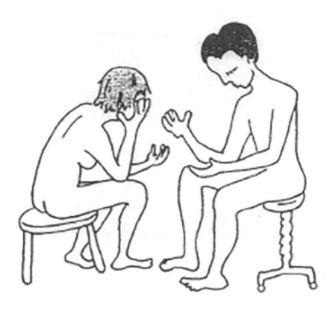

Figure 4 Both patient and carer stripped of their resources, present to each other, naked and empty-handed, as two human beings. Reproduced with permission.[30]

'Slowly, I learn about the importance of powerlessness.
I experience it in my own life and I live with it in my work.
The secret is not to be afraid of it – not to run away.
The dying know we are not God.
All they ask is that we do not desert them.'[29]

REFERENCES

1　Royal College of Physicians (2015) Acute care resource. End-of-life care in the acute care setting. www.rcplondon.ac.uk

2　Leadership Alliance for the Care of Dying People (2014) One chance to get it right Improving people's experience of care in the last few days and hours of life.

3　NICE (2015) Care of dying adults in the last days of life. www.nice.org.uk/guidance/ng31

4　General Medical Council (2008) Consent: patients and doctors making decisions together. www.gmc-uk.org/guidance

5　General Medical Council (2010) Treatment and care towards the end of life: good practice in decision making. www.gmc-uk.org/guidance

6　Anonymous (2005) Mental Capacity Act 2005: Elizabeth II. Chapter 9 Reprinted May and December 2006; May 2007. www.opsi.gov.uk/acts/acts2005/20050009.htm

7　Anonymous (2000) Adults with Incapacity (Scotland) Act. www.scotland-legislation.hmso.gov.uk/legislation/scotland/acts2000

8　National Council for Palliative Care / National End of Life Care Programme (2008) Advance Decisions to Refuse Treatment A Guide for Health and Social Care Professionals. www.endoflifecareforadults.nhs.uk/eolc/files/NHS_NEoLC_ADRT_082008.pdf

9 Mental Capacity Act (2005) www.legislation.gov.uk/ukpga/2005/9/pdfs/ukpga_20050009_en.pdf

10 University of Nottingham (2008) *Advance care planning: a guide for health and social care staff.* www.ncpc.org.uk/sites/default/files/AdvancedCarePlanning.pdf

11 Anonymous (2015) *Identifying a deprivation of liberty: a practical guide. The Law Society.* www.lawsociety.org.uk

12 Cheshire West and Chester Council and P & Q Surrey County Council (2014) UKSC 9.

13 Clark D *et al.* (2014) Imminence of death among hospital inpatients: Prevalent cohort study. *Palliative Medicine.* **28:** 474–479.

14 Prognostic Indicator Guidance Prognostic Indicator Guidance Sept 2011. www.goldstandardsframework.org.uk

15 National Emergency Care and Treatment Plan. www.resus.org.uk/consultations/emergency-care-and-treatment-plan/

16 Taylor R and Chadwick S (2015) Palliative care in hospital: Why is it so difficult? *Palliative Medicine.* **29:** 770–773.

17 Virdun C *et al.* (2015) Dying in the hospital setting: A systematic review of quantitative studies identifying the elements of end-of-life care that patients and their families rank as being most important. *Palliative Medicine.* **29:** 774–796.

18 Glare P *et al.* (2003) A systematic review of physicians' survival predictions in terminally ill cancer patients. *British Medical Journal.* **327:** 195–198.

19 Stone PC and Lund S (2007) Predicting prognosis in patients with advanced cancer. *Annals of Oncology.* **18:** 971–976.

20 Carey I *et al.* (2015) Improving care for patients whose recovery is uncertain. The AMBER care bundle: design and implementation. *BMJ Supportive and Palliative Care.* **5:** 405–411.

21 Sinclair A *et al.* (2013) End of life diabetes care: A strategy document commissed by diabetes UK. *Clinical care recommendations 2nd edition.* www.diabetes.org.uk/end-of-life-care

22 Blinderman CD and Billings JA (2015) Comfort care for patients dying in the hospital. *New England Journal of Medicine.* **373:** 2549–2561.

23 Bruera E *et al.* (2013) Parenteral hydration in patients with advanced cancer: a multicentre, double-blind, placebo-controlled randomized trial. *Journal of Clinical Oncology.* **31:** 111–118.

24 Navigante AH *et al.* (2006) Midazolam as adjunct therapy to morphine in the alleviation of severe dyspnea perception in patients with advanced cancer. *Journal of Pain and Symptom Management.* **31:** 38–47.

25 Campbell ML and Yarandi HN (2013) Death rattle is not associated with patient respiratory distress: is pharmacologic treatment indicated? *Journal of Palliative Medicine.* **16:** 1255–1259.

26 Wee B and Hillier R (2012) Interventions for noisy breathing in patients near to death. *Cochrane Database of Systematic Reviews.* **1:** CD005177.

27 Lokker ME *et al.* (2014) Prevalence, impact, and treatment of death rattle: a systematic review. *Journal of Pain and Symptom Management.* **47:** 105–122.

28 Mercadante S (2014) Death rattle: critical review and research agenda. *Supportive Care in Cancer.* **22:** 571–575.

29 Mota Vargas R *et al.* (2016) The transformation process for palliative care professionals: The metamorphosis, a qualitative research study. *Palliative Medicine.* **30:** 161–170.

30 Cassidy S (1988) *Sharing the darkness.* Darton, Longman and Todd, London, pp. 61–64.

FURTHER READING

NHS *Deciding Right* App (2016) Available from: Apple iTunes, Google Play and NHS app site.

15. CHILDREN: GENERAL ASPECTS

INTRODUCTION

Across the UK, the prevalence of life-threatening or life-limiting illness in 0–19 year olds is 30–45 per 10,000 population and is increasing.[1]

Although there are differences, paediatric and adult palliative care are generally similar (Table 1). In the UK, there are about 50 children's hospices, and Paediatric Palliative Medicine is a recognized subspecialty.

Table 1 A comparison of adult and children's palliative care

	Adult	Children's
Referral	Generally at points of symptom crisis, when disease-specific treatments exhausted, or at end of life	Often at the point of diagnosis, sometimes antenatally
Conditions	Mostly cancer, prognosis relatively predictable	Diverse conditions (Table 2), sometimes multisystem, and associated with major disabilities; prognosis less predictable
Admissions	Most for symptom management or terminal care	Focus on respite care in hospice, at home or elsewhere, e.g. special school, day centre, rehabilitation facility, nursing home
Physiotherapy, occupational therapy	Generally short-term interventions in response to specific needs	Generally long-term support with preventive and therapeutic aims
Duration	Weeks → months	Months → years

Respite care plays a major role in paediatric palliative care. It provides:
- a break for carers
- an opportunity to review health and social care need
- valuable social interaction
- access to leisure facilities
- peer support
- sibling support.

Table 2 Categories of conditions likely to require paediatric palliative care[2]

Category	Description
1	Life-threatening conditions for which curative treatment may be feasible but can fail
	e.g. cancer, irreversible heart, liver, or kidney failure
	Access to palliative care services may be necessary when treatment fails or during an acute crisis, irrespective of the duration of threat to life. On reaching long-term remission or following successful curative treatment there is no longer a need for palliative care services
2	Conditions where premature death is inevitable
	e.g. cystic fibrosis, muscular dystrophy
	There may be long periods of intensive treatment aimed at prolonging life and allowing participation in normal activities
3	Progressive conditions without curative treatment options
	e.g. Batten's disease, mucopolysaccharidoses
	Treatment is exclusively palliative and may commonly extend over many years
4	Irreversible but non-progressive conditions causing severe disability, leading to susceptibility to health complications and likelihood of premature death
	e.g. severe cerebral palsy, multiple disabilities such as following brain or spinal cord injury, complex health care needs, high-risk of unpredictable life-threatening event or episode

COLLABORATIVE COMMUNICATION

The ability to communicate with children appropriately is an essential skill in paediatric palliative care. It allows them to express concerns, hopes and desires, and should involve them in decision-making.

Collaborative communication is required between health professionals and the child, family, other carers and relevant services. Achieving a consensus about care and to avoid conflict requires a diplomatic approach which balances:
- the emergent autonomy of the child
- the ethics and legislation around capacity
- involvement of parents
- involvement of other carers.[3]

Family dynamics are complex, and each family is unique:
- parents are generally closely involved and must know that they are being:
  ▷ listened to
  ▷ kept fully informed
  ▷ involved in decision-making
- parents and other regular carers should be considered expert care providers.

Shared decision-making with the family facilitates:
- routine care
- advance care planning
- positive outcomes in bereavement.

Challenges in collaborative communication and decision-making

Several challenges may be present:
- *managing uncertainty:* uncertainty around prognosis may lead to a lack of consensus on goals of care
- *accepting that cure is impossible:* the trajectory of many life-limiting illnesses in children often includes unexpected reversals, idiosyncratic responses to therapy, and periods of relative stability. Parents whose child has previously survived 'against the odds' may be reluctant to acknowledge an inevitable fatal outcome and may pursue desperate attempts to prevent it
- *recognizing denial:* despite clear explanations and objective evidence indicating a child's poor prognosis, parents may still seemingly deny what is happening. However, denial can be a helpful coping mechanism, giving parents the emotional energy to support their child
- *recognizing that death is near:* this facilitates:
  ▷ optimal end of life care
  ▷ the avoidance of aggressive curative treatments which would most likely increase suffering and prolong dying
- *recognizing and challenging collusion:* e.g. when professionals and parents fail to share information adequately with a child in the belief that sharing might cause distress. However, avoiding discussions with a child can lead to isolation and misunderstanding, compound distress, and prevent them accessing comfort and the assurance they may require
- *recognizing and facilitating communication in situations of 'mutual pretence' or 'conspiracy of silence':* e.g. when both child and parent have an awareness of potentially distressing information but wish to protect one another by avoiding discussion.

In addition, older children and their families need to be adequately prepared for the transition to the adult sector; moving from an emphasis on a collaborative approach to an emphasis on self-advocacy and more independent decision-making (see p.292). It is important to acknowledge that previously parents have generally made decisions, managed what, when and how their children have been involved in discussions and set information boundaries.

The emerging young adult and the family may prefer to continue using a familiar and comfortable pattern of communication though this requires confirmation. Parents cannot be expected simply to 'step down' abruptly after years of close involvement and the young person may not welcome sudden independence.

Legislation around capacity and decision-making

Health professionals should be aware of the legal implications of the Mental Capacity (England and Wales) Act 2005[4] and the Adults with Incapacity (Scotland) Act 2000[5] so that they can prepare families for the changing emphasis in decision-making as a child matures:
- over-16s are assumed to be competent to make their own decisions; they must be given any support required in order to have capacity to do so
- under-16s may have the capacity to consent depending on their maturity and ability to understand what is involved. General Medical Council guidance suggests that doctors 'encourage young people to involve their parents in making important decisions, but…should usually abide by any decision they have the capacity to make themselves'[6]
- under-18s are not permitted to make an Advance Decision to Refuse Treatment or create a Lasting Power of Attorney (see p.261).

A child's capacity to make decisions evolves over time and at different rates according to their cognitive ability, developmental level and experience. There is a need to check how they prefer to receive information, and how involved they wish to be in discussions and decision-making; this should be rechecked from time to time. Involvement can be facilitated by:
- listening and responding to them
- using techniques to increase understanding, e.g. play therapy
- giving them opportunities to develop their own opinion and voice.

Some children may have little or no views about proposed care, e.g. because of immaturity or because their disability limits understanding; some may want to be involved but not necessarily as the sole decision-maker.[7]

Particularly for children with cognitive and/or communication difficulties:
- verbal information should be clear, simple and truthful, and given in small amounts at many sittings
- alternative methods should be considered, e.g. written, audio, pictorial, film, web-based formats, computers/laptop or tablet devices, body or sign-language, speech/communication boards, voice synthesizers, text-to-speech or eye-tracking technology
- communication can be facilitated by specialist support staff, e.g. speech and language therapists, play therapists, learning disability teams.

ETHICAL CONSIDERATIONS

Salient issues include:
- autonomy, consent, confidentiality and information sharing (see above)
- planning care in the child's best interests which respects their emerging capacity to make reasonable decisions; this is particularly difficult when the child and the parents disagree
- quality of life judgements
- end-of-life decisions: withdrawal of life-sustaining treatments, CPR, mechanical ventilation, clinically-assisted nutrition and hydration.

It is important to try to resolve disagreements through skilled communication. Sometimes help may be necessary from, among others, Patient Advice and Liaison Service (PALS), Clinical Ethics Service or Chaplaincy. Where differences cannot be resolved, the Court's intervention may be required to decide if a proposed course of action is in the child's best interests.

Conflict may arise about the appropriateness of treatment based on differing assumptions about the quality of life of the child, particularly when there is severe neuro-disability and/or cognitive disability.[7,8] Health professionals need to guard against making judgments about quality of life based on how the child was when first admitted to hospital and at their sickest. Families and carers are generally better judges because they have a longitudinal perspective, incorporating better times.

EDUCATION

School or college for children with life-limiting illness may be a welcome refuge from the world of hospitals and illness.[9]

An uncertain prognosis can create tension by interfering with planning long-term educational goals. However, all children should have an equal opportunity to realize their own potential. Further, attending school or college is not just about education; it also provides the opportunity for:[9]

- having a 'normal' routine
- developing friendships
- social, emotional and spiritual growth
- enhancing quality of life through positive contributions to school life, achieving goals and fulfilling ambitions
- affirming that the child is of value with the capacity for growth and a purposeful future, however short that may be.

Thus, illness permitting, a return to school or college should be supported whenever possible, even for short periods.

Local authorities support the educational attainment of a child with health needs whether attending mainstream or special schools and colleges. Some educational establishments provide individualized educational programmes, e.g. adapting standard curricula, basing examinations on life or employment skills, or realizing independent living. Home tutoring may be an option.[10] For those spending significant time in hospital, hospital teachers are available.

Many children with life-limiting illnesses also have complex health requirements, significant social care needs and special educational needs, and will need extra support with:

- communication and interaction (many may be non-verbal)
- cognitive problems including learning disability
- social, emotional and mental health needs
- sensory and physical needs.

Increasingly, children with additional educational needs attend mainstream establishments. When greater levels of support are required, there are specifically resourced special schools and colleges, which can:
- support day attendance or may be residential
- provide access to comprehensive healthcare services, e.g.:
  - ▷ community paediatrician-led clinics and visits
  - ▷ occupational therapy
  - ▷ physiotherapy
  - ▷ wheelchair services
  - ▷ speech and language therapy
  - ▷ school nurses.

All under-25s with disability need a personalized Education, Health and Care plan in place to facilitate the integration of education, health and care services.[11] These are made collaboratively involving the child/young person, parents/carers and the educational professionals, with input from health professionals when required, and should be able to respond to changing needs.

WITHDRAWAL OF INTENSIVE MEDICAL CARE

Increasingly children's palliative care services facilitate the transfer from acute hospital settings to the child's home or a hospice where timely withdrawal of intensive medical care can be carried out in a supportive environment. For example, discontinuation of ventilation with steps in place to prevent avoidable complications and with psychological support for the whole family.[12]

TRANSITIONING INTO ADULT SERVICES

Medical advances have resulted in more children with life-limiting illnesses reaching adulthood. In response, some children's palliative care services have extended their care provision to people up to 35 years of age. Nonetheless, a significant number exceed the upper age range and require a transition to adult services.

Young people and their families need to be pro-actively prepared for the transition to adult services so as to minimize the risks of disrupted care and to have realistic expectations of what can and cannot be achieved. Unsupported or poorly managed transition to adult services can result in poor health and social outcomes regarding management of the illness, social participation, educational achievement, and quality of life.[13]

Transition from childhood to adulthood is challenging. At present, a seamless transition between paediatric and adult care is generally lacking. It is particularly stressful for those with more complex health needs who have been dependent on a wide range of health and social services. Transition includes moving from people and teams in children's services, with whom there will generally be a strong and trusting relationship, to adult services with new specialists and teams, different systems and an unfamiliar approach.

Developmental challenges

Changes during adolescence can impact significantly on a young person's experiences of disease, treatment or access to care. These include:

- physical (biological and sexual), cognitive, behavioural, psychological and social development
- establishing own identity and self-image (including sexuality); involves developing independence from parents, seeking autonomy, challenging authority and experimenting with different, often risk-taking, behaviours along with forming relationships outside the family, particularly with peers
- developing the ability to think abstractedly and become curious about existential questions.

A life-threatening illness may interrupt normal development and result in problems with:

- delayed puberty, loss of fertility, disturbed or altered sexual development
- body changes and altered body image
- self-esteem
- parental relationships
- social rejection, isolation and withdrawal.

In comparison with healthy peers, young people with life-threatening illness may also:

- have relatively under-developed psychosocial skills which can impact on decision-making, autonomy, self-management and determination
- have restricted cognitive development and learning as a result of the disease process, school absences, medication, pain, depression or fatigue
- have varying degrees of readiness or capability in engaging with the process of transition to adult services.

Holistic transition

The unstable nature of many life-limiting and life-threatening illnesses, with the associated difficulty in prognostication, makes appropriate transition planning difficult. There are various initiatives in the UK to help improve transition.[14-16] Identifying an adult lead clinician or team to facilitate the transition and take over co-ordination of care is vital. The GP may be able to continue, or be supported in, playing a significant role.

Ideally, transition planning should start at about the age of 14, guided by local policies, procedures and guidelines. However, plans for transition to adult services may have been delayed because death was expected sooner. To avoid this, parallel planning is appropriate, i.e. plans for transition incorporate both the expectation of life and also the possibility of deterioration and death.

Holistic transition requires consideration of:

- health care:
  ▷ identify community health provision, e.g. primary care teams, learning disability teams, district nurses, etc.

> ▷ involve adult hospices for palliative and end-of-life care
> ▷ consider the physical environments, e.g. accessibility, age-appropriateness
> ▷ consider secondary care provision, e.g. admissions procedures, admission 'passports', ward environments, clinics
> ▷ engage in discussions and documentation around advance care planning (see p.259)

- social care:
  - ▷ identify appropriate respite provision
  - ▷ consider how complex 24/7 home care packages will transition to adult services
  - ▷ provide access to benefits advice, education around personal finance and personal budgets
- education:
  - ▷ support access to further and higher education including attainment of life-skills, assisted technology, apprenticeships and work-based learning
  - ▷ ensure the development of Education, Health and Care plans where indicated (see p.291)
- work and leisure:
  - ▷ identify suitable day care, social and leisure provision including access to arts, sports, holidays, social networks and support groups
  - ▷ consider involvement of local employment agencies
  - ▷ look at opportunities for vocational training
- independent living:
  - ▷ find appropriate accommodation to support independent living
  - ▷ consider shared accommodation.

Technology dependence/equipment needs

Commonly, there are multiple pieces of equipment which need servicing, repairing, reviewing or replacing as the child grows. When a young person moves into adult services, equipment often comes from different sources. Careful planning is required so that access and support continues uninterrupted.

A collaborative approach

Collaborative work between primary, secondary and tertiary care, across statutory and voluntary sectors, in the community and in schools is necessary to improve the process of transition for young people and families. Children's and adult services should consider:
- sharing knowledge of local services in both sectors
- sharing knowledge of transition guidelines/frameworks
- identifying a named professional who can be a point of contact point during transition and co-ordinate the process (separate from the lead clinician co-ordinating the healthcare transition)
- sharing up-to-date, relevant information and documentation with the young person, parents, carers and other professionals
- integrating services when possible, e.g. joint clinics, sharing staff and skills across both sectors.

REFERENCES

1 Fraser LK et al. (2011) *Life-limiting conditions in children in the UK.* Univeristy of Leeds. www. togetherforshortlives.org.uk/assets/0000/1100/Leeds_University___Children_s_Hospices_ UK_-_Ethnicity_Report.pdf

2 Harrop E and Edwards C (2013) How and when to refer a child for specialist paediatric palliative care. *Archives of Disease in Childhood Education and Practice Edition.* **98**: 202–208.

3 Wright B et al. (2009) Clinical dilemmas in children with life-limiting illnesses: decision making and the law. *Palliative Medicine.* **23**: 238–247.

4 Mental Capacity Act (2005) www.legislation.gov.uk/ukpga/2005/9/pdfs/ukpga_20050009_ en.pdf

5 Adults with Incapacity (Scotland) Act (2000) www.legislation.gov.uk/asp/2000/2004/contents

6 General Medical Council (2013) *0-18 years guidance:Young people who have capacity. Paragraph 29.* www.gmc-uk.org/guidance/ethical_guidance/children_guidance_29_capacity_to_consent.asp

7 Larcher V et al. (2015) Making decisions to limit treatment in life-limiting and life-threatening conditions in children: a framework for practice. *Archives of Disease in Childhood.* **100**: S1–S23.

8 Feudtner C and Nathanson PG (2014) Pediatric palliative care and pediatric medical ethics: opportunities and challenges. *Pediatrics.* **133**: S1–S7.

9 Craig F et al. (2012) Schooling of children with life-limiting or life-threatening illness. *European Journal of Palliative Care.* **19**: 131–135.

10 Department of Education (2013) *Ensuring a good education for children who cannot attend school because of health needs.* www.gov.uk/government/uploads/system/uploads/attachment_data/ file/269469/health_needs_guidance__-_revised_may_2013_final.pdf

11 Special Educational Needs and Disabilities (SEND) Reforms (2014) *0 to 25 SEND code of practice: a guide for health professionals.* www.gov.uk/government/uploads/system/uploads/ attachment_data/file/357645/Health_professionals_guide_to_the_SEND_code_of_ practice_-_Sept357614.pdf

12 Association for Children's Palliative Care (2011) *A care pathway to support extubation within a children's palliative care framework.* www.togetherforshortlives.org.uk/professionals/ resources/2433_the_extubation_care_pathway_2010

13 Colver A and Longwell S (2013) New understanding of adolescent brain development: relevance to transitional healthcare for young people with long term conditions. *Archives of Disease in Childhood.* **98**: 902–907.

14 Department of Health (2011) *Self-review tool for quality criteria for young people friendly health services.* www.gov.uk/government/publications/self-review-tool-for-quality-criteria- for-young-people-friendly-health-services

15 Nagra A (2012) *Ready Steady Go.* University Hospital Southampton NHS Foundation Trust. www.uhs.nhs.uk/OurServices/Childhealth/TransitiontoadultcareReadySteadyGo/ Transitiontoadultcare.aspx

16 NICE (2016) Transition from children's to adult's services for young people using health or social are services. *NICE Guideline* NG43. www.nice.org.uk

FURTHER READING

Care Quality Commission (2014) *From the pond into the sea: Children's transition to adult health services.* www.cqc.org.uk/sites/default/files/CQC_Transition%20Report.pdf

Carter BS and Levetown M (2004) *Palliative Care for Infants, Children and Adolescents: A Practical Handbook.* The Johns Hopkins University Press, Baltimore and London.

Child and young person's advanced care plan collaborative. www.cypacp.nhs.uk

16. CHILDREN: SYMPTOM MANAGEMENT

Many symptoms and difficulties experienced by children at the end of life are comparable with those in adults, and the approach to management is the same: a holistic approach incorporating both non-drug and drug interventions. This chapter highlights those more commonly encountered in paediatric palliative care.

POSITIONING

Many children need specific postural management. Pro-active and experienced physiotherapists, occupational therapists and community teams with the full involvement of the family/other carers are essential. Round-the-clock postural management is important in relation to:
- joint care
- prevention of contractures and pressure sores
- improving bone density
- management of pain and discomfort
- maximizing mobility
- respiratory and swallowing difficulties
- management of constipation and recurrent urinary tract infections
- facilitating communication, and cognitive and functional skills
- enabling access to and participation in educational and recreational activities

A postural management programme may involve standing programmes, attention to overnight positioning, provision of appropriate armchairs, wheelchair services, regular passive or active exercise, and care plans regarding manual handling.

PAIN

Pain management is essentially the same as in adults (see p.83).[1] However, in children pain evaluation may be more difficult:
- because expression of pain is influenced by age and developmental stage
- for some a change in behaviour or non-verbal indicators may be the only clues, particularly in those who are pre-verbal, non-verbal, cognitively impaired, or just frightened

- testimony from the family and caregivers is generally invaluable
- a trial of analgesia may help to distinguish pain from other causes of distress.

Pain evaluation tools have been developed for children, although there is no 'gold standard'.[2] The Wong and Baker faces visual rating scale is widely used: 'Face 0 is very happy because he doesn't hurt at all... Face 6 hurts as much as you can imagine'.[3]

The use of intranasal and buccal routes for opioids is more common in children. For example, diamorphine can be used buccally by mixing the injection powder in water for injections (unauthorized route) or intranasally (authorized for severe acute pain in the over-2s).

SPASTICITY AND MUSCLE SPASMS

Spasticity is a condition in which muscles are continuously contracted resulting in stiffness or tightness of the muscles.

Generally, it is caused by damage to areas in the CNS controlling voluntary movement. In children, cerebral palsy is the most common cause.[4] Other causes include traumatic brain injury, stroke, neurodegenerative disease and spinal cord injury.

A pro-active management approach is required to:
- reduce pain and muscular spasms
- improve posture
- minimize contractures and deformity
- facilitate mobility and dexterity
- support speech and communication.[5]

Spasticity ranges in intensity from a mild feeling of muscle tightness to uncontrollable severely painful limb spasms. These can be rapid in onset, occur spontaneously or following trivial stimulation, and can last several minutes. Triggers and exacerbating factors include infection, pain, fracture.

The clinical features of spasticity can be subtle and non-specific, including reports of:
- 'not being quite right'
- mild changes in dexterity, problems with dressing, difficulty remaining seated or 'sliding from chair'
- discomfort or pain
- anxiety
- fatigue
- weight loss or poor nutritional status (persistent muscle contraction expends calories)
- altered behaviour.

Management includes stretching and exercise programmes, along with optimizing posture, bladder, bowel and skin care regimens. The involvement of carers is essential.

Drugs used include diazepam and baclofen (see p.372). For severe spasticity not responding to usual approaches, options include:

- botulinum toxin injected into affected muscles (under general anaesthetic)
- tenotomies, particularly for wrists and lower limbs
- intrathecal baclofen.

SEIZURES

Causes of seizures include:
- primary neurological conditions, e.g. brain tumour
- systemic illness, acute or chronic
- biochemical derangement.

Watching a child have a seizure can be frightening for parents, carers and health professionals. Seizures impact on quality of life both physically (risk of injury, aspiration, hospitalization) and psychologically (anxiety, embarrassment). The emotional burden for parents and carers of children with uncontrolled or unpredictable seizures can be considerable.

Challenges include:
- making the diagnosis: various behaviours can mimic seizures, particularly in children with severe neurological conditions, e.g. arching or posturing with pain, exaggerated startle reactions, dystonia, myoclonus
- identifying and managing any precipitating factors, e.g. fever, sleep deprivation, drugs, biochemical derangement, CNS infection
- knowledge of anti-epileptic pharmacology, particularly undesirable effects, drug interactions, routes of administration
- developing a seizure care plan, including training for family/carers so that they can manage seizures at home; this may well improve outcome, decrease anxiety and prevent hospital admissions (Figure 1).

The management of seizures, status epilepticus and the approach in the last days of life are similar to adults (p.203).

Name *Joe Davies*   **DoB** *February 16, 2004*   **Weight** *40kg*

Maintenance anti-epileptics: *clobazam, levetiracetam, sodium valproate*

Seizure type 1: *Tonic clonic seizures*

Triggers: *Fever*

Warning signs: *May look slightly startled/restless immediately beforehand*

Presentation: *Facial twitching (R side)*

                Limb jerking (usually R side)

                Generalized increased tone (all 4 limbs)

Frequency: *Variable from daily to once weekly*

Duration: *Has had episodes of status epilepticus lasting 45+ minutes*

Ever suffered from status epilepticus? *Yes*

Rescue medication and when to use:

First line: *Diazepam 7.5mg PR*   after 5 minutes

Second line: *Diazepam 7.5mg PR*   after a further 10 minutes

Third line: *Paraldehyde 3.5ml PR*   after a further 15 minutes

Response to rescue medication: *Hopefully stops fitting, but may be drowsy for a while afterwards and may need CPAP*

Is oxygen required? *Yes sometimes*

Usual recovery period and support needed: *May remain drowsy. Place in a safe recovery position. May need oxygen ± CPAP. Consider intercurrent illness.*

If no response to rescue medication should emergency services be contacted?

No: Call Dr Brown (pager 123) re possible phenobarbital loading

Who else should be contacted?   *Parents: Peter & Mary Davies*

                           Home 01234 556789

                           Mob. 09718 112233

Seizure type 2: (Complete as many as required when there are multiple types of seizure which require different rescue medication protocols).

Figure 1 Example of a hospice inpatient Seizure Care Plan for a 12 year-old boy with generalized seizures as a result of hypoxic brain injury at birth

INBORN ERRORS OF METABOLISM

Individual inborn errors of metabolism are relatively rare but collectively are a significant cause of morbidity and mortality. Many are inherited by autosomal recessive or sex-linked genes.

They vary widely in presentation, specific management and prognosis, depending on which body systems are affected (Table 1). Most present in childhood; some are diagnosed antenatally or through neonatal screening programmes, e.g. phenylketonuria. Milder forms may present in adulthood. Generally, the conditions are multisystem, progressive and life-limiting.

Table 1 Examples of inborn errors of metabolism

Metabolism affected	Example	Features
Carbohydrate	Pompe disease Glycogen storage disease type II	Progressive muscle weakness, cardiomyopathy, hepatomegaly, cardiac and respiratory failure; treated with enzyme replacement
Amino acid	Non-ketotic hyperglycinaemia Caused by carnitine transporter deficiency	Cardiomyopathy and muscle weakness; treated with carnitine supplementation. Intercurrent illness may cause encephalopathy, hypoglycaemia and worsening cardiomyopathy
Organic acid	Lesch-Nyan syndrome Disorder of purine metabolism causing over-production of uric acid	Self-injury, dystonia and renal failure; treatment includes drugs to reduce uric acid (e.g. allopurinol), adequate hydration, and protective splints or straps
Lysosomal storage	Hurler's disease Mucopolysaccharidosis type I	Organomegaly, mental regression, bony changes, kyphosis; treatment includes enzyme replacement and haematopoietic stem cell transplant
Mitochondrial	Leigh's disease	Intestinal dysmotility, seizures, dementia, hearing and visual loss, peripheral neuropathy, autonomic dysfunction, central hypoventilation, cardiomyopathy and cardiac conduction defects; treatment includes vitamins (e.g. thiamine)

Multiprofessional management includes:
- correct-the-correctable, e.g. use of dietary treatment or drugs (vitamins, enzyme replacement) to prevent or delay deterioration
- optimize supportive care, e.g. nutritional, respiratory, cardiac, renal and liver support
- manage complications, e.g. dystonia, spasticity, seizures.

Stressors such as fever, vomiting or diarrhoea can trigger an acute life-threatening decompensation marked by, for example, hypoglycaemia, seizures, encephalopathy.

An affected child should have individualized standard and emergency protocols which will include resuscitation and supportive measures as well as disease-specific treatments. More information is available on the website of the British Inherited Metabolic Disease Group (www.bimdg.org.uk/guidelines/guidelines-child.asp).

PRESCRIBING IN CHILDREN

For specialist guidance on prescribing for children and neonates generally, and more specifically in palliative care, see Further reading (p.305).

Extra care is required when prescribing for children:
- consider non-drug options, and prescribe only if there is a definite indication
- become familiar with a limited range of drugs and their effects in children
- simplify regimens as much as possible
- try to avoid the need to administer drugs at school
- check dose calculations (often based on weight or surface area)
- consider rounding down to the nearest practical dose.

Children are at increased risk of medication errors because of:
- lack of evidence base
- the rarity of their conditions
- the need to calculate and adjust the dose for the age and/or weight of the child
- the lack of suitable dose formulations
- variations in recommendations
- inconsistent presentation of dose information (e.g. microgram/kg per dose, microgram/kg/h, mg per dose, total 24h dose).

Particular care is required when prescribing in the neonatal period (<1 month) because of immature renal and liver function, immature reticular activating system, and higher volumes of distribution.

Flexible personalized regimens make it easier for the child, increasing adherence and minimizing disruption to schooling and sleep. However, regular timing is important for some drugs, e.g. IV antibacterials.

As in adult palliative care, there are many occasions when it is necessary to prescribe drugs 'off-label', i.e. beyond their authorized indications and/or routes of administration.

Deciding the dose

Paediatric dosing is based on the physiological characteristics of the child, and the pharmacokinetics of the drug. Body weight is generally a better determinant of dose than age. Body surface area mirrors physiological processes most closely and is used for certain drugs, e.g. cytotoxics.

Drug formulation and administration

Most children are able to take medicines orally, and many continue to do so throughout their illness. A liquid may be easier to administer than tablets or capsules, particularly for young children and those with dysphagia. However, tablets may be preferable to large volumes of unpleasant tasting liquids.

Many tablets (but *not* m/r ones) can be split, cut or crushed to aid dosing or administration. Although not recommended by the manufacturers, some matrix (*but not reservoir*) patches can be cut.

The use of alternative routes of administration (buccal, intranasal, inhaled, PR, SC, IV) is relatively common in children. These routes avoid both degradation by gastric acid and first-pass metabolism by the liver. Some children already have a central venous line which can be used for continuous drug infusions.

IM administration is particularly distressing for children, and should generally be avoided. SC administration may be appropriate and acceptable for children, and is the route of choice for continuous infusions if there is no permanent central venous access.

Many seriously ill children are fed by nasogastric tube or gastrostomy, and these provide an alternative route of drug administration. However, there is a risk that drugs may continue to be administered via a feeding tube even when no longer necessary. Regular review is essential.

Pharmacokinetics and pharmacodynamics

Compared with adults, under-12s tend to absorb and metabolize drugs differently.

Neonates (<1 month)

Relatively low renal and hepatic clearances, and higher volumes of distribution, result in a *longer halflife* for many drugs. This may necessitate lower doses at longer intervals. Neonates have less fat and muscle, and increased bio-availability. Drugs primarily metabolized by the liver should be administered with extreme care in those under 2 months. There is a higher risk of respiratory depression with opioids (see below).

Immaturity also affects pharmacodynamics, e.g. paradoxical reactions to benzodiazepines have been observed in neonates, particularly in premature infants, probably related to the delayed maturation of GABA receptors.

Infants and children (1 month–12 years)

Relatively high drug clearances and normal volumes of distribution result in a *shorter halflife* for many drugs. This may necessitate relatively higher doses at shorter intervals. On the other hand, midazolam and morphine, for example, have longer halflives in infants (as in neonates).

Specific cautions when prescribing for children

Anti-epileptics

Many children with life-limiting conditions are on complicated anti-epileptic regimens. Interactions are common, variable and unpredictable, and may increase toxicity. Anti-epileptics also have significant interactions with other drugs (see, p.345). Specialist paediatric neurology advice is recommended when titrating or reducing anti-epileptics in children.

Generally, anti-epileptic medication should *not* be stopped in the terminal phase, although absorption and administration may prove unpredictable. An alternative route of administration, and the addition or substitution of SC midazolam or phenobarbital may be necessary. Some anti-epileptics (e.g. carbamazepine, clonazepam, diazepam, lorazepam, phenobarbital and valproate) can be given PR, but may require dose adjustment.

Corticosteroids

In paediatric palliative care, the commonest reason for prescribing a corticosteroid is headache and vomiting caused by raised intracranial pressure associated with an intracranial tumour. Compared with adults, children seem to experience a more rapid onset of undesirable effects, particularly cushingoid facies, proximal myopathy, weight gain, and changes in mood and behaviour.

Consequently, short courses are preferred, e.g. dexamethasone ≤500microgram/kg/day for 3–5 days (for symptoms related to raised intracranial pressure), repeated as necessary. This often provides adequate symptom relief and causes less toxicity than continuous dosing. However, continuous dosing is sometimes unavoidable.

Codeine

Codeine is no longer recommended for the management of pain in children because of genetic variability in metabolism, affecting efficacy, undesirable effects and safety. In particular, ultra-rapid metabolizers are vulnerable to potentially fatal respiratory depression.

Strong opioids

Strong opioids can generally be used safely in children, just as in adults, although careful explanation to parents and carers may be required to allay fears.

Fentanyl and buprenorphine TD patches are widely used as convenient long-acting opioid formulations. However, because of a risk of fatal respiratory depression in opioid-naïve children, they should be used only after initial dose titration with an oral product. Pyrexia accelerates the rate of diffusion from the patch.

In neonates (<1 month), late respiratory depression has been reported, >4h after administration of immediate-release morphine. Compared with doses in children aged 2–12 years, the recommended doses per kg are lower in the under-2s, and much lower in neonates.

Of the undesirable effects of opioids, pruritus and urinary retention are possibly more common, and nausea less common than in adults.

Phenothiazines

Although evidence is sparse, children may have an age-related increased risk of dystonic reactions with D_2 antagonists, e.g. phenothiazines and metoclopramide. Such drugs should be used with caution in the under-20s.

REFERENCES

1 Zernikow B et al. (2006) Paediatric cancer pain management using the WHO analgesic ladder-results of a prospective analysis from 2265 treatment days during a quality improvement study. European Journal of Pain. 10: 587–595.
2 von Baeyer CL and Spagrud LJ (2007) Systematic review of observational (behavioral) measures of pain for children and adolescents aged 3 to 18 years. Pain. 127: 140–150.
3 Wong D and Baker C (1988) Pain in children: comparison of assessment scales. Pediatric Nursing. 14: 9–17.
4 Ronan S and Gold JT (2007) Nonoperative management of spasticity in children. Childrens Nervous System. 23: 943–956.
5 Delgado MR et al. (2010) Practice parameter: pharmacologic treatment of spasticity in children and adolescents with cerebral palsy (an evidence-based review). Neurology. 74: 336–343.

FURTHER READING

British National Formulary for Children (2015–2016). London: BMJ Group and Pharmaceutical Press. www.bnf.org
Hain R and Jassal S (2010) Paediatric Palliative Medicine. Oxford University Press, Oxford.
Jassal S and Hain RD (2014) Association for Paediatric Medicine Master Formulary. www.appm.org.uk/10.html
Neonatal Formulary 7 (2014) www.neonatalformulary.com

17. CHILDREN: BEREAVEMENT

INTRODUCTION

Although the focus of this chapter is on the death of a parent, the content is relevant for any significant loss.

Every year in the UK, more than 20,000 children experience a parental death.[1] Indeed, by the age of 16, about 1 in 20 children will have experienced the death of one or both of their parents.[2] The death of a parent is one of the most stressful events for a child to experience. In later life, it increases the risk of:

- physical ill-health
- psychological and social problems
- psychiatric disorders, particularly depression and anxiety, possibly precipitated by further losses later in life
- self-harm, suicidal thoughts, attempted suicide.

However, the impact is not always negative; some bereaved children develop:

- increased independence
- a determination to do better at school
- a greater ability to understand the distress of others
- an increased appreciation of family relationships and of life.

GRIEF IN CHILDREN

Grief is a normal physical, emotional, behavioural and cognitive response to a significant loss. It is healthy and predictable, and improves over time. The onset may be delayed by weeks or months; and it typically manifests on and off for months or years.

A positive outcome for the child is strongly related to the surviving parent's mental health, coping style, and levels of warmth, discipline and communication.[2,3] *Thus, providing support to the remaining parent or carer is crucial.*

Other factors influencing the duration and intensity of grief include:

- closeness of the relationship with the dead parent
- family circumstances (parental conflict, separation, divorce → poorer outcome)
- circumstances of the death (suicide, unexpected death → poorer outcome)

- previous experiences of loss
- personality and coping style (mainly determined by early attachments)
- availability of support from other adults and/or children's bereavement service.

Expressions of grief

Although the expression of grief in children is similar to that in adults (see p.67), it is influenced by their understanding of death. This varies with age, gender, stage of emotional development, and verbal and cognitive abilities. As they grow older and their understanding of death and perceptions of the world change, children may revisit grief or re-explore the death from a different perspective. Times of change and reaching significant milestones (e.g. moving school, attending the school prom, choosing a university, leaving home) may also retrigger grief.

Physical responses

It is common for grieving children to have somatic complaints:
- disturbed sleep, e.g. difficulty going to sleep, hypersomnia, nightmares
- pain, e.g. stomach ache, headaches
- feeding difficulties, loss of appetite, compulsive eating
- regression to urinary or faecal incontinence, bed wetting, constipation.

There may be difficulty sleeping unless an attachment figure is nearby.

Emotional responses

In addition to the responses seen in adults, children commonly fear:
- other loved ones or they themselves might also die
- changes in lifestyle, e.g. need to move home, reduced family income
- abandonment.

They may also be burdened by guilt, a sense of responsibility for the parent's death.

Normal coping skills for children include distraction and diversion, and this may make it seem that a child has recovered from or has not been affected by the bereavement. There is often an episodic quality to their grief:
- switching from being very sad one moment to being excited and happy the next
- sadness accompanied by a desire to rapidly return to normal activities.

Knowing that these are common responses is helpful to parents and carers. Further, although still distressed, some children try to protect the surviving parent by giving the impression that they have got over their loss.[4,5]

Behavioural responses

Children's behaviour commonly changes when grieving (Box A; Table 1).[4,6] Regressive behaviour is common and generally indicates that a child is seeking security. Children are more likely than adults to 'act out' their feelings. This can result in unprovoked anger or aggression towards other children, which may simply be put down to 'being naughty' or 'misbehaving'. Awareness and acceptance by the surviving parent and other carers will help the child adjust. Age-appropriate behavioural boundaries should be maintained.

Box A Behavioural responses to loss in children and young people	
Argumentativeness	Nightmares
Attention-seeking	Poor school work
Bed wetting	Refusing to go to school
Clinginess	Regression
Daydreaming	Restlessness
Difficulty bonding with new carers	Temper tantrums
Difficulty concentrating	Withdrawal
Mood swings	

PREPARATION FOR THE DEATH OF A PARENT

A lower level of anxiety and a better long-term adjustment to bereavement is linked to adequate preparation after a parent is given a life-threatening diagnosis.

Children observe, hear, listen to and know much more than adults often realize. Even pre-verbal and non-verbal children can tell from the distress of the adults around them that something upsetting is happening. Avoiding discussions about what is uppermost in a child's mind may result in them feeling confused, isolated, and imagining things worse than probable reality. For parents experiencing anticipatory grief, it will be extremely challenging for them to respond effectively to a child's questions and emotional needs.

Age-appropriate advice about how to have conversations about dying, the best language to use and the amount of information to convey is invaluable (Box B).

Box B Useful books for when a parent becomes seriously ill (ISBN)
For parents: As big as it gets (9780953912391)
For teenagers: A monster calls (9781406361803)
For primary school children: The secret C (9780955953927)

CHILDREN'S UNDERSTANDING OF DEATH

Children's understanding of death develops gradually. Their developmental stage is the predominant determinant of their ability to understand causality and the irreversible nature of death, along with the implications of separation (Table 1).

Verbally- and cognitively-able children acquire the concept of death earlier than less able children, as do those as young as 8 if they have previously known another person who has died.

Table I Age-related understanding of death and possible manifestations[3-8]

Age	Understanding of death	Possible manifestations
Infants and toddlers	No cognitive understanding of death May react to distress expressed by those around them	Reactions to loss may progress through protest and crying → despair → detachment and indifference Separation anxiety, increased dependency → need reassuring company and physical contact Continuing to search for the dead parent Needing to be told repeatedly that the dead parent is not returning.
Preschool	See death as temporary and reversible May understand illness primarily as contagion Often believe that their actions can impact on the world around them and that, in some way, they may have caused the death	Seemingly callous or insensitive questions generated from a concrete and literal interpretation of the world, e.g. they may ask for a replacement parent Apparent inconsistencies in their understanding, e.g. may acknowledge that they know their parent is dead, but then subsequently ask when they are returning Misconceptions may need addressing, e.g. assure the child that the death is not related to anything they have said or done.
5–8 years	Begin to understand that death: • is irreversible; those who have died cannot return • means the end of thinking, feeling, hearing, seeing, speaking, eating, moving • is universal; it eventually happens to everyone including themselves	Anger towards the dead parent and/or towards those unable to prevent the death Increased dependence on the surviving parent → resists separation from them even for short periods When the child understands that death means the end of thinking, feeling and moving → stops worrying about the dead parent being lonely or cold Fears about death and concerns about the safety of other loved ones.

continued

Table I. Contd.

Age	Understanding of death	Possible manifestations
8–12 years	Develop a full understanding of the nature of death and its causes	A wish to be dead; requires careful exploration but generally reflects a desire to be with the dead parent and not to commit suicide
		Need for assurance that they cannot catch the dead parent's illness
	May develop a morbid curiosity; often interested in the physical details of the dying process	Comfort from imagining an afterlife in which the dead parent continues to enjoy favourite activities and/or continues to watch over and care for them.
Adolescents	Have an adult understanding of death	Normal to have difficulty talking to the surviving parent
		Rejection of adult rituals and family activities
	Develop the ability to think abstractedly; often curious about the existential implications of death	Try to solve problems themselves or seek support from trusted peers or adults other than the surviving parent
		Feeling that no one understands them
		Engaging in high risk activities in order to fully challenge their own mortality
		Strong emotional reactions or difficulty in identifying and expressing feelings
		Taking on new family roles and responsibilities because of expectations (e.g. 'Be strong for your mother', 'You're the man of the house now'); these are likely to be burdensome.

DIFFICULT CONVERSATIONS

Repetitive distressing questioning from younger children is normal, and guidance to parents about this is available (see Box B). Older children often ask very direct questions, e.g. 'Are you going to die?' It is important to be truthful and acknowledge that death is a possibility. Information needs to be:

- age-appropriate
- possibly given progressively in small amounts, preferably child-led, in response to their questions
- repeated as necessary
- unambiguous: use 'dying', 'death', 'dead', not potentially confusing euphemisms such as 'gone to sleep', 'we've lost him'.

Parents should be assured that it is all right to cry in front of a child. Shielding them from expressions of grief may result in a child feeling isolated within the sadness they have sensed and to conclude that it is unacceptable to show emotions. This can limit access to the comfort they need.

OTHER CONSIDERATIONS

Viewing the body

Children may find seeing the body after death a helpful experience allowing confirmation of death, and a chance to say goodbye. Sensitive preparation, including clear descriptions of the coffin, the room, the body and what to expect, allows the child to make an informed choice about whether to view the body.

Check several times before the viewing to allow them to change their mind. They should be accompanied by a trusted adult, given time and opportunities to ask questions. They may wish to take something special to leave in the coffin.

Attending the funeral

Decisions about a child's attendance should be made on an individual basis, and involve the child when possible. A child can be supported in making an informed choice about attending a funeral if they are provided with clear explanations about the arrangements for the day, and what they may see (children may be shocked to see other people crying).

Being excluded may add to any existing feelings of guilt, isolation and abandonment. Conversely, being placed in an intensely emotional situation without adequate warning may leave lasting traumatic memories. Check several times before the funeral to allow them to change their mind.

To enable relatives to mourn at the funeral, it can be helpful to have someone present who is less directly affected by the death to support the child.

Actively reminiscing

Talking about the dead parent can help a child maintain a positive connection with them. Keeping and sharing special memories, mementos and photographs all help ensure that the dead parent is an important part of the child's ongoing life-story.

School and other activities

School can provide security and routine but can also be a place where children feel different and isolated. There may also be concerns about school work and exams. Other regular activities and special events are generally helpful to the child and also to the family.

Teasing and bullying

This is a common experience for bereaved children. It may stem from fear: the other children trying to distance themselves from the possibility of such a thing happening to them by seeing the affected child as somehow different. Work with the school to help normalize the situation for the child's classmates and enable them to become more supportive.

BEREAVEMENT SUPPORT

A central need is giving the child permission to express sorrow in age-appropriate ways, e.g. music, art, play, fantasy, activity, sport, long walks, silence.

Information and support are available from various organizations (Box C).

Box C Some organizations providing information and support	
For parents	
Cancer Counselling Trust	www.cancercounselling.org.uk
Cruse Bereavement Care	www.cruse.org.uk/children
Macmillan Cancer Support	www.macmillan.org.uk
Parentline Plus	www.parentlineplus.org.uk
Winston's Wish	www.winstonswish.org.uk
For children and young people	
Childline	www.childline.org.uk
Cruse (bereavement)	www.hopeagain.org.uk
Get Connected	www.getconnected.org.uk
Macmillan Youth Line	www.macmillan.org.uk
Riprap	www.riprap.org.uk
Siblinks (for siblings)	www.siblinks.org

Parental education

Parents benefit by learning about children's grief in general, helping them to understand their child's behaviour, and providing advice about how best to handle it.

Books

Books and other age-appropriate literature are generally helpful to children of all ages (Box D):
- child characters who are coping with loss in stories can provide bereaved children with role models
- reading together enables adults to gain valuable insights into the thoughts and feelings of the child
- focused storytelling can be used to draw out grief-related feelings and concerns.

Widening the family's support network

Widening the family support network is helpful for both children and parents. Encourage parents to share the responsibility of managing their child's grief with other relatives and trusted adults. Formal channels include school teachers, school nurses, parent support advisors, family support workers, and social workers.

Formal bereavement support

Not all grieving children need formal therapy. Children's bereavement services with counselling and support groups are mostly in the voluntary sector with limited resources. Activities include play, art, music, and family therapies. If formal support is needed but unavailable, bereavement support for the surviving parent is a priority.

CHILDREN WITH LEARNING DISABILITIES

Children with learning disabilities are at greater risk of a poorer outcome, and should be offered formal bereavement support. This reflects a more dependent relationship with the dead parent and a higher background risk of mental health problems. As with other children, the response to bereavement will reflect their understanding of death and loss (Table 1), and the general approach to supporting them and their remaining parent will be broadly similar.

When the child is unable to express their feelings, grief may go unrecognized, particularly when the response to loss presents as physical symptoms or as altered behaviour, e.g. irritability, lethargy, inappropriate speech and hyperactivity, anger, 'attention seeking'. Explanation to carers that these behaviours are normal responses to grief is important; likewise, avoiding the over-use of drugs and behaviour-modifying therapies.

It is important to ensure that the child receives consistent information and support in all settings: home, school, respite care. If difficulty in communication limits counselling or therapy, the use of touch, talking truthfully, familiar people and familiar routines are all helpful.

Box D Useful books for bereaved children (ISBN)

Explaining death

For children and adults together:

Always and Forever (9780575051836)

The original velveteen rabbit (9781405210546)

Waterbugs and dragonflies: explaining death to young children (9780826464583)

We need to talk about the funeral (9781906125011)

What do we think about death? (9780750232180)

Why do people die? (9780818406287)

When a parent dies

For teenagers:

A Monster Calls (9781406361803)

How it feels when a parent dies (9780575051836)

When parents die (9780722531310)

For pre-school/primary school children:

Is daddy coming back in a minute? Explaining sudden death to pre-school children in words they can understand (9780957474505)

Muddles, puddles and sunshine (9781903458969)

When a close family member or friend dies

For adults:

Helping children cope with grief (9780859695596)

For children and adults together:

A birthday present for Daniel: A child's story of loss (9781573929462)

For all age ranges:

Michael Rosen's sad book (9781406317848)

Remembering grandad (9780192723680)

The Soul Bird (9781849010320)

For primary school children:

Emma says goodbye: a child's guide to bereavement (9780745927596)

The day the sea went out and never came back (helping children) (9780863884634)

I wish I could hold your hand: a child's guide to grief and loss (9780915166824)

REFERENCES

1 Childhood Bereavement Network. *Key Statistics.* www.childhoodbereavementnetwork.org. uk/research/key-statistics.aspx
2 Aynsley-Green A *et al.* (2012) Bereavement in childhood: risks, consequences and responses. *BMJ Supportive and Palliative Care.* **2**: 2–4.
3 Dowdney L (2008) Children bereaved by parent or sibling death. *Psychiatry.* **7**: 270–275.
4 Black D (1998) Coping with loss. Bereavement in childhood. *British Medical Journal.* **316**: 931–933.
5 Himebauch A *et al.* (2008) Grief in children and developmental concepts of death #138. *Journal of Palliative Medicine.* **11**: 242–244.
6 Stuber ML and Mesrkhani VH (2001) 'What do we tell the children?': understanding childhood grief. *Western Journal of Medicine.* **174**: 187–191.
7 Barnado's Northern Ireland (2006) How to explain death to children and young people and help them cope. www.barnados.org.uk/child_bereavement_booklet_explaining_death.pdf
8 D'Antonio J (2011) Grief and loss of a caregiver in children. *Journal of Psychological Nursing.* **49**: 17–20.

FURTHER READING

Barnardo's Cymru. Swansea Children Matter. (2008) *Helping children manage bereavement.* www.fis.carmarthenshire.gov.uk/pdf/barnardo1.pdf
British Psychological Society Division of Educational and Child Psychology (2004) Loss, separation and bereavement. *Educational and Child Psychology* **21 (3)**.
Winston's Wish Charter for Bereaved Children: www.winstonswish.org.uk

18. THE ESSENTIAL PALLIATIVE CARE FORMULARY

This chapter overviews the principles of prescribing and features selected drugs used in palliative care. For advice about prescribing in children, see p.302.

The content is derived from the 5th edition of the Palliative Care Formulary (*PCF*), where greater detail and references are provided. *PCF*, with the latest updates, can also be accessed on www.palliativedrugs.com.

PCF highlights off-label indications and routes, and deals extensively with the administration of multiple drugs by Continuous Subcutaneous Infusion (CSCI).

GENERAL PRINCIPLES

Safe prescribing

Safe prescribing is a skill, and is crucial to success in symptom management. It requires good communication with patients, carers, and other professionals. Poor communication contributes to many preventable drug errors and much patient dissatisfaction.

Good communication includes clear documentation (e.g. allergies, co-morbidities, prescription writing). The use of a patient's 'logbook' is to be encouraged; this would include important contact names and telephone numbers.

Safe prescribing practice is particularly important in palliative care where polypharmacy, debility, co-morbidities (e.g. renal impairment), involvement of many health professionals, and the use of higher risk medications are among the many factors which make patients particularly vulnerable to problems with adherence (compliance), undesirable effects, drug errors, drug interactions and other potentially preventable burdens.

Safe prescribing includes avoiding doses which force patients to take more tablets, and/or open more containers than would be the case if the dose is 'rounded up' to a more convenient single tablet size.

Think before you ink!

When prescribing any drug, particularly for patients already taking several other drugs, it is important to ask:

'What is the treatment goal?'

'How can it be monitored?'

'What is the risk of undesirable effects?'

'What is the risk of drug interactions?'

'Can any of the patient's other drugs be stopped?'

Keep it simple!

Many palliative care patients are taking 5–6 different drugs concurrently. Patients with diabetes and those with COPD may be taking 8–12 different ones. Drugs should be reviewed regularly and stopped if no longer necessary, e.g. long-term prophylactic medication such as statins, antihypertensives, oral hypoglycaemics.

A home medicines chart (Figures 1 and 2) helps to rationalize drug administration. Generally, the drug which needs to be taken most frequently should act as the 'anchor' drug and, as far as possible, other drugs linked to its administration times.

It should be noted that:

- antacids reduce the absorption of many drugs, e.g. azithromycin, e/c products, itraconazole, quinolone antibacterials, and tetracyclines, and should ideally be taken 2h before or after these drugs
- for PO administration of antibacterials there is generally no need to be exact about the 'every 8 hours' or 'every 6 hours' timing of administration
- patients with opioid-induced nausea are sometimes advised to take metoclopramide 30min before the opioid but, in practice, almost always both drugs can be taken at the same time.

Only if absolutely necessary should patients be asked to separate out drugs in relation to food. For example:

- if drug absorption is significantly affected by food (Box A)
- with drugs which are known to be gastric irritants (Box B).

In addition:

- drugs for diabetes and pancreatin should always be taken as recommended in relation to food/meal times
- in order to increase the contact time of the drug with the mucosa, food should not be taken immediately after drugs which are absorbed through the buccal mucosa (e.g. transmucosal fentanyl) or those used topically to treat oral ulceration or oropharyngeal candidosis.

Box A Optimal absorption of drugs in relation to food[a 7,8]

Take on an *empty* stomach[b]
Antibacterials
  demeclocycline[c]
  doxycycline[c]
  flucloxacillin
  itraconazole *liquid[d]*
  phenoxymethylpenicillin
  tetracycline[c]
  rifampicin
  voriconazole
Bisphosphonates[c]
  ibandronic acid[c]
  sodium clodronate[c]
Propantheline

Take *with* or *just after* food
Cefuroxime
Itraconazole *capsules[d]*
Nitrofurantoin

a. these lists are limited to drugs featured in *PCF*
b. generally 30min before first food or drink of the day or 1h before and 2h after food at other times of the day
c. also avoid antacids, iron, zinc or milk for 2h before or after each dose to improve absorption
d. itraconazole liquid requires an empty stomach for full absorption, whereas food significantly improves the absorption of itraconazole capsules.

Box B Drugs for which food *may* reduce the risk of nausea/vomiting or gastric irritation[a]

Baclofen
Corticosteroids
Etamsylate (not UK)
Metronidazole
NSAIDs[b]
Iron

Potassium
Spironolactone
Tinidazole
Venlafaxine
Zinc

a. this list is limited to drugs featured in *PCF*
b. no substantial evidence.

Clear written instructions

Drug regimens should be written out in full for patients and/or families to work from on a purpose-designed chart, including the following:
• name of drug (generic and, if appropriate, also brand)
• formulation and strength

- reason for use ('for pain', 'for bowels', etc.)
- dose (x mL, y tablets)
- frequency and times to be taken.

For examples, see Figure 1 and Figure 2. Advice should also include specific details about how to obtain further supplies. An alternative system will be necessary if both the patient and the immediate family cannot read.

Monitoring medication

It is often difficult to predict the optimum dose of a symptom relief drug, particularly opioids, laxatives and psychotropics. Further, undesirable effects put drug adherence in jeopardy. Thus, arrangements must be made for monitoring the effects of medication. The responsibility for monitoring must be clearly stated: shared decision-making is a definite risk factor for medication errors and problematic polypharmacy.

Compromise is sometimes necessary

It may be necessary to compromise on complete relief in order to avoid unacceptable undesirable effects. Antimuscarinic effects, e.g. dry mouth and visual disturbance, may limit dose escalation. Also, with inoperable bowel obstruction, it may be more realistic to aim to reduce the incidence of vomiting to once or twice a day rather than to seek complete control.

Rescue ('as needed') medication

Patients need advice about what to do for intermittent symptoms, particularly episodic pain. Generally, it is good practice to err on the side of generosity in relation to the recommended frequency of p.r.n. medication. However, it does depend on the class and formulation of the drug in question, and whether the patient is an inpatient or at home.

In all circumstances, it is important that the dose and permitted frequency is stated clearly on the patient's medication chart (see Figures 1 and 2), and also verbally explained to the patient and the family.

Patients taking regular modified-release (m/r) strong opioid medication at home

The *corresponding* immediate-release formulation should also be prescribed q1h p.r.n. in an appropriate dose (see p.92).

Patients taking regular immediate-release strong opioid medication at home

The *same* immediate-release opioid analgesic formulation should also be prescribed routinely q1h p.r.n. in an appropriate dose (see p.92).

With regular immediate-release strong opioids, if a patient needs an *occasional* rescue dose, say, 40min or less before the next regular dose is due, it may suffice to give the next regular dose early. However, some specialists say that the p.r.n. dose should be given followed by the regular dose in due course.

Hospice Home Care

Name Linda Barton   **Age** 58   **Date** 7 July 2015

Tablets/Medicines	2am	On waking	10am	2pm	6pm	Bed time	Purpose
MORPHINE (Oramorph 2mg in 1mL)		10mL	10mL	10mL	10mL	20mL	pain relief
METOCLOPRAMIDE (10mg tablet)		1	1		1	1	anti-sickness
NAPROXEN (500mg tablet)			1			1	pain relief
LANSOPRAZOLE (30mg capsule)			1				to protect stomach
SENNA (7.5mg/5mL liquid)			10mL			10mL	for bowels
TEMAZEPAM (20mg tablet)						1	for sleep

If troublesome pain: take an extra 10mL of MORPHINE between regular doses.

If bowels remain constipated: increase SENNA to 15mL twice a day.

[Use this space for adding additional information, e.g. further advice about 'rescue' medication]

- Keep this chart with you so you can show your doctor or nurse this list of what you are taking.
- Ask for a fresh supply of your medication 2–3 days before you need it.
- Sometimes your medication may be supplied in different strengths or presentations. If you have any concerns about this, check with your pharmacist.
- In an emergency, phone_____ and ask to speak to _____

Figure I Example of a patient's home medication chart (q4h).

Hospice Home Care

Name *Nicolas Crowthorne*   **Age** *65*   **Date** *7 July 2015*

Tablets/Medicines	Breakfast	Midday meal	Evening meal	Bedtime	Purpose
MORPHINE (MST 60mg tablet)	1			1	pain relief
NAPROXEN (500mg tablet)	1			1	pain relief
LANSOPRAZOLE (30mg capsule)	1				to protect stomach
SENNA (7.5mg/5mL liquid)	10mL			10mL	for bowels
HALOPERIDOL (1.5mg tablet)				1	anti-sickness

If troublesome pain: take MORPHINE SOLUTION (2mg in 1mL) 10mL, up to every hour.
If bowels remain constipated: increase SENNA to 15mL twice a day.

[Use this space for adding additional information, e.g. further advice about 'rescue' medication]

- Keep this chart with you so you can show your doctor or nurse this list of what you are taking.
- Ask for a fresh supply of your medication 2–3 days before you need it.
- Sometimes your medication may be supplied in different strengths or presentations. If you have any concerns about this, check with your pharmacist.
- In an emergency, phone_____ and ask to speak to _____

Figure 2 Example of a patient's home medication chart (q.d.s.).

Patients taking regular analgesic medication other than a strong opioid

Paracetamol and NSAIDs are often prescribed at the maximum recommended dose. In this case, an immediate-release opioid analgesic should be prescribed *q2h p.r.n.*, e.g. a low dose of a strong opioid.

For recommendations for anti-emetics, laxatives, and psychotropics, see their respective sections.

ANALGESICS

NON-OPIOIDS

Paracetamol

Paracetamol is a synthetic centrally-acting non-opioid analgesic and antipyretic. Actions include inhibition of cyclo-oxygenase (COX)-2, interaction with opioid and cannabinoid systems, and activation of descending serotoninergic inhibitory pain pathways. Evidence of synergy between paracetamol and NSAIDs suggests differing analgesic mechanisms.

The following features distinguish paracetamol from NSAIDs:
- undesirable effects are relatively uncommon
- does not injure the gastric mucosa, although it may cause non-specific dyspepsia
- is well-tolerated by patients with peptic ulcers
- does not affect plasma uric acid concentration.

Paracetamol has no effect on platelet function. It can be taken by two thirds of patients who are hypersensitive to aspirin. The main drawback with paracetamol is the frequency of administration, generally q.d.s., and its potential for hepatotoxicity. The latter can arise from both deliberate and unintentional overdose. Risk factors for hepatotoxicity include:
- old age
- poor nutritional status
- fasting/anorexia
- chronic alcohol use.

NSAIDs and paracetamol can be used together with an additive effect. Evidence of benefit from paracetamol used in combination with an opioid in *cancer pain* is mixed. At best, about one third of patients obtain a clinically important additive effect. Given that paracetamol 1g q.d.s. is a considerable tablet burden for some patients, a pragmatic solution is a 48h therapeutic trial, with long-term use restricted to those in whom there is definite benefit.

Dose and use

In palliative care, typical PO doses for adults range from 500mg–1g q.d.s. However, in patients with risk factors for paracetamol hepatotoxicity (see above), it is safer to opt for a submaximal dose, e.g. 500mg q.d.s. Bio-availability is lower PR, but in practice the same dose as PO is generally given.

IV doses of paracetamol (rarely used in palliative care) are dependent on body weight and the presence/absence of risk factors for hepatotoxicity. Massive iatrogenic IV overdose leading to hepatic failure, sometimes fatal, has been reported (see *PCF*).

NSAIDs

NSAIDs are of particular benefit for pains associated with inflammation, including postoperative pain and most forms of cancer pain. The efficacy of NSAIDs in pure neuropathic pain is less well established. All NSAIDs are antipyretic.

NSAIDs inhibit cyclo-oxygenase (COX), an important enzyme in the arachidonic acid cascade which results in the production of tissue and inflammatory prostaglandins (PGs). COX exists in two forms (Figure 3). Both forms have a physiological ('constitutive') role in certain tissues (particularly COX-1) and both play a role in inflammation (particularly COX-2, which is massively induced in a few hours by inflammation, dehydration or trauma). The increased production of pro-inflammatory prostaglandins results in *peripheral* and *central sensitization* of sensory neurons to noxious stimuli.

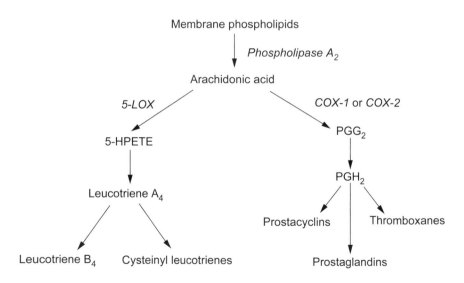

COX = cyclo-oxygenase; 5-HPETE = hydroperoxyeicosatetrenoic acid; LOX = lipoxygenase; PG = prostaglandin.

Figure 3 Products of arachidonic acid metabolism involved in inflammation.

COX-2 also produces anti-inflammatory PGs and is required for both peptic ulcer and bone healing. NSAIDs are now generally classified on the basis of their relative ability to inhibit COX-1 and COX-2. In addition to inhibiting COX, there are probably other mechanisms by which NSAIDs contribute towards analgesia.

NSAIDs can cause serious undesirable effects, notably related to the GI tract, kidneys, and CVS. In some patients, NSAIDs cause bronchospasm. The importance of these effects varies. However, in end-stage disease, the benefit of greater comfort generally far outweighs the potential harm from GI or thrombotic complications. On the other hand, worsening heart failure after an infarct or disability from a stroke would be a high price to pay. Thus, in order to minimize harm:
- select the safest drug for each patient (see below)
- use the smallest effective dose for the shortest possible time
- prescribe appropriate gastroprotection, e.g. a PPI.

The renal risks of different NSAIDs (including coxibs) are similar, and thus are not a factor in determining choice. In practice, the choice is generally between four NSAIDs (Box C and Table 1). *Low-dose* ibuprofen (≤1,200mg/24h) is a good all-round first choice.

Box C Choice of NSAID

First choice

Ibuprofen in *low dose* (≤1,200mg/24h) carries a low risk of GI toxicity and possibly a low risk of a major cardiovascular event.

In *high dose* (2,400mg/24h), ibuprofen's GI toxicity is comparable with naproxen and its cardiovascular toxicity is comparable with diclofenac. It is thus generally *not* advisable to use ibuprofen in *high dose* (2,400mg/24h).

Patients with a high risk of upper GI complications

Celecoxib (200mg/24h) is the first-line choice for patients at *high risk* of upper GI complications, e.g. recent bleed, and for whom the use of an NSAID is considered essential. Gastroprotection is recommended, e.g. standard dose PPI.

Celecoxib has no effect on bleeding time, and is thus also a good choice in patients with thrombocytopenia (e.g. from chemotherapy or other cause) for whom an NSAID is considered essential.

Diclofenac (150mg/24h), like celecoxib, has a low risk of upper GI complications, but also a higher risk of major cardiovascular events (see below).

Patients with a high risk of a major cardiovascular event

Naproxen (1g/24h) is the drug of choice for patients with cardiovascular risk factors (no increased risk).

Celecoxib (200mg/24h) and diclofenac (150mg/24h) have the highest risk of major cardiovascular events; their *use in patients with cardiovascular disease is contra-indicated*, and should be discouraged in patients with cardiovascular risk factors.

Table 1 PO doses of NSAIDs

NSAID[a]	Class	Starting dose	Maximum recommended dose
Celecoxib	Selective COX-2 inhibitor	100mg b.d. *or* 200mg once daily	200mg b.d.
Diclofenac *sodium*	Preferential COX-2 inhibitor	50mg b.d.–t.d.s.	50mg t.d.s.
Ibuprofen	Non-selective COX inhibitor	400mg t.d.s.	800mg t.d.s.
Naproxen	Non-selective COX inhibitor	250–500mg b.d.	500mg b.d.[b]

a. for patients with a high risk of GI complications, prescribe a PPI for gastroprotection
b. 500mg t.d.s. is sometimes used for a limited period, but is higher than the manufacturer's recommended maximum daily dose.

It is often recommended that NSAIDs are taken with/after food. However, there is no evidence that food reduces the incidence of upper GI complications. As far as possible, NSAIDs should be avoided in end-stage heart failure. Patients with hypertension and/or with cardiac, hepatic or renal impairment may deteriorate, and should be monitored carefully.

In patients who can no longer reliably take PO medication, diclofenac 50mg PR t.d.s. or 75mg/24h CSCI can be given instead. However, in someone taking a strong opioid and who is expected to die within 1–2 days, it is generally possible to discontinue the NSAID without provoking a resurgence of pain.

WEAK OPIOIDS

Codeine is the archetypical weak opioid. However, the division of opioids into 'weak' and 'strong' is somewhat arbitrary because opioids manifest a spectrum of potencies, not two discrete categories. Other opioids generally categorized as 'weak' include dihydrocodeine and tramadol (Table 2). All three can be considered to be equipotent by mouth with an approximate relative potency 1/10 that of PO morphine.

Table 2 Weak opioids

Drug	Status	Duration of analgesia (h)[a]	Starting dose	Maximum recommended dose
Codeine	Pro-drug[b]	4–6	30–60mg q4h	60mg q4h
Dihydrocodeine	Active drug	3–4	30mg q6–q4h	60mg q4h
Tramadol	Pro-drug[b]	4–6	50mg q.d.s.	400mg/24h

a. when used in typical doses for mild–moderate pain
b. in relation to opioid effect which is dependent on conversion to morphine (for codeine) or O-desmethyltramadol (for tramadol)

There is no pharmacological need for weak opioids. Low doses of morphine can generally be used instead. Weak opioids are no longer part of the WHO Analgesic ladder for children, and many centres also avoid their use in adults. However, weak opioids remain a practical necessity in many countries because of restricted availability (or non-availability) of oral morphine and other strong opioids.

If a weak opioid is to be used, there is little to choose between codeine and its alternatives in terms of efficacy but the following should be noted:

- codeine is a pro-drug and has little or no analgesic effect until metabolized to morphine mainly via CYP2D6, a hepatic oxidase enzyme. Thus, in poor metabolizers (decreased enzyme activity, seen in up to 10% of Caucasians), it is essentially ineffective. In contrast, in ultra-rapid metabolizers (increased enzyme activity) it is potentially toxic. In children this may have contributed to rare postoperative deaths. Codeine is now contra-indicated in children <12 years and is subject to restrictions in 12–18 year olds
- tramadol has both opioid and non-opioid analgesic effects (mono-amine reuptake inhibition). It is less constipating than codeine and dihydrocodeine, but causes more vomiting, dizziness and anorexia. Further, if used with another drug which affects serotonin metabolism or availability, it can lead to serotonin toxicity, particularly in the elderly. It lowers seizure threshold. Tramadol's opioid effects are dependent on its conversion to O-desmethyltramadol via CYP2D6 and in poor metabolizers there will be a reduced analgesic effect.

The following general rules should be observed:

- a weak opioid should be added to, not substituted for, a non-opioid analgesic
- it is generally inappropriate to switch from one weak opioid to another weak opioid
- if a weak opioid is inadequate when given regularly, change to morphine or an alternative strong opioid.

STRONG OPIOIDS

Strong opioids (morphine and its alternatives) are essential drugs in palliative care; their use should be dictated by therapeutic need and response, not by brevity of prognosis.

When carefully titrated against a patient's pain, strong opioids do *not* cause clinically significant respiratory depression. The risk of respiratory depression is further reduced in cancer patients with pain because generally they:

- have previously been taking a weak opioid (i.e. are not opioid-naïve)
- take medication PO (slower absorption, lower peak concentration)
- undergo gradual dose titration (less likelihood of an excessive dose being given).

Naloxone, an opioid antagonist, is rarely needed in palliative care. The relationship of the therapeutic dose to the lethal dose of a strong opioid (the therapeutic ratio) is greater than commonly supposed. For example, patients who take a double dose of morphine at bedtime are no more likely to die during the night than those who do not.

The undesirable effects of strong opioids are listed in Box D.

Box D Undesirable effects of strong opioids when used for analgesia

Common initial
Nausea and vomiting[a]
Drowsiness
Lightheadedness/unsteadiness
Delirium (acute confusional state)

Common ongoing
Constipation
Nausea and vomiting[a]
Dry mouth

Possible ongoing
Suppression of hypothalamic-
pituitary axis
Suppression of immune system

Less common
Neurotoxicity
    hyperalgesia
    allodynia
    myoclonus
    cognitive failure/delirium
    hallucinations
Sweating
Urinary retention
Postural hypotension
Spasm of the sphincter of Oddi
Pruritus

Rare
Respiratory depression
Psychological dependence

---

a. generally, opioid-related nausea and vomiting is transient and improves after 5–7 days.

Generally, tolerance to strong opioids is not a practical problem. Psychological dependence (addiction) to morphine is rare in patients with cancer pain. Caution in this respect should be reserved for patients with a present or past history of substance abuse; but even then strong opioids should be used when there is clinical need. Physical dependence does not prevent a reduction in the dose if the patient's pain ameliorates, e.g. as a result of radiotherapy or a nerve block.

Strong opioids are not the panacea for cancer pain; generally they are best administered with an NSAID (or, when contra-indicated, paracetamol). Myofascial pain (e.g. persistent muscle cramp and trigger point-related pain) does not respond well to opioids and, however severe, should be treated by alternative measures (e.g. a muscle relaxant, physiotherapy, trigger point injection). Some neuropathic pains respond poorly to opioids, but are relieved when an adjuvant analgesic is added (e.g. an antidepressant or anti-epileptic).

However, even the combined use of non-opioid, opioid and adjuvant analgesics does not guarantee success, particularly if psychosocial dimensions are ignored. Other reasons for poor relief include:
- underdosing (failure to up-titrate the dose or administer doses at the correct time interval)
- poor patient adherence (patient not taking medication)
- poor alimentary absorption (e.g. because of vomiting)
- opioid-induced hyperalgesia (Box E)
- genetic variation in the μ-opioid receptor (altered response to morphine).

> **Box E** Opioid-induced hyperalgesia (OIH)
>
> In some patients, opioids can paradoxically exacerbate pain. This opioid-induced hyperalgesia (OIH) can occur in both acute and chronic pain and appears to result from sustained sensitization of the nervous system in which excitatory neurotransmitters and the NMDA-receptor-channel complex play important roles.
>
> In patients with cancer, OIH may manifest in various ways:
> - rapidly developing tolerance to opioids
> - short-lived benefit from increased doses
> - a change of pain pattern, i.e. worsening pain which becomes more diffuse, extending beyond the distribution of the initial pain.
>
> There may be allodynia (pain elicited from ordinary non-painful stimuli, e.g. stroking skin with cotton) and other manifestations of opioid-induced neural hyperexcitability: myoclonus, seizures, delirium.
>
> Susceptibility to OIH appears to vary widely and genetic make-up probably plays an important part in its development.
>
> *Specialist advice should be sought.* The mainstay of treatment includes:
> - a progressive and rapid reduction in the dose of the causal opioid
> - use of a multimodal approach to analgesia, i.e. non-opioids, e.g. NSAID or paracetamol, and adjuvant analgesics, e.g. gabapentin.

Although similar considerations exist regarding the use of strong opioids for chronic non-cancer pain, benefits are generally lower and risks higher, e.g. in rates of addiction and fatal overdose. Thus, specialist advice should be followed (e.g. Faculty of Pain Medicine guidelines) and/or sought from chronic pain teams.

These concerns have led to the introduction of m/r opioid products which reduce abuse potential: attempts to crush and dissolve the tablet result in the formation of an insoluble precipitate or releases a sequestered opioid antagonist which negates misuse by injection.

Morphine

Morphine by mouth is the global strong opioid of choice for moderate–severe cancer pain (Box F). It is available in immediate-release and m/r formulations. Immediate-release morphine is administered as a tablet or aqueous solution. An increasing range of m/r formulations is available, i.e. tablets, capsules, suspensions. Most are administered b.d., some once daily.

The main metabolites of morphine are morphine-3-glucuronide (M3G) and morphine-6-glucuronide (M6G). M3G is not analgesic but M6G is more potent than morphine. Both glucuronides accumulate in renal failure. This results in a prolonged duration of action, with a danger of severe sedation and respiratory depression if the dose or frequency of administration is not reduced.

Box F Starting a patient on PO morphine

The starting dose of morphine is calculated to give a greater analgesic effect than the medication already in use:

- if the patient was previously receiving a weak opioid regularly (e.g. codeine 240mg/24h or equivalent), give 10mg q4h or m/r 20–30mg q12h, but less if suspected to be a poor codeine metabolizer
- if changing from an alternative strong opioid (e.g. fentanyl, methadone) a much higher dose of morphine may be needed
- if the patient is frail and elderly, or opioid-naïve, a lower dose helps to reduce initial drowsiness, confusion and unsteadiness, e.g. 5mg q4h
- because of accumulation of an active metabolite, a lower and/or less frequent regular dose may suffice in mild–moderate renal impairment, e.g. 5–10mg q8h–q6h (but the use of a 'renally safer' opioid is generally advisable with moderate–severe renal impairment).

When adjusting the dose of morphine, p.r.n. use should be taken into account; increments should not exceed 33–50% every 24h. As a general rule, the p.r.n. dose must be increased when the regular dose is increased.

As with all opioids, patients must be monitored for undesirable effects, particularly nausea and vomiting, and constipation. Depending on individual circumstances, an anti-emetic should be prescribed for regular or p.r.n. use, e.g. haloperidol 1.5mg stat & at bedtime and, routinely, a stimulant laxative prescribed, e.g. senna 15mg at bedtime–b.d.

Upward titration of the dose of morphine stops when either the pain is relieved or unacceptable undesirable effects occur. In the latter case, it is generally necessary to consider alternative measures. The aim is to have the patient free of pain and mentally alert after the initial drowsiness has cleared.

Because of poor absorption, m/r morphine may not be satisfactory in patients troubled by frequent vomiting or those with diarrhoea or an ileostomy.

Scheme 1: immediate-release morphine solution or tablets
- give morphine q4h 'by the clock' and allow p.r.n. doses 1/10–1/6 of the 24h dose q2–4h
- after 1–2 days, recalculate q4h dose by dividing the total used in previous 24h (regular + p.r.n. use) by 6
- continue q4h and p.r.n. doses
- increase the regular dose until there is adequate relief throughout each 4h period, taking p.r.n. use into account
- a double dose at bedtime obviates the need to wake the patient for a dose during the night
- >90% of patients achieve satisfactory pain relief within 5 days.

Box F Contd.

Scheme 2: immediate-release morphine and modified-release (m/r) morphine
- begin as for Scheme I
- when the q4h dose is stable, replace with m/r morphine q12h, or once daily if a 24h product is prescribed
- the q12h dose will be three times the previous q4h dose; a q24h dose will be six times the previous q4h dose, rounded to a convenient number of tablets or capsules
- continue to provide immediate-release morphine solution or tablets for p.r.n. use; give 1/10–1/6 of the 24h dose q2–4h.

Scheme 3: m/r morphine and immediate-release morphine
- generally start with m/r morphine 20–30mg q12h, or 10mg q12h in frail elderly patients
- use immediate-release morphine solution or tablets for p.r.n. medication; give 1/10–1/6 of the 24h dose q2–4h
- if necessary, increase the dose of m/r morphine every 2–3 days until there is adequate relief throughout each 12h period, guided by p.r.n. use.

Two-thirds of patients never need >30mg q4h (or m/r morphine 100mg q12h); the rest need up to 200mg q4h (or m/r morphine 600mg q12h), and occasionally more.

If changing from PO to IV/SC, give 1/3–1/2 of the PO dose. Alternatively, morphine may be given PR (same dose as PO).

For potential intolerable effects of morphine and their management see Table 3.

Diamorphine

Diamorphine hydrochloride (di-acetylmorphine, heroin) is available for medicinal use only in the UK. It is much more soluble than morphine sulfate or hydrochloride and large amounts can be given in a very small volume.

Diamorphine was traditionally used by palliative care units as the alternative to morphine when injections were necessary. However, following a protracted supply problem and increases in cost of diamorphine, many now use morphine as their standard parenteral strong opioid, unless the need for high doses means that solubility is an issue when providing a continuous SC infusion (CSCI) using a portable battery-driven syringe driver.

When changing to SC diamorphine, give 1/3 of the PO dose of morphine, and adjust as necessary, e.g. m/r morphine 30mg b.d. PO = morphine 60mg/24h PO → diamorphine 20mg/24h CSCI.

Table 3 Potential intolerable effects of morphine[a]

Type	Effects	Initial action	Comment
Gastric stasis	Epigastric fullness, flatulence, anorexia, hiccup, persistent nausea	Prescribe a prokinetic, e.g. metoclopramide 10mg t.d.s.	If the problem persists, change to an alternative opioid, with less impact on the GI tract
Sedation	Intolerable persistent sedation	Reduce dose of morphine; consider a psychostimulant, e.g. methylphenidate 5mg b.d.	Sedation may be caused by other factors; stimulant rarely appropriate
Cognitive failure	Agitated delirium with hallucinations	Prescribe an antipsychotic, e.g. haloperidol 500microgram stat & q2h p.r.n.; reduce dose of morphine and, if no improvement, switch to an alternative opioid	Some patients develop intractable delirium with one opioid but not with an alternative opioid
Myoclonus	Multifocal twitching ± jerking of limbs	Prescribe a benzodiazepine, e.g. diazepam/midazolam 5mg or lorazepam 500microgram stat & q1h p.r.n.; reduce dose of morphine but increase again if pain recurs	Uncommon with typical oral doses; more common with high dose IV and spinal morphine
Neurotoxicity	Abdominal muscle spasms, symmetrical jerking of legs; whole-body allodynia, hyperalgesia (manifests as excruciating pain)	Prescribe a benzodiazepine, e.g. diazepam/midazolam 5mg or lorazepam 500microgram stat & q1h p.r.n.; reduce dose of morphine; consider changing to an alternative opioid	A rare syndrome in patients receiving intrathecal or high dose IV morphine; occasionally seen with typical oral and SC doses

continued

Table 3 Contd.

Type	Effects	Initial action	Comment
Vestibular stimulation	Movement-induced nausea and vomiting	Prescribe an antihistaminic antimuscarinic anti-emetic, e.g. cyclizine 50mg t.d.s. or promethazine 25mg t.d.s–q.d.s.	If intractable, try levomepromazine or switch to an alternative opioid
Pruritus	Whole-body itch with systemic morphine; localized to upper body or face/nose with spinal morphine	With systemic opioids, prescribe PO H_1-antihistamine (e.g. chlorphenamine 4mg stat; if beneficial continue with 4mg t.d.s. or p.r.n. for 2–3 days). Possibly switch opioids, e.g. morphine → oxycodone.	Pruritus after systemic opioids is uncommon. It can sometimes be caused by cutaneous histamine release and be self-limiting but the most distressing cases are chronic and antihistamine-resistant. Centrally-acting opioid antagonists also relieve the pruritus but will also antagonize analgesia
Histamine release	Bronchoconstriction → breathlessness	Treat as for anaphylaxis; change to a chemically distinct opioid immediately, e.g. methadone	Rare

a. all strong opioids tend to cause the same undesirable effects although to a varying degree.

Alternative strong opioids

Other strong opioids are used mainly when:

- the patient has intolerable undesirable effects with morphine (Table 3)
- there is little or no benefit from morphine (in a pain anticipated to be opioid-responsive); occasionally, a genetic mutation of the μ-opioid receptor results in reduced analgesia from morphine
- the TD route is preferable (buprenorphine, fentanyl) because of:
  - ▷ difficulty in swallowing
  - ▷ dislike of oral medication
  - ▷ lack of adherence to oral regimen
  - ▷ convenience
- there is a 'phobia' to morphine
- there are specific circumstances where morphine is best avoided (e.g. renal failure).

Differences in intrinsic activity, receptor site affinity, and non-opioid effects (Table 4) may partly explain why some patients report better pain relief after switching opioids. Similarly, the pattern and severity of undesirable effects may be altered, e.g. when switching from morphine to oxycodone or TD fentanyl. The initial dose of the second opioid depends on the relative potency of the two drugs (Table 4).

Oxycodone and hydromorphone have a place in patients who are intolerant of morphine. Methadone is harder to use safely because of its long and variable halflife, and generally should be prescribed only by palliative care and pain relief specialists.

Buprenorphine and fentanyl are both available as transdermal (TD) patches in a range of strengths which provide pain relief for several days. Guidelines for their use are available in the SPC and the *PCF*. After removal of a patch, there is a reservoir of the opioid sequestered in body fat; this will be released slowly over the next few days.

Although convenient, TD formulations are more expensive than standard morphine preparations and they are not generally considered for first-line use except in specific circumstances, e.g. patients with dysphagia.

Fentanyl is available in several transmucosal (TM) formulations for use in the mouth or nose for cancer-related episodic pain. Because of different pharmacokinetic characteristics, TM fentanyl products are *not* interchangeable. They are all much more expensive than immediate-release PO strong opioids. Generally, the use of TM fentanyl formulations should be restricted to patients for whom PO strong opioids (including a trial of a PO solution if necessary) are too slow in onset of action or cause prolonged undesirable effects.

Opioid switching ('rotation')

Dose conversion ratios are *never* more than an approximate guide. When switching from one opioid to another, careful monitoring is necessary to avoid both underdosing and excessive dosing.

Table 4 Alternative strong opioids (for more details, see individual drug monographs in PCF)

	Opioid receptor affinity			Non-opioid properties	Duration of action[a]	Potency relative to PO morphine[b]
	Mu	Kappa	Delta			
Buprenorphine	pA	Ant	Ant	None	6–9h 72h TD	80 SL 100 (75–115) TD
Fentanyl	A	–	–	None	3–4h 72h TD	100 (150) TD
Hydromorphone	A	–	–	None	4–5h	4–5 (7.5)
Morphine	A	–	–	None	4–6h	1
Methadone	A	–	A(?)	Blocks presynaptic re-uptake of serotonin; NMDA-receptor-channel blocker	4–6 single dose; 8–12h repeat doses	5–10[c]
Oxycodone	A	A	–	None	4–6h 12h m/r	1.5 (2)

Key: A = strong agonist; pA = partial agonist; Ant = strong antagonist; – = no activity; IV = intravenous; SC = subcutaneous; SL = sublingual; TD = transdermal.

a. PO unless stated otherwise

b. numbers in parenthesis are the manufacturer's preferred ratios

c. variable long halflife leads to accumulation and a variable relative potency, occasionally as high as 30:1.

Switching from morphine (or other strong opioid) to an alternative is undertaken in an attempt to improve analgesia and/or reduce undesirable effects. Before switching, it is worth considering if other options may be more appropriate, e.g. the use of adjuvant analgesics or modifying the management of the undesirable effects.

Switching is reported necessary in about one third of patients prescribed morphine PO. The threshold for switching is probably lower when alternative strong opioids are readily available. Examples of when switching may be appropriate include:
- poor adherence (→ TD fentanyl)
- intolerable undesirable effects, e.g. *intractable* constipation (→ TD fentanyl)
- significant decline in the patient's renal function (morphine → methadone, TD fentanyl or TD buprenorphine)
- opioid-induced hyperalgesia or other manifestations of neurotoxicity, e.g. cognitive failure/delirium, hallucinations, myoclonus, allodynia.

In cases of neurotoxicity, hydromorphone, oxycodone and methadone have all been substituted successfully for morphine. Similarly, in the presence of inadequate pain relief and intolerable undesirable effects, TD buprenorphine has been substituted successfully for TD fentanyl, and vice versa.

When converting from morphine to an alternative strong opioid, or vice versa, the initial dose depends on the relative potency of the two drugs (Table 5).

Table 5 Approximate potency of opioids relative to morphine; PO and immediate release formulations unless stated otherwise[a]

Analgesic	Potency relative to morphine	Duration of action (h)[b]
Codeine	} 1/10	3–6
Dihydrocodeine		
Tramadol	1/10	4–6
Oxycodone	1.5 (2)[c]	3–4
Methadone	5–10[d]	8–12
Hydromorphone	4–5 (5–7.5)[c]	4–5
Buprenorphine (SL)	80	6–8
Buprenorphine (TD)	100 (75–115)[c]	Formulation dependent
Fentanyl (TD)	100 (150)[c]	72

a. multiply dose of opioid in the first column by relative potency in the second column to determine the equivalent dose of morphine sulfate/hydrochloride; conversely, divide morphine dose by the relative potency to determine the equivalent dose of another opioid
b. dependent in part on severity of pain and on dose; often longer lasting in very elderly and those with renal impairment
c. the numbers in parenthesis are the manufacturers' preferred ratios; for explanation of divergence, see individual drug monographs in *PCF*
d. a single 5mg dose of methadone is equivalent to morphine 7.5mg, but a variable long plasma halflife and broad-spectrum receptor affinity result in a much higher than expected relative potency when administered regularly, sometimes much higher than the range given above; it is essential to read the methadone monograph in *PCF*.

Providing precise guidance on switching opioids is difficult because the reasons for switching are varied, as are the patient's circumstances. Certainly, a dose reduction of at least 50% would seem prudent when switching at high doses (e.g. morphine or equivalent doses of $\geq$1g/24h), in elderly or frail patients, because of intolerable undesirable effects (e.g. delirium), or when there has been a recent rapid escalation of the first opioid (possibly causing opioid-induced hyperalgesia). In such circumstances, p.r.n. doses can be relied on to make up any deficit while re-titrating to a satisfactory dose of the new opioid.

A separate strategy is necessary for methadone (see *PCF*).

Combining opioids

It is generally considered bad practice to prescribe more than one opioid for simultaneous use. Thus, for example, regular morphine is best backed up by p.r.n morphine for episodic pain.

However, there are circumstances when this may be necessary, for example TD fentanyl backed up by p.r.n. morphine. Also, someone with good pain relief from a regular weak opioid may have a supply of morphine for back-up use in case of severe episodic pain.

ANTIDEPRESSANTS

Authorized uses include depression, anxiety and panic disorders.

Off-label uses include neuropathic pain, bladder spasm, drooling, paraneoplastic sweating and pruritus.

Antidepressants are classified according to their principal actions (Table 6) which generally enhance neurotransmission by one or more mono-amines.

Tricyclic antidepressants (TCAs) are a *chemical* class of drugs, their modes of action are not always identical; thus they are not a discrete *pharmacological* class.

The term 'dual inhibitor' refers to serotonin and noradrenaline (norepinephrine), the two mono-amines traditionally associated with the pathophysiology of depression. More recently the significance of dopamine has been recognized, and has led to attempts to modulate all three mono-amines in refractory depression.

The analgesic effects of antidepressants relate to enhanced mono-amine transmission in descending pain modulation pathways (see p.93). Sodium-channel blockade and NMDA-glutamate-receptor antagonism may also play a part.

For important cautions, interactions and undesirable effects see Tables 7 and 8.

Use of antidepressants in palliative care

Neuropathic pain

Benefit from noradrenergic and dual re-uptake inhibitors is comparable. SSRIs are inferior to TCAs. Amitriptyline and nortriptyline are commonly used; the latter is better tolerated than amitriptyline (Table 9).

Table 6 Classification of selected antidepressants according to principal action

Class	Examples
Mono-amine re-uptake inhibitors	
Serotonin and noradrenaline/ norepinephrine (SNRIs; 'dual inhibitors')	Amitriptyline, venlafaxine, duloxetine
Serotonin (selective serotonin re-uptake inhibitors, SSRIs)	Sertraline, citalopram, paroxetine, fluoxetine
Noradrenaline/norepinephrine (NRIs)	Nortriptyline, lofepramine, desipramine, reboxetine
Noradrenaline/norepinephrine and dopamine (NDRIs)	Bupropion
Psychostimulant-antidepressants	Dextroamfetamine, methylphenidate, modafinil
Receptor antagonists[a]	Trazodone (α_1, $5HT_2$) Mirtazapine (central α_2, $5HT_2$, $5HT_3$)
Mono-amine oxidase inhibitors (MAOIs)[b]	Phenelzine, tranylcypromine

a. these block receptors that inhibit mono-amine release
b. included for completeness; use by non-psychiatrists is not recommended.

Table 7 Important cautions with antidepressants

Context	Danger
History of mania	Antidepressants may precipitate a recurrent episode
Suicidal ideation	Risk of suicide, particularly in those ≤25 years
Epilepsy	Dose-dependent reduction in seizure threshold; lowest risk with SSRIs
Parkinson's disease	SSRIs can worsen extrapyramidal symptoms and TCAs can worsen autonomic dysfunction (a blockade) and cognitive impairment
QT prolongation	Citalopram and escitalopram contra-indicated
Drug interactions	Fluoxetine, fluvoxamine and paroxetine are potent inhibitors of cytochrome P450; conversely the metabolism of several antidepressants may be affected by P450 inhibitors and inducers
	Risk of serotonin toxicity when two serotoninergic drugs are prescribed concurrently or concurrent drug interacts to increase serotonin levels

The efficacy and tolerability of TCAs are comparable with duloxetine and anti-epileptics (gabapentin or pregabalin), and so other factors influence which is the more appropriate first-line choice, e.g. concurrent low mood, poor sleep.

Frequently a TCA or other antidepressant and an anti-epileptic are combined (see p.345).

Table 8 Undesirable effects of antidepressants

System	Undesirable effect
CNS	Nausea (e.g. SSRIs)
	Sedation (e.g. some TCAs, mirtazapine)
	Agitation, restlessness, insomnia (e.g. SSRIs, some TCAs)
	Weight gain (e.g. amitriptyline, mirtazapine)
	Sexual dysfunction (variable, but *not* with mirtazapine)
	Serotoninergic effects (e.g. MAOIs, SSRIs, SNRIs)
Cardiovascular	Postural hypotension (e.g. TCAs)
	QT prolongation dose-related with citalopram and escitalopram, affected by presence of other risk factors; important not to exceed dose recommendations or combine with other drugs which either prolong QT or interact to increase plasma concentration
GI tract	GI bleeding; risk tripled by SSRIs; safer alternatives include NRIs (e.g. nortriptyline) and mirtazapine
	Dry mouth, constipation (e.g. TCAs)
	Diarrhoea (e.g. SSRIs)
Biochemical	SIADH (syndrome of inappropriate ADH secretion; may occur with all antidepressants)
Miscellaneous	Antimuscarinic effects (p.350), particularly TCAs

Table 9 PO doses of TCAs for neuropathic pain

TCA	Starting dose	Titration	Maximum recommended dose
Amitriptyline[a]	10mg at bedtime	Increase to 25mg after 3–7 days. If necessary, increase by 25mg every 1–2 weeks	150mg at bedtime (seldom required)
Nortriptyline	10–25mg at bedtime	Increase by 10mg/day every 3–5 days up to 50mg, or double dose from 25mg to 50mg after 2 weeks	150mg at bedtime (seldom required)

a. if helpful but poorly tolerated, consider switching to nortriptyline; switch on a mg for mg basis.

Depression

For general approach, see p.189.

For typical doses and titration, see Quick Clinical Guide: Depression, p.192.

Generally:
- sertraline or citalopram are good first-line choices; they have fewer drug interactions, lower risk in overdose, and are marginally better tolerated

- second-line options include an alternative SSRI or mirtazapine; generally, the first-line SSRI can be directly substituted; taper higher doses of paroxetine (>20mg) or sertraline (>50mg) before switching
- methylphenidate, with its rapid onset, is preferable in patients with a very short prognosis, e.g. 2–4 weeks
- consider use of amitriptyline or nortriptyline when depression and neuropathic pain co-exist; slower titration reduces risk of intolerance and discontinuation

Minimum duration of treatment *after full remission* depends on the presence of risk factors for relapse, i.e. previous depression, severe prolonged episode, degree of treatment resistance, and the presence of residual symptoms:

- no risk factors, 6 months
- one risk factor, 1 year
- ≥2 risk factors, ≥2 years.

In palliative care, this means that treatment is likely to be until death. However, if an antidepressant is discontinued after long-term use (>8 weeks), reduce the dose slowly over 4 weeks to avoid a discontinuation reaction (withdrawal syndrome). Symptoms vary but include flu-like symptoms, insomnia, nausea, dizziness, sensory disturbances (paraesthesia, sensations of electric shock), restlessness, anxiety and agitation.

Other uses

In palliative care, antidepressants have several other, mostly off-label uses (Table 10); generally *not* first-line, seek specialist advice.

Table 10 Antidepressants: other uses

Symptom	Example of antidepressant used	Comment	Cross-reference
Anxiety and panic disorders	Citalopram, sertraline (authorized use)	Consider if prognosis = months, and general supportive measures (± a benzodiazepine) are insufficient	p.185
Bladder spasm, urge incontinence	Amitriptyline, duloxetine, imipramine	Antimuscarinic drugs	p.174, 176
Drooling	Amitriptyline	Antimuscarinic drugs	p.351
Insomnia	TCAs, mirtazapine, trazodone;	Sedative drugs	p.194
Hot flushes	Venlafaxine, SSRIs	Menopausal or related to hormone therapy in breast and prostate cancers	See *PCF*
Paraneoplastic sweating	Amitriptyline	Consider if an NSAID is ineffective	p.324
Pruritus	Sertraline, paroxetine, mirtazapine	Particularly for cholestatic pruritus	p.228

ANTIDIARRHOEALS

Loperamide, is a potent μ-opioid receptor agonist (μ agonist). Its general lack of CNS effects makes it a popular first-line choice for the control of diarrhoea in:
- acute and chronic diarrhoea
- patients with an ileostomy (to improve faecal consistency)
- patients with ileo-anal pouches (to improve night-time continence).

Loperamide should be avoided in ulcerative, infective and antibiotic-associated colitis, and conditions associated with a risk of ileus, megacolon or toxic megacolon.

Like other μ agonists, loperamide increases intestinal transit time by decreasing propulsive activity and increasing non-propulsive activity via its effect on the myenteric plexus in the longitudinal muscle layer. Loperamide also increases anal sphincter tone, stimulates absorption of water and electrolytes and, unlike other opioids, has an anti-secretory action.

As an antidiarrhoeal, loperamide is about 50 times more potent than codeine, and is longer-acting. However, its maximum therapeutic impact may not manifest for 16–24h. If taken regularly long-term for chronic diarrhoea (see below), a twice daily regimen is generally adequate. The following are approximately equivalent:
- loperamide 2mg b.d.
- codeine phosphate 60mg q.d.s.

CNS effects and reduced consciousness have been rarely reported, e.g. in severe hepatic impairment or following excessive doses in children.

Dose and use

Ensure that the diarrhoea is not secondary to faecal impaction.

Acute diarrhoea

- start with loperamide 4mg PO stat
- continue with 2mg after each loose bowel action for up to 5 days
- maximum recommended dose 16mg/24h.

Chemotherapy- or radiotherapy-induced diarrhoea

- if mild–moderate, give 4mg stat and 2mg after each loose bowel action
- if not responding to doses of 24mg/24h, switch to octreotide (see p.131)
- if severe, use octreotide first-line.

Chronic diarrhoea

If symptomatic treatment is appropriate, the same initial approach is used for 2–3 days, after which a prophylactic b.d. regimen is instituted based on the needs of the patient during the previous 24h, plus 2mg after each loose bowel action. The effective dose varies widely. In palliative care, it is occasionally necessary to increase the dose to as much as 32mg/24h; *this is twice the recommended maximum daily dose.*

ANTI-EMETICS

The choice of an anti-emetic in palliative care is guided by the probable cause of the nausea and vomiting (see p.119) and the mechanism by which the drug acts (see Chapter 8, Figure 1, p.121). The most appropriate anti-emetic should be prescribed both regularly and as needed (see Quick Clinical Guide: Management of nausea and vomiting, p.123).

In palliative care, metoclopramide, haloperidol (p.352) and cyclizine are commonly used first-line anti-emetics. Domperidone is an alternative for metoclopramide; and, in the medical mangement of inoperable bowel obstruction, cyclizine is often replaced by an antisecretory drug, e.g. hyoscine *butylbromide*, octreotide.

Corticosteroids and levomepromazine (p.352) are useful options when first-line anti-emetics fail to relieve nausea and vomiting. Dexamethasone is generally added to an existing regimen, whereas levomepromazine is generally substituted. Occasionally it is necessary to use dexamethasone and levomepromazine concurrently.

$5HT_3$ antagonists were developed primarily for use alongside chemotherapy. They have a definite but limited role in palliative care (p.123).

Occasionally, benzodiazepines (p.356) and anti-epileptics (p.345) are used as anti-emetics, generally in specific circumstances, e.g. lorazepam with chemotherapy, valproate with meningeal carcinomatosis.

Metoclopramide

Metoclopramide is a prokinetic anti-emetic. It acts, in part, by antagonizing D_2-receptors:
- in the chemoreceptor trigger zone (CTZ) in the brain stem
- at the gastro-oesophageal and gastroduodenal junctions, and thereby counteracts the gastric 'dopamine brake' associated with nausea from any cause (Figure 4).

Prokinetics act by triggering a cholinergic system in the wall of the GI tract (Figure 4). Opioids impede this action, and antimuscarinics block it competitively. *Thus, the concurrent use of a prokinetics and an antimuscarinic should be discouraged*; although domperidone will still act as D_2-antagonist in the CTZ even if its GI prokinetic effect is blocked. However, if D_2-antagonism alone is needed, haloperidol (p.355) is generally a better choice because of the advantage of once daily administration.

Prokinetics are used in various situations in palliative care (Box G).

Dose and use

- start with metoclopramide 10mg PO t.d.s.–q.d.s. or 30–40mg/24h CSCI and 10mg PO/SC p.r.n.
- in severe delayed gastric emptying, occasionally increased to a maximum of 100mg/24h PO/CSCI.

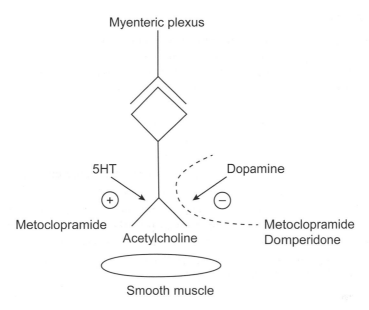

Myenteric plexus

5HT   Dopamine

Metoclopramide   Metoclopramide
         Acetylcholine   Domperidone

Smooth muscle

(+) stimulatory effect of 5HT triggered by metoclopramide; (−) inhibitory effect of dopamine; − − − blockade of dopamine inhibition by metoclopramide and domperidone.

Figure 4 Schematic representation of drug effects on antroduodenal co-ordination via a postganglionic effect on the cholinergic nerves from the myenteric plexus.

Box G Indications for prokinetics in palliative care

Gastro-oesophageal reflux
Delayed gastric emptying
Hiccup
 	
Gastroparesis
   dysmotility dyspepsia
   paraneoplastic autonomic neuropathy
   spinal cord compression
   diabetic autonomic neuropathy
 	
Functional GI obstruction
   drug-induced, e.g. opioids
   cancer of head of pancreas
   linitis plastica (locally diffuse mural infiltration by cancer)

Domperidone

Domperidone, like metoclopramide, is a prokinetic anti-emetic. It acts by antagonizing D_2-receptors:

- in the chemoreceptor trigger zone (CTZ) in the brain stem
- at the gastro-oesophageal and gastroduodenal junctions, and thereby counteracts the gastric 'dopamine brake' associated with nausea from any cause.

Compared with metoclopramide, negligible amounts of domperidone penetrate the blood-brain barrier which results in a negligible risk of extrapyramidal effects and less drowsiness and loss of mental acuity. Thus, domperidone is the prokinetic and anti-emetic of choice in Parkinson's disease, including nausea caused by levodopa and bromocriptine.

Domperidone use is associated with an increased risk of serious ventricular arrhythmia/sudden cardiac death, possibly further increased in those >60 years old or receiving higher doses (>30mg/24h). As a consequence, the MHRA advises clinicians to:

- use domperidone *only* for nausea and vomiting, at the lowest effective dose, for the shortest possible time (generally ≤1 week)
- limit it to a maximum dose of 10mg t.d.s.
- avoid it in patients:
  - ▷ where cardiac conduction is, or could be, impaired
  - ▷ with underlying cardiac disease, e.g. CHF
  - ▷ with severe hepatic impairment
  - ▷ concurrently receiving drugs known to be CYP3A4 inhibitors and/or cause QT prolongation
- advise patients to seek prompt medical attention should symptoms such as syncope or cardiac arrhythmias occur.

However, many palliative care patients have been treated with domperidone for extended periods. The risk:benefit balance should be determined on an individual patient basis, taking circumstances and other options into account. For example, if a patient with end-stage CHF requires a long-term anti-emetic, domperidone may be preferable to cyclizine (also pro-arrhythmic) or metoclopramide (risk of extrapyramidal effects).

Dose and use

- start with 10mg PO b.d.
- increase to 10mg t.d.s., the new recommended maximum dose.

Previously, doses were increased to 20mg b.d. or 10mg q.d.s., with 20mg q.d.s. the old maximum recommended dose.

Cyclizine

Cyclizine is an antihistaminic anti-emetic. It acts by:

- decreasing the excitability of the inner ear labyrinth
- blocking conduction in the vestibular-cerebellar pathways
- acting directly on the vomiting centre in the brain stem.

Cyclizine is effective in many causes of vomiting, including opioid-induced. However, in practice metoclopramide (see p.342) and haloperidol (see p.355) are often used in preference, sometimes because of more specific indications or to avoid drowsiness and antimuscarinic effects (see Box H, p.350).

Elderly patients are more susceptible to sedative and central antimuscarinic effects, e.g. postural hypotension, memory impairment, extrapyramidal reactions. Additional caution is required in patients with narrow-angle glaucoma, severe heart failure or urinary tract obstruction as all may be exacerbated by cyclizine.

Dose and use

In the UK, cyclizine is generally the antihistaminic antimuscarinic anti-emetic of choice. Depending on circumstances, cyclizine is generally given PO or SC:

- 50mg PO b.d.–t.d.s. & 50mg p.r.n.
- 100–150mg/24h CSCI & 50mg SC p.r.n.
- usual maximum daily dose 200mg PO and CSCI.

For CSCI dilute cyclizine with WFI; cyclizine is *incompatible* with 0.9% saline and will precipitate.

ANTI-EPILEPTICS

Authorized uses include neuropathic pain, epilepsy, mania and anxiety.

Off-label uses include paraneoplastic sweats and hot flushes, refractory hiccup, refractory cough, nausea and vomiting, and uraemic itch. Generally, anti-epileptics are used in these situations when more established treatments are ineffective.

Anti-epileptic drugs, through various mechanisms, inhibit rapidly firing neurones and can thereby impact on symptoms arising from excessive neuronal activity in any part of the nervous system. Anti-epileptics are classified according to their principal actions (Table 11).

For important cautions and undesirable effects see Tables 12 and 13.

Table 11 Classification of selected anti-epileptics according to principal action

Class	Examples
Membrane stabilizers	
Sodium channel blocker	Carbamazepine, lamotrigine, oxcarbazepine, phenytoin, topiramate
Reduced neurotransmitter release	
$\alpha 2\delta$ ligand	Gabapentin, pregabalin
SV2A ligand	Levetiracetam
GABAmimetic	Benzodiazepines, phenobarbital
Polymodal	Valproate

Table 12 Important cautions with anti-epileptics

Context	Danger
Drug interactions	Carbamazepine, phenobarbital and phenytoin are potent inducers of cytochrome P450, conversely the metabolism of carbamazepine and phenytoin may be affected by P450 inhibitors and inducers
	Gabapentin, pregabalin and levetiracetam have no clinically significant pharmacokinetic interactions
Risk of suicide	Anti-epileptics may cause suicidal thoughts or behaviour
Atrioventricular block	Carbamazepine, oxcarbazepine may cause complete block
Heart failure	Oxcarbazepine, pregabalin cause fluid retention
Hepatic impairment	Most anti-epileptics, excluding gabapentin, pregabalin and vigabatrin
Renal impairment	Most anti-epileptics; specific dose adjustment advice available for gabapentin and pregabalin (see SPC)
Skin rash with a previous anti-epileptic	Cross-reactive hypersensitivity can occur
HLA B*1502 status	Increased risk of Stevens-Johnson syndrome with carbamazepine, oxcarbazepine and phenytoin; test before prescribing in Han or Hong Kong Chinese and Thais
Bone marrow suppression	Possible increased risk with carbamazepine

Table 13 Undesirable effects of anti-epileptics

System	Undesirable effect
CNS	Drowsiness, cognitive impairment, dizziness, diplopia, ataxia
Psychiatric	Agitation, lability, depression, psychosis
Biochemical	Abnormal LFTs (rarely severe)
Haematological	Folate deficiency with enzyme-inducers, e.g. phenytoin. Rarely, agranulocytosis, aplastic anaemia
GI tract	Pancreatitis
Skin	Transient rashes common (particularly carbamazepine, lamotrigine, oxcarbazepine), more likely when rashes with other anti-epileptics, higher starting doses and rapid titration. Rarely, severe, e.g. Stevens-Johnson syndrome; risk increased by an HLA type (see Table 12)

Use of anti-epileptics in palliative care

Neuropathic pain

The efficacy and tolerability of anti-epileptics and antidepressants are comparable, and so other factors influence which is the more appropriate first-line choice, e.g. concurrent low mood, poor sleep.

Frequently an anti-epileptic and a TCA or other antidepressant are combined (see p.337). Note:

- gabapentin or pregabalin are first-line choices; they are authorized for neuropathic pain and have few drug interactions
- valproate is used in some centres, generally second line
- carbamazepine is an authorized first-line treatment for trigeminal neuralgia.

For dosing information, see Table 14.

Table 14 PO doses of commonly used anti-epileptics for neuropathic pain

Anti-epileptic	Starting dose	Titration	Maximum recommended dose
Gabapentin[a,b]	100–300mg at bedtime	Increase by 100–300mg/24h every 2–3 days Typical dose 600mg t.d.s.	1,200mg t.d.s.
Pregabalin[a,b]	25–75mg b.d.	Increase by 50–150mg/24h every 3–7 days	300mg b.d.; necessary in about one third
Valproate	150–200mg m/r at bedtime	Increase by 150–200mg/24h every 2–3 days; with doses >1g/24h give b.d.	1g b.d.

a. the starting and maximum doses should be reduced in adults with renal impairment and those on haemodialysis (see SPC)
b. in elderly and frail patients, use the smaller initial dose and slower titration.

Epilepsy

Seizures caused by brain lesions, e.g. cerebral tumour, multiple sclerosis, are, by definition focal, even if obscured by rapid secondary generalization:

- a maintenance anti-epileptic should be started after a first seizure
- carbamazepine or lamotrigine are suitable first-line anti-epileptics, but both require slow titration over several weeks
- in patients with a short prognosis, levetiracetam, oxcarbazepine or valproate are preferable (Table 15)
- if the first choice treatment fails, add a second anti-epileptic; when the second one is at an adequate or maximally tolerated dose, the first one is slowly withdrawn (see p.348)
- if monotherapy fails, seek specialist advice

- if surgery is likely, discuss with neurosurgeon before starting valproate because of an association with abnormal haemostasis in vitro
- for patients in the last days of life, midazolam (typically 20–30mg/24h CSCI) is generally used first-line because of familiarity, concurrent symptoms and compatibility with other drugs given by CSCI (see p.356); phenobarbital is sometimes used instead.

Table 15 PO doses of commonly used anti-epileptics for focal seizures in palliative care

Anti-epileptic	Starting dose	Titration	Maximum recommended dose
First-line alternatives			
Valproate[a]	150–200mg m/r b.d.	Increase by 150–200mg b.d. every 3 days; most require ≤750mg b.d.	1,250mg b.d.
Oxcarbazepine[b]	150mg b.d. (75mg b.d. in elderly and frail patients)	Increase by 75–150mg weekly	1,200mg b.d.
Second-line: switch to alternative first-line drug or prescribe			
Levetiracetam[a,b]	250–500mg b.d.	Increase after 2 weeks to 500mg b.d.; otherwise increase by 500–1,000mg/24h every 2 weeks	1,500mg b.d.

a. can be titrated rapidly, IV/SC if necessary
b. dose adjustment required in renal impairment, see SPC.

For the management of convulsive status epilepticus, see p.204.

Non-convulsive status epilepticus (NCSE) is characterized by seizure activity on an EEG but without associated tonic-clonic activity. Presentations include delirium or coma. Treatment is less urgent than for convulsive status epilepticus. In a case series, most responded to levetiracetam (none to phenytoin, only one to valproate).

Other uses

In palliative care, anti-epileptics have several off-label uses (Table 16); generally *not* first-line, seek specialist advice.

Stopping anti-epileptics

Abrupt cessation of long-term anti-epileptics risks causing rebound seizures, even if their use was for indications other than epilepsy. Gabapentin and pregabalin can be tapered steadily over 1–2 weeks. Other anti-epileptics, particularly benzodiazepines and barbiturates, should be tapered *over several months*.

For patients unable to swallow PO medication, consider substituting a SC alternative. For valproate and levetiracetam, the dose is the same SC/IV as PO. In the last days of life, the more sedative midazolam is often used (see p.348).

Table 16 Off-label uses of anti-epileptics

Symptom	Example of anti-epileptic used	Comment	Cross-reference
Hot flushes and paraneoplastic sweating	Gabapentin	For flushes associated with treatment of breast and prostate cancers, or the menopause	See *PCF*
Nausea and vomiting	Carbamazepine, valproate, levetiracetam	Of benefit if CNS cause, e.g. meningeal carcinomatosis, seizures	p.119
Refractory cough	Gabapentin	Consider for chronic cough (>8 weeks) despite resolution of initial cause	p.155
Refractory hiccup	Gabapentin		p.166
Terminal agitation	Phenobarbital	Occasionally used to control refractory agitation in imminently dying patients	p.254
Uraemic itch	Gabapentin, pregabalin		p.230

ANTIMUSCARINICS

Antimuscarinics are mostly used as:
* smooth muscle antispasmodics, e.g. for bladder or rectal spasm, intestinal colic
* antisecretory drugs, e.g. for drooling, death rattle, bowel obstruction.

Antimuscarinics are either natural belladonna alkaloids (atropine, hyoscine) or semi-synthetic/fully synthetic derivatives. They are further classified as:
* tertiary amines, e.g. atropine, hyoscine *hydrobromide,* oxybutynin, tolterodine
* quaternary ammonium compounds, e.g. glycopyrronium, hyoscine *butylbromide.*

Tertiary amines, particularly the naturally-occurring alkaloids, have central effects. At typical therapeutic doses, hyoscine *hydrobromide* causes CNS depression and atropine conversely causes CNS stimulation. However, at toxic doses, all the tertiary amines can cause CNS stimulation, resulting in agitation and delirium. Unlike most causes of delirium, this is best treated with a benzodiazepine (see p.356).

To reduce the risk of central effects, quaternary ammonium compounds which do not cross the blood-brain barrier have been developed, e.g. glycopyrronium. More selective drugs are also available, e.g. oxybutynin and tolterodine which are relatively selective for muscarinic receptors in the urinary tract.

Peripheral antimuscarinic effects are a class characteristic (Box H), and have been summarized as:

'Dry as a bone, blind as a bat, red as a beet, hot as a hare, mad as a hatter.'

Box H Peripheral antimuscarinic effects

Visual
Mydriasis
Loss of accommodation } blurred vision (may impair driving ability)

Cardiovascular
Tachycardia, palpitations
Extrasystoles } also related to noradrenaline (norepinephrine) potentiation and a quinidine-like action
Arrhythmias

Gastro-intestinal
Dry mouth (inhibition of salivation)
Heartburn (relaxation of lower oesophageal sphincter)
Constipation (decreased intestinal motility)

Urinary tract
Hesitancy of micturition
Retention of urine

Skin
Reduced sweating
Flushing

Many other drugs have antimuscarinic effects, e.g. chlorphenamine, cyclizine, phenothiazines, tricyclic antidepressants. These could exacerbate toxicity, particularly in debilitated elderly patients. As far as possible, the concurrent use of two drugs with antimuscarinic properties should be avoided.

Because antimuscarinics competitively block the final common (cholinergic) pathway through which prokinetics (domperidone, metoclopramide) act, concurrent prescription of a prokinetic and an antimuscarinic should generally be avoided.

Antimuscarinics relax the lower oesophageal sphincter and may exacerbate acid reflux. Both antimuscarinics and opioids cause constipation (by different mechanisms) and, if used together, will result in an increased need for laxatives, and may even result in paralytic ileus (not a concern when purposely combined in terminally ill patients with inoperable bowel obstruction). Narrow-angle glaucoma may be precipitated in those at risk, particularly the elderly.

Dose and use

By injection, there is no good evidence to recommend one antimuscarinic in preference to another. However, because atropine tends to stimulate the CNS rather than sedate, an alternative antimuscarinic should be used if available, e.g. glycopyrronium, hyoscine.

Antispasmodic

Antimuscarinics are used to relieve smooth muscle spasm in the bladder and rectum. For bladder spasm, trial more selective drugs first, e.g. oxybutynin and tolterodine.

Antispasmodic and antisecretory

Antimuscarinics are used to reduce intestinal colic and intestinal secretions, particularly gastric, associated with inoperable bowel obstruction in terminally ill patients (Table 17).

Table 17 Antisecretory and antispasmodic drugs: typical SC doses

Drug	Stat and p.r.n. doses	CSCI dose/24h
Glycopyrronium	200microgram	600–1,200microgram
Hyoscine *butylbromide*	20mg	20–300mg[a]
Hyoscine *hydrobromide*[b]	400microgram	1,200–2,000microgram

a. death rattle 20–60mg, some centres use up to 120mg; intestinal obstruction 60–300mg
b. atropine doses are generally the same as hyoscine hydrobromide.

Antisecretory

Drooling (and sialorrhoea)

Seen particularly in patients with ALS/MND, advanced Parkinson's disease and with various disorders of the head and neck. First-line options include:
- hyoscine *hydrobromide*, e.g. 1mg/3 days TD
- amitriptyline (a tricyclic antidepressant with prominent antimuscarinic effects), e.g. 10–25mg PO at bedtime
- glycopyrronium (tablets and special order oral solutions are available but expensive), e.g. 200microgram q8h
- atropine, e.g. 1% ophthalmic solution, 4 drops on the tongue or SL q4h p.r.n.

In relation to the latter, drop size varies with applicator and technique. Thus, the dose varies from 200–500microgram per drop (800microgram–2mg/dose). It is important to titrate the dose upwards until there is an adequate effect.

Death rattle (noisy respiratory secretions)

Parenteral antimuscarinics are widely used to reduce death rattle (noisy rattling breathing) in those close to death (see Quick Clinical Guide, p.280).

ANTIPSYCHOTICS

Authorized uses include psychosis, mania and bipolar disorders.

Off-label uses include nausea and vomiting, delirium, terminal agitation, refractory hiccup, refractory depression.

Antipsychotics act predominantly through D_2 receptor antagonism, countering symptoms of dopamine excess, e.g. delusions and hallucinations. However, this can also cause dopamine depletion-related extrapyramidal reactions, i.e. drug-induced movement disorders (see Table 19).

Therapeutic and undesirable effects vary between antipsychotics because of differences in their affinity for the D_2 and multiple other receptors, notably α-adrenergic, muscarinic and serotoninergic. Interactions with non-dopaminergic receptors can be beneficial, e.g. by reducing the risk of dopamine depletion symptoms or contributing towards anti-emetic and antidepressant effects. Conversely, they may result in additional undesirable effects, e.g. antimuscarinic (see p.349), sedation, cognitive impairment.

Antipsychotic classification reflects their varying propensity to cause dopamine depletion symptoms. The risk is a spectrum (in descending order):
* typical:
  ▷ butyrophenones (*highest risk*), e.g. haloperidol
  ▷ phenothiazines, e.g. chlorpromazine, levomepromazine, prochlorperazine
* atypical:
  ▷ less sedating, e.g. risperidone
  ▷ more sedating (*lowest risk*), e.g. olanzapine, quetiapine.

Although extrapyramidal reactions account for more discontinuations with typical compared with atypical antipsychotics, overall discontinuation rates for undesirable effects or lack of efficacy are comparable.

For important cautions, interactions and undesirable effects see Tables 18–19.

Neuroleptic (antipsychotic) malignant syndrome

Neuroleptic (antipsychotic) malignant syndrome (NMS) is an idiosyncratic life-threatening reaction seen in <1% of those prescribed an antipsychotic. Because it is caused by dopamine depletion, it is more accurate and helpful to consider it an *acute dopamine depletion syndrome* (Box 1).

Most cases occur within 2 weeks of starting treatment or a dose increase. NMS can also occur in patients with Parkinson's disease if long-term treatment with levodopa or D_2 agonists are abruptly discontinued.

Table 18 Important cautions with antipsychotics

Context	Danger
Increased risk of stroke	2–3 times higher in elderly patients, greatest in those with dementia. Mechanism unknown
Epilepsy	Dose-dependent reduction in seizure threshold. Risk approximates to the degree of sedation, e.g. chlorpromazine (higher), haloperidol (lower)
Parkinsonism and Parkinson's disease	All antipsychotics can cause parkinsonism or worsen existing parkinsonism of any cause. Risk is lowest with clozapine and quetiapine
QT prolongation	Droperidol, haloperidol and pimozide are contra-indicated, specific cautions with chlorpromazine, levomepromazine and sulpiride
Drug interactions	The metabolism of some antipsychotics may be affected by cytochrome P450 inhibitors and inducers, e.g. haloperidol, olanzapine, risperidone, quetiapine

Table 19 Undesirable effects of antipsychotics

System	Undesirable effect
CNS	Extrapyramidal reactions (parkinsonism, akathisia, dystonia, tardive dyskinesia)
	Sedation
Endocrine	Hyperprolactinaemia resulting in amenorrhoea, galactorrhoea, gynaecomastia, sexual dysfunction, osteoporosis; more common with typicals and risperidone
	Metabolic effects (weight gain, dyslipidaemia, type 2 diabetes mellitus); more common with atypicals, particularly olanzapine, quetiapine and clozapine. Consider monitoring weight, glucose and lipids at baseline and 3-monthly thereafter
Cardiovascular effects	QT prolongation: dose-related, affected by presence of other risk factors, including concurrent use with other drugs that prolong QT or interact to increase the antipsychotic plasma concentration; highest risk with chlorpromazine, droperidol, haloperidol, levomepromazine, pimozide and sulpiride
	Venous thrombo-embolism
	Postural hypotension (α-adrenergic antagonism), particularly clozapine, phenothiazines and quetiapine
Miscellaneous	Antimuscarinic effects: more with phenothiazines and clozapine
	Neuroleptic (antipsychotic) malignant syndrome (see below)
	Agranulocytosis in about 1% of patients taking clozapine, generally after 3–6 months

Box I Acute dopamine depletion syndrome; also known as neuroleptic (antipsychotic) malignant syndrome

Clinical features

Essential:
- severe (lead-pipe) muscle rigidity; possibly progressing to immobilization
- pyrexia ± sweating

Additional:
- muteness → stupor
- tachycardia and elevated/labile blood pressure (autonomic instability)
- leukocytosis
- raised plasma creatine phosphokinase ± other evidence of muscle injury, e.g. myoglobinuria.

Management

Specific measures:
- discontinuation of the causal drug
- prescription of a muscle relaxant, e.g. a benzodiazepine
- in severe cases, prescription of bromocriptine, a D_2 agonist, halves mortality.

Hypoxia, acidosis and renal failure require appropriate acute management.

Outcome

The syndrome is self-limiting if the causal antipsychotic drug is discontinued.

Resolves in 1–2 weeks; but 4–6 weeks if caused by a depot antipsychotic.

Death occurs in <20% of cases, mostly from respiratory failure.

Subsequent prescription of an antipsychotic carries a 30–50% risk of recurrence.

Use of antipsychotics in palliative care

Nausea and vomiting

The D_2 antagonism of all antipsychotics is likely to provide anti-emetic activity in the area postrema (chemoreceptor trigger zone; see p.342). Where specific action at this site is required (e.g. most chemical causes of nausea), a selective dopaminergic agent such as haloperidol is used (Table 20).

However, many antipsychotics bind to other receptors involved in emesis and, to a variable extent, are broad-spectrum anti-emetics (see p.342). Levomepromazine and olanzapine are the most widely used (Table 20).

Table 20 Doses of commonly used antipsychotics for nausea and vomiting

Antipsychotic	Starting dose	Titration	Maximum recommended dose
Haloperidol[a]	PO: 500microgram– 1.5mg stat, at bedtime, & p.r.n.	Increase after 2 days if p.r.n. doses still necessary.	PO/SC: 10mg/24h
	SC: 2.5–5mg/24h, & 1mg SC p.r.n.		
Levomepromazine[b]	6–6.25mg PO/SC stat, at bedtime, & p.r.n.	Increase after 2 days if p.r.n. doses still necessary.	50mg/24h at bedtime, or 25mg b.d.
		Generally limited by drowsiness	
Olanzapine[c]	1.25–2.5mg PO/SC stat, at bedtime, & p.r.n.	Increase after 2 days if p.r.n. doses still necessary.	5mg b.d
		If necessary, increase to 5mg at bedtime	

a. as a general rule, the dose of haloperidol is halved when switching from PO to SC
b. some centres use a lower starting dose, i.e. 3mg PO
c. injection not available in the UK.

Other uses

In palliative care, antipsychotics have several other off-label uses (Tables 21 and 22). Apart from delirium and terminal agitation, they are generally *not a* first-line drug, seek specialist advice.

Delirium

Antipsychotics should be considered alongside non-drug measures in agitated, hypo-active and mixed delirium (see p.196).

When antipsychotics alone are insufficient, or when sedation is also required, e.g. for the initial management of a hyperactive agitated patient, a benzodiazepine can be added (see p.356).

Note: although benzodiazepines can paradoxically worsen agitation, they are preferable for delirium related to alcohol withdrawal, antimuscarinic toxicity, neuroleptic malignant syndrome or Parkinson's disease.

The efficacy and tolerability of the antipsychotics in Table 21 are comparable.

Table 21 PO doses of commonly used antipsychotics for delirium

Antipsychotic	Starting dose	Titration	Maximum recommended dose
Haloperidol[a]	500microgram stat & q2h p.r.n.	If necessary, increase progressively, e.g. 1mg → 1.5mg etc.	5mg p.r.n
		Maintenance dose is based on initial cumulative dose needed to settle the patient, typically ≤5mg/24h	
Olanzapine	2.5mg stat, p.r.n. & at bedtime	If necessary, increase to 5mg–10mg at bedtime	10mg at bedtime
Risperidone	1mg at bedtime & p.r.n.	If necessary, increase by 1mg every other day	4mg at bedtime
		Typical maintenance dose 1mg at bedtime	

a. consider a higher starting dose (1.5–3mg) when patient distress is severe and/or immediate danger to self or others, possibly combined with a benzodiazepine.

Table 22 Off-label uses of antipsychotics

Symptom	Example	Comment	Cross-reference
Terminal agitation	Haloperidol, levomepromazine	Levomepromazine generally used when sedation is desired	p.254
Refractory hiccup	Chlorpromazine, haloperidol	Generally third-line after metoclopramide ± anti-foaming agent, and baclofen or gabapentin	p.166
Refractory depression	Olanzapine, quetiapine	An adjunct, particularly when switching antidepressants has been unsuccessful; generally added to an SSRI	p.193

BENZODIAZEPINES

Authorized uses include insomnia, anxiety and panic disorder, myoclonus, seizures, skeletal muscle spasm, alcohol withdrawal.

Off-label uses include breathlessness, acute psychotic agitation, terminal agitation, nausea and vomiting, restless legs syndrome.

Benzodiazepines work by enhancing the action of GABA, the major inhibitory neurotransmitter of the nervous system.

Contra-indications (*all irrelevant in the imminently dying*) include acute severe pulmonary insufficiency, untreated sleep apnoea syndrome, severe hepatic impairment, myasthenia gravis.

Tolerance and dependence are unlikely to be a problem when used for ≤4 weeks. Other undesirable effects and risk of drug interactions necessitate appropriate caution, particularly for those at greater risk, e.g. the elderly and frail patients (Tables 23 and 24).

Table 23 Important cautions with benzodiazepines

Context	Danger
Benzodiazepines with long halflives accumulate with repeated use, e.g. diazepam	Undesirable effects may manifest only after several days or weeks
Mild–moderate hepatic impairment	Increased risk of undesirable effects
Renal impairment	Increased risk of undesirable effects
Chronic respiratory disease	Risk of respiratory depression; flumazenil, a specific antagonist, is used to reverse life-threatening respiratory depression
Psychological and physical dependence	Closely monitor patients with a history of substance abuse; if long-term treatment is discontinued, taper gradually to avoid withdrawal symptoms
Drug interactions	The metabolism of some benzodiazepines is affected by cytochrome P450 inhibitors and inducers, e.g. diazepam, midazolam

Table 24 Undesirable effects of benzodiazepines

System	Undesirable effect
CNS	Drowsiness, impaired psychomotor skills, fatigue, cognitive impairment and hypotonia → unsteadiness/ataxia and falls
	Paradoxical arousal, agitation and aggression; risk factors include alcohol misuse; use an antipsychotic instead

Use of benzodiazepines in palliative care

Apart from insomnia, diazepam or midazolam cover most situations when a benzodiazepine is needed.

Although the manufacturers recommend giving diazepam in divided doses, its long plasma halflife means that administration at bedtime is generally satisfactory, and easier for the patient.

In practice, midazolam (intermittent SC or by CSCI) is mostly used in the last hours or days of life when PO medication is difficult. An oromucosal solution for buccal administration (primarily used to treat seizures) is an alternative if injections are unavailable. The contents of an ampoule for injection can also be used for buccal administration.

Insomnia

Initial management includes correcting contributory factors when possible, e.g. pain, delirium, and non-drug measures (see p.194). Where drug treatment is required, use a benzodiazepine with a short halflife, ideally for <4 weeks, e.g. temazepam (halflife 8–15h) 10–20mg PO at bedtime.

Alternatively, use a non-benzodiazepine such as zopiclone (halflife 3.5h) 7.5mg (or 3.75mg initially if elderly or frail) PO at bedtime. Others options include sedating antidepressants (e.g. doxepin, mirtazapine, trazodone; see p.340) and melatonin.

Anxiety and panic disorder

- if prognosis is <4 weeks, prescribe diazepam 2–10mg PO at bedtime and p.r.n. or lorazepam 0.5–1mg PO b.d. and p.r.n.
- if prognosis is >4 weeks, prescribe an SSRI (see p.192) *initially with diazepam*. With severe anxiety or panic, consider mirtazapine instead.

Myoclonus

In the imminently dying, give SC midazolam 2.5–5mg p.r.n. or CSCI 10–20mg/24h.

Seizures

Benzodiazepines are first-line treatment for acute seizures, including status epilepticus (see p.204). Because of the development of tolerance, long-term use is limited to epilepsy refractory to other measures (see p.345).

Skeletal muscle spasm and spasticity

Benzodiazepines are used for the *short-term* management of pain due to skeletal muscle spasm such as acute low back pain, e.g. diazepam 2–5mg PO at bedtime and p.r.n. For long-term use (>4 weeks), consider baclofen instead (p.372).

Midazolam 10mg/24h CSCI, can be used to relieve muscle spasm or spasticity in the last days of life.

Alcohol withdrawal

Use SC midazolam as for seizures (see p.204).

Other uses

In palliative care, benzodiazepines have several off-label uses (Table 25); generally *not* first-line, seek specialist advice.

Table 25 Selected off-label uses of benzodiazepines

Symptom	Example of drug used	Comment	Cross-reference
Breathlessness	Diazepam PO or, close to death, midazolam SC (generally with morphine)	Benzodiazepines main role is when breathlessness is exacerbated by anxiety	p.145
Acute psychotic agitation	Lorazepam 2mg PO/IM every 30min until the patient is settled	Haloperidol is normally drug of first-choice	p.356
Nausea and vomiting	Lorazepam SL or Midazolam CSCI	Sometimes used with chemotherapy and postoperatively	p.119

Switching between benzodiazepines

Dose conversion is not straightforward and switching is best avoided if possible (Table 26). Equivalent doses are always approximations, and appropriate caution is required. Particularly when switching at a high dose, it is prudent to use a 30–40% lower dose than predicted and to ensure that both flumazenil and additional benzodiazepine doses are available for p.r.n. use.

Table 26 Approximate equivalent PO anxiolytic-sedative doses

Drug	Dose
Clonazepam	250microgram
Diazepam	5mg
Lorazepam	500microgram
Midazolam	5mg (PO not UK)
Temazepam	10mg

When converting from PO diazepam to SC midazolam, the dose should be halved (e.g. diazepam 5mg PO → midazolam 2.5mg SC). However, because the bio-availability of midazolam is about half that of diazepam, starting PO doses are the same.

BISPHOSPHONATES

Include ibandronic acid, pamidronate disodium and zoledronic acid.

Authorized uses vary between products but include tumour-induced hypercalcaemia, prophylaxis to reduce skeletal-related events (SRE) associated with osteolytic bone metastases (hypercalcaemia, pain, fracture), osteoporosis and Paget's disease.

Off-label uses include metastatic bone pain and the primary prevention of bone loss in patients treated for breast or prostate cancer.

Bisphosphonates are analogues of pyrophosphate, a naturally occurring regulator of bone metabolism. They have a high affinity for calcium ions and are rapidly bound to hydroxyapatite in bone where they remain for months. Bisphosphonates are released and taken up by osteoclasts, interfering with their function and/or survival. Thus, bisphosphonates help counter the cancer-related increase in number and activity of osteoclasts which contributes towards hypercalcaemia and bone pain.

For important cautions and undesirable effects see Tables 27 and 28.

Renal toxicity

Bisphosphonates can affect renal function in ~10% of patients following usual doses of zoledronic acid or pamidronate. In about 3%, increases in plasma creatinine lead to treatment delay or discontinuation; increases in creatinine levels >3 times the upper limit of normal are seen rarely.

Onset of decreased renal function varies, but often within 2 months of starting treatment. Mild impairment tends to recover a few days–several months after discontinuing the bisphosphonate. In those with renal failure, the damage is generally permanent.

Life-threatening renal failure caused by toxic acute tubular necrosis also rarely occurs, generally when there are additional risk factors (e.g. dehydration, pre-existing renal impairment, concurrent use of other nephrotoxic drugs).

The risk of renal toxicity is reduced by:
- using the recommended dose and infusion rate
- ensuring adequate hydration
- monitoring renal function and adjusting the dose of bisphosphonate as appropriate or discontinuing treatment if there is deterioration
- avoiding the concurrent use of other nephrotoxic drugs.

Renal toxicity is uncommon with ibandronic acid and it is authorized for use in severe renal failure. Denosumab is an option in this setting (see Box J, p.364).

Jaw osteonecrosis

All bisphosphonates (and denosumab) increase the risk of jaw osteonecrosis. The jaw bones may be particularly susceptible because of the combination of repeated low-level local trauma (e.g. from chewing, dentures) and ease of infection from microbes. This increases demand for bone repair which the bisphosphonate-inhibited bone cannot meet, resulting in localized bone necrosis.

Although reported after as little as 4 months of bisphosphonate use, patients generally have been receiving bisphosphonates for ≥1 year. Other risk factors include dental procedures, poor dental health, blood clotting disorders, anaemia, and possibly chemotherapy and corticosteroids.

Osteonecrosis can present as an asymptomatic bony exposure, or with orofacial pain, trismus, offensive discharge from a cutaneous fistula, chronic sinusitis because of an oro-antral fistula and numbness in the mandible or maxilla. There may be osteomyelitis.

Table 27 Important cautions with bisphosphonates

Context	Danger
Renal impairment	Increased risk of undesirable effects; correct hypovolaemia before treatment and monitor renal function; adjust dose according to SPC
Calcium and vitamin D deficiency	Unless being treated for tumour-related hypercalcaemia, daily oral supplements of calcium and vitamin D are recommended
Dental procedures	Risk of osteonecrosis of the jaw (see below)
Drug interactions	Risk of hypocalcaemia increased with aminoglycosides (also hypomagnesaemia) and loop diuretics (also dehydration)
	Risk of renal impairment increased with other nephrotoxic drugs and thalidomide in multiple myeloma

Table 28 Undesirable effects of bisphosphonates

System	Undesirable effect
Gastro-intestinal	Particularly with PO formulations: anorexia, dyspepsia, nausea, vomiting, abdominal pain, diarrhoea or constipation
Skeletal	Atypical femoral fractures (usually in patients treated for >5 years for osteoporosis)
Endocrine	Asymptomatic hypocalcaemia, hypomagnesaemia, hypophosphataemia; symptomatic hypocalcaemia (e.g. tetany)
Renal	Deterioration in renal function (see below).
	Pamidronate: collapsing focal segmental glomerulosclerosis, nephrotic syndrome
Miscellaneous	Very common: transient pyrexia and flu-like symptoms, e.g. fatigue, headache, arthralgia, myalgia, bone pain. Generally resolve within 1–2 days and lessen with repeat doses; treat with paracetamol or NSAID
	Common: jaw osteonecrosis (see below)
	Rare: ocular inflammation (see below), angioedema, anaphylaxis, bronchospasm

Osteonecrosis may show as mottling on a plain radiograph, and be confused with bone metastases on a bone scan. Pathological fracture can occur.

Long-term outcomes are generally poor and thus, prevention is an important part of the recommended approach:

- *preventive dental treatment* before commencing long-term bisphosphonates, e.g. treat infection, teeth extractions
- *encourage good dental hygiene* including regular dental cleaning by a dentist or dental hygienist
- avoid invasive dental procedures during treatment
- *minimize trauma*, e.g. patients with dentures should wear soft liners.

If osteonecrosis occurs:

- *discontinue the bisphosphonate* but new lesions may continue to appear
- *treat infection*, e.g. antimicrobials, chlorhexidine mouthwash, periodic minor debridement and wound irrigation (major debridement is avoided as it may worsen the situation)
- *avoid major surgery* unless there is no alternative, e.g. due to sequestered bone, pathological fracture, or oro-antral fistula.

If urgent treatment precludes a prior dental examination, a dental referral and any treatment should be undertaken within 1–2 months for patients expected to receive long-term bisphosphonates.

Ocular toxicity

Rarely ocular inflammation can occur, causing eye pain, redness, swelling, abnormal vision or impaired eye movement. Typically, the onset is within 2 days of the first or second infusion and affects both eyes.

An urgent ophthalmology assessment is required, followed by appropriate treatment. Patients with mild reactions, e.g. those which settle quickly without treatment, can generally continue to receive the same bisphosphonate. For those with more severe reactions, e.g. uveitis or scleritis, specialist advice should be sought from the ophthalmologist ± endocrinologist.

Use of bisphosphonates in palliative care

Bisphosphonates are generally given IV. Ibandronic acid is also available as a PO product authorized for prophylactic use to reduce the incidence of skeletal-related events (see SPC). To maximize absorption and to minimize undesirable gastro-oesophageal effects, patients should receive specific instruction on its administration (see SPC/PIL).

Unless being treated for tumour-related hypercalcaemia, daily oral supplements of elemental calcium 500mg and vitamin D 400 units are recommended, e.g. Calcichew® D3 Forte.

Because zoledronic acid is more effective and now available as a generic, it is replacing pamidronate as bisphosphonate of first choice. For dosing of pamidronate, see SPC.

Tumour-induced hypercalcaemia

Stop and think! Are you justified in correcting a potentially fatal complication in a moribund patient?

For zoledronic acid:
- patients should be well hydrated
- give 4mg IVI in 100mL 0.9% saline or 5% glucose over 15min
- if plasma calcium does not normalize, repeat after 1 week
- measure plasma creatinine before each dose; no dose adjustment is needed in mild–moderate renal impairment for patients being treated for hypercalcaemia.

Onset of effect is <4 days, with a maximum effect about 4–7 days. Normocalcaemia is restored in 90% of patients with a duration of effect of 4 weeks.

If the IV route is inaccessible, consider denosumab SC (Box J). Alternatively, pamidronate can be administered by CSCI, together with SC hydration, e.g. 90mg in 1L 0.9% saline over 12–24h.

In palliative care, treatment with a bisphosphonate is unlikely to be started in patients with hypercalcaemia and severe renal impairment (creatinine clearance <30mL/min). However, if appropriate, seek specialist renal/endocrinology advice and consider using denosumab (Box J) or ibandronic acid IV (see Bondonat SPC).

Prophylactic use to reduce the incidence of skeletal-related events (SRE) in patients with myeloma or bone metastases

An established use in patients with:
- breast cancer with bone metastases
- myeloma whether or not bone lesions are evident.

Bisphosphonates are also recommended for the relief of pain from bone metastases in patients with hormone-resistant prostate cancer when analgesia and radiotherapy have failed. No consensus exists for other cancers, although it is reasonable to consider their use in any patient with a prognosis of >4 months and multiple bone metastases.

Bisphosphonates are generally continued for as long as they are tolerated, or there is a substantial decline in the patient's performance status.

For zoledronic acid:
- patients should be well hydrated
- give 4mg IVI in 100mL 0.9% saline or 5% glucose over 15min every 3–4 weeks; with appropriate support, these can be given in the home setting
- for dose in patients with renal impairment, see Table 29
- measure plasma creatinine before each dose; withhold treatment if creatinine increases by:
  - ≥44micromol/L in patients with a normal baseline creatinine concentration (i.e. <124micromol/L) or
  - ≥88micromol/L in patients with a raised baseline creatinine concentration (i.e. >124micromol/L)
- treatment may be resumed at the same dose as before when plasma creatinine returns to within 10% of the baseline value
- discontinue treatment permanently if plasma creatinine fails to improve after 4–8 weeks.

For pamidronate, see SPC.

Box J Denosumab

Indications: for patients for whom bisphosphonates are contra-indicated or poorly tolerated; refractory hypercalcaemia of malignancy (off-label).

Contra-indication: untreated severe hypocalcaemia.

Pharmacology

Denosumab is a human monoclonal antibody which reduces osteoclast number and function, thereby decreasing bone resorption and cancer-induced bone destruction.

Denosumab is superior to zoledronic acid in preventing SRE in metastatic bone cancer. It can be used in renal impairment without dose adjustment. Its long-term efficacy and safety are unknown.

Undesirable effects

Very common (>10%): breathlessness, diarrhoea.

Common (<10%, >1%): hypocalcaemia, hypophosphataemia, hyperhidrosis, osteonecrosis of jaw (comparable with zoledronic acid).

Uncommon (<1%, >0.1%): cellulitis, drug hypersensitivity.

Dose and use

See SPC; can be given SC. The manufacturer recommends daily supplementation with at least 500mg calcium and 400 IU Vitamin D unless the patient is hypercalcaemic.

Table 29 Dose reduction for zoledronic acid in patients with cancer involving the bones and mild–moderate renal impairment[a,b,c]

Baseline creatinine clearance (mL/min)	Recommended dose (mg)
>60	4 (i.e. no reduction)
50–60	3.5
40–49	3.3
30–39	3

a. manufacturer's recommendations for patients with multiple myeloma or bone metastases
b. no data exist for severe renal impairment (creatinine clearance <30mL/min) because these patients were excluded from the studies
c. reduced doses are diluted in 100mL 0.9% saline or 5% glucose and given IVI over 15min; see SPC for preparation details.

Metastatic bone pain

Bisphosphonates have been used for metastatic bone pain when more conventional methods have been exhausted. Benefit is more likely in patients with breast cancer or myeloma, and with an IV bisphosphonate.

For zoledronic acid, use same doses as in prophylaxis (see above). In patients not responding to a first treatment, a second can be tried but, if still no response, discontinue. If helpful, repeat every 4 weeks for as long as benefit is maintained.

For pamidronate suggested (off-label) regimens include:
- pamidronate disodium 90mg IVI (50% of patients respond, generally within 1–2 weeks); if helpful repeat 60–90mg every 3–4 weeks for as long as benefit continues
- pamidronate disodium 120mg IVI, repeat p.r.n. every 2–4 months.

CORTICOSTEROIDS

Corticosteroids have a potent anti-inflammatory effect which may be of benefit in many settings in advanced cancer (Box K).

Box K Off-label indications for systemic corticosteroids in advanced cancer

This list of off-label uses is not exhaustive and inclusion does not mean that a systemic corticosteroid is necessarily the treatment of choice. The evidence-base for some indications is only 'expert opinion'.

Specific

Spinal cord compression

Nerve compression

Breathlessness:
    pneumonitis (after radiation therapy)
    lymphangitic carcinomatosis
    tracheal compression/stridor

Superior vena caval obstruction

Obstruction of hollow viscus:
    bronchus
    ureter
    GI

Radiation-induced inflammation

Discharge from rectal tumour (can give either PO or PR)

Paraneoplastic fever

Nausea and vomiting in cancer resistant to standard measures (see p.123)

Hypercalcaemia associated with cancer (an adjunct to SC calcitonin)

Pain relief [a]

Pain associated with spinal cord or nerve compression

Pain caused by a tumour in a confined organ or body cavity, e.g. raised intracranial pressure

Anticancer hormone therapy

Breast cancer

Prostate cancer

Haematological malignancies

Lymphoproliferative disorders

General ('tonic')

To improve appetite

To enhance sense of wellbeing

---

a. RCT evidence is mixed, but overall suggests that the use of corticosteroids for cancer pain *per se* outside of the above indications has little benefit.

The anti-inflammatory action of corticosteroids is broader than the more specific impact of NSAIDs on prostaglandin synthesis (see p.324). Thus, as anti-inflammatory agents, corticosteroids are potentially more effective than NSAIDs. However, certainly when used long-term, corticosteroids are likely to cause more numerous and more serious undesirable effects (Box L).

Dexamethasone and prednisolone are both frequently used. Dexamethasone, with high glucocorticoid activity but insignificant mineralocorticoid effect, is particularly suitable for high-dose anti-inflammatory therapy. It is 7 times more potent than prednisolone, i.e. 2mg of dexamethasone is approximately equivalent to 15mg of prednisolone, and it has a longer duration of action (36–54h vs. 12–36h).

Dose and use

Given the many and significant undesirable effects of corticosteroids, and the potentially deleterious effect of rapid withdrawal, corticosteroids should be prescribed cautiously:

Box L Undesirable effects of corticosteroids

Glucocorticoid effects

Adrenal suppression[a]

Avascular bone necrosis

Cataract (seen with long-term systemic or inhaled steroids)

Diabetes mellitus or deterioration of glycaemic control in known diabetics

Infection (increased susceptibility)

Muscle wasting and weakness

Osteoporosis

Peptic ulceration (if given with an NSAID)

Psychiatric disturbances:
  anxiety
  bipolar disorder
  delirium
  depression
  mania
  paranoid ('steroid') psychosis
Suppression of growth (in child)

Mineralocorticoid effects

Hypertension

Potassium loss

Sodium and water retention → oedema

Cushingoid features

Acne

Bruising

Hirsuitism

Lipodystrophy after ≥8 weeks of treatment in 30–70% of patients (reversible on stopping treatment):
  buffalo hump
  increased abdominal fat
  moon face
  reduced subcutaneous fat in limbs
Striae

---

a. patients taking >10mg prednisolone (or equivalent) daily for 3 weeks who develop any significant intercurrent illness, trauma or surgical procedure require a temporary increase in corticosteroid dose (or, if stopped within the past 3 months, a temporary re-introduction).

- for defined symptoms potentially responsive to corticosteroid therapy
- always bearing in mind potential benefit vs. risk
- at a low–moderate dose, titrated to clinical effect
- for a time-limited trial
- discontinued if no clinical/symptomatic benefit seen *or*
- weaned to the lowest effective dose.

Dexamethasone and prednisolone can be given in a single daily dose each morning. However, when 'tablet burden' or injection volume is an issue, higher doses of dexamethasone (i.e. >8mg) can be halved and administered as a morning and a lunchtime dose. Giving doses later in the day should generally be avoided, as this increases the risk of corticosteroid-induced insomnia. Nonetheless, even with morning doses, temazepam or diazepam at bedtime is sometimes needed to counter insomnia or agitation.

The initial dose of dexamethasone varies according to indication (Table 30).

Table 30 Typical PO and SC/IV starting doses for dexamethasone, expressed as dexamethasone base[a]

Indication	Typical PO dose	SC/IV dose (volume)	
		3.3mg/mL formulation[b]	3.8mg/mL formulation[b]
Anorexia[c]	2–6mg	1.7–5mg (0.5–1.5mL)	1.9–5.7mg (0.5–1.5mL)
Anti-emetic[d]	8–16mg	6.6–13.2mg (2–4mL)	7.6–15.2mg (2–4mL)
Obstruction of hollow viscus	8–16mg	6.6–13.2mg (2–4mL)	7.6–15.2mg (2–4mL)
Raised intracranial pressure	8–16mg	6.6–13.2mg (2–4mL)	7.6–15.2mg (2–4mL)
Spinal cord compression	16mg	13.2mg (4mL)	15.2mg (4mL)

a. generally given once daily in the morning (see text)
b. for pragmatic purposes, both 3.3mg and 3.8mg dexamethasone *base* of the injectable formulations can be considered approximately equivalent to dexamethasone *base* 4mg PO
c. prednisolone 15–40mg each morning is an alternative
d. also see Quick Clinical Guide, p.123.

'Tonic' use

The non-specific 'tonic' use of corticosteroids is based on their general physiological effects. Thus, in patients with advanced cancer, treatment with a corticosteroid may result in increased appetite, reduced nausea and improved well-being.

Obstruction

In obstructive syndromes (see Box K), corticosteroids may help by reducing inflammation at the site of the obstruction, thereby increasing the lumen of the obstructed hollow viscus. Dexamethasone (e.g. 6.6–13.2mg/24h SC) may improve bowel obstruction. High-dose dexamethasone (e.g. 20–40mg/24h PO) may relieve stridor patients with cancer-related upper airway obstruction.

Brain metastases

Dexamethasone 4–8mg/24h PO provides temporary symptomatic relief for patients with mild symptoms related to raised intracranial pressure from cerebral oedema. For those with severe symptoms or at risk of herniation, doses of ≥16mg/24h PO are recommended.

Symptom relief from dexamethasone reduces over time and undesirable effects increase. Thus, ideally, the dose of dexamethasone should be reduced after one week and discontinued after 2–4 weeks.

However, unless patients receive additional treatment (e.g. palliative radiotherapy), they will experience a recurrence of their symptoms at some point as the dose of dexamethasone is decreased. Thus, it may be necessary to taper more slowly or continue 'maintenance' dexamethasone indefinitely in some patients.

Whole brain radiotherapy may cause nausea, vomiting, headache, fever and a transient worsening of neurological symptoms. Dexamethasone should be continued for one week after treatment and then tapered over 2–4 weeks.

Spinal cord compression

Spinal cord compression must be treated as an emergency (see p.241). Because corticosteroids inhibit inflammation, stabilize vascular membranes, and reduce spinal cord oedema, their use in spinal cord compression often results in a dramatic reduction in pain, and an early improvement in the patient's physical status.

A typical regimen for dexamethasone would be:
- a stat dose of 16mg PO (sometimes initially given IV)
- continue with 16mg PO each morning for a further 3–4 days
- maintain on 8mg PO each morning until the completion of radiotherapy
- taper (and discontinue) over 2 weeks after the completion of radiotherapy.

If there is neurological deterioration during the dose reduction, the dose should be increased again to the previous satisfactory dose, and maintained at that level for a further 2 weeks before attempting to taper the dose again. About 1/4 require maintenance dexamethasone in order to preserve neural function.

Stopping corticosteroids

If after 7–10 days the corticosteroid fails to achieve the desired effect, generally it should be stopped. It is often possible to stop corticosteroids abruptly (Box M).

> **Box M** Recommendations for withdrawing systemic corticosteroids
>
> **Abrupt withdrawal**
>
> Systemic corticosteroids may be stopped abruptly in those whose disease is unlikely to relapse *and* have received treatment for <3 weeks *and* are not in the groups below.
>
> **Gradual withdrawal**
>
> *Gradual* withdrawal of systemic corticosteroids is advisable in patients who:
> - have received more than 3 weeks treatment
> - have received prednisolone >40mg/24h or equivalent, e.g. dexamethasone 4–6mg
> - have had a second dose in the evening
> - have received repeated treatments
> - are taking a short course within 1 year of stopping long-term treatment
> - have other possible causes of adrenal suppression.
>
> During corticosteroid withdrawal the dose may initially be reduced rapidly (e.g. halving the dose daily) to physiological doses (prednisolone 7.5mg/24h or equivalent) and then more slowly (e.g. 1–2mg per week) to allow the adrenals to recover and to prevent a hypo-adrenal crisis (malaise, profound weakness, hypotension, etc.). The patient should be monitored during withdrawal in case of deterioration.
>
> **Moribund patients**
>
> For patients who are close to death and no longer able to swallow tablets, it is generally acceptable to discontinue corticosteroids abruptly. Sometimes a maintenance SC dose may be indicated to prevent distress from symptomatic hypo-adrenalism.

LAXATIVES

Constipation is common in palliative care. Generally, the cause is multifactorial and includes the use of constipating drugs. Opioids cause constipation by increasing ring contractions, decreasing propulsive intestinal activity, and by enhancing the resorption of fluid and electrolytes (see p.125).

Laxative use aims to:
- restore the amount of water in the faeces by:
  - ▷ reducing bowel transit time
  - ▷ increasing faecal water
  - ▷ increasing the ability of the faeces to retain water
- improve rectal evacuation by improving faecal consistency and promoting peristalsis.

Laxatives should be prescribed regularly (see Quick Clinical Guide: Opioid-induced constipation, p.127). An appreciation of how different laxatives work guides laxative choice.

There are two broad classes of laxatives: those acting predominantly as faecal softeners and those acting predominantly as bowel stimulants (Table 31). *However, a stimulant laxative, by reducing bowel transit time, will also have a softening effect.*

Table 31 Classification of commonly used laxatives

Class of laxative[a]	General mode of action	Example
Faecal softeners		
Surface-wetting agents	Act as a detergent, lowering surface tension, thereby allowing water and fats to penetrate hard, dry faeces	Docusate sodium[a]
Osmotic laxatives	Water is retained in the gut lumen with a subsequent increase in faecal volume	Lactulose syrup, magnesium hydroxide suspension, macrogols (e.g. Movicol®)
Stimulant laxatives	Act via direct contact with the submucosal and myenteric plexus in the large bowel, resulting in rhythmic muscle contractions and improved intestinal motility. Also increase water secretion into the bowel lumen	Bisacodyl, dantron, senna, sodium picosulfate
Lubricants	Coat the surface of the stool to make it more slippery and easier to pass	Arachis oil
Bulk-forming agents (fibre)	Increases faecal bulk through water-binding and increasing bacterial cell mass. This causes intestinal distension and thereby stimulates peristalsis; only a limited role in palliative care	Ispaghula (psyllium) husk (e.g. Fybogel®, Regulan®)

a. reflects predominant action. Stimulant laxatives can also act as faecal softeners and vice versa, e.g. docusate, at doses >400mg/24h also has a stimulant effect.

Note:
- the concurrent prescription of several different laxatives should be avoided
- patient preference and drug tolerability should be taken into account; adherence with laxative therapy is sometimes limited by palatability, undesirable effects (e.g. colic, flatulence), volume required, and polypharmacy
- laxative doses should be titrated every 1–2 days according to response up to the maximum recommended or tolerable dose before changing to an alternative
- although traditionally a combination of a bowel stimulant with a faecal softener has been recommended in palliative care patients, a stimulant laxative alone, e.g. bisacodyl or senna, is generally adequate (see Quick Clinical Guide: Opioid-induced constipation, p.127).

Some patients also need rectal measures (suppositories, enemas, digital evacuation) either because of failed oral treatment or electively, e.g. in bedbound frail elderly patients, paraplegics.

Generally, rectal interventions should be avoided in patients who are neutropenic or thrombocytopenic because of the risk, respectively, of infection or bleeding.

Methylnaltrexone, a peripherally-acting opioid antagonist, should be considered only when the optimum use of laxatives is ineffective (see p.127).

PO formulations of strong opioids containing opioid antagonists are being developed. Although primarily designed to deter misuse (e.g. by crushing and injecting IV) some may help antagonize the constipating effect of the opioid.

Dose and use

See Quick Clinical Guide: Opioid-induced constipation, p.127.

Faecal softeners

Surface-wetting agents

Docusate

Dose varies according to individual need:
- generally start with 100mg PO b.d.
- if necessary, increase to 200mg b.d.–t.d.s.

Docusate can also be used as an enema (see below).

Osmotic laxatives

Lactulose

Useful in patients who experience intestinal colic with stimulant laxatives, or who fail to respond to stimulant laxatives alone:
- start with 15mL PO once daily–b.d. and adjust according to need
- for hepatic encephalopathy, start with 30–50mL t.d.s. and adjust the dose to produce 2–3 soft evacuations per day.

Some patients find lactulose nauseating, and it may cause abdominal bloating.

Macrogols

Macrogols are generally supplied as powder in sachets. A concentrated oral liquid is also available. All formulations need to be dissolved or diluted in water to 125–250ml; follow manufacturers' recommendations.

Macrogol 3350 can also be used for faecal impaction:
- start with 8 sachets on day 1, each dissolved in 125mL of water, and taken in <6h (total 1L)
- if necessary, repeat on days 2 and 3; most patients do not need the full dose on day 2
- patients with cardiovascular impairment should restrict intake to 2 sachets/h, i.e. 250mL/h.

Stimulant laxatives

Bisacodyl

- if *not* constipated:
  ▷ generally start with 5mg at bedtime
  ▷ if no response after 24–48h, increase to 10mg at bedtime
- If already constipated:
  ▷ generally start with 10mg at bedtime
  ▷ if no response after 24–48h, increase to 20mg at bedtime
  ▷ if no response after a further 24–48h, consider adding a second daytime dose
  ▷ if necessary, consider increasing to a maximum of 20mg t.d.s.

Senna

- if *not* constipated:
  ▷ generally start with 15mg at bedtime
  ▷ if no response after 24–48h, increase to 15mg at bedtime and each morning
- if already constipated:
  ▷ generally start with 15mg at bedtime and each morning
  ▷ if no response after 24–48h, increase to 22.5mg at bedtime and each morning
  ▷ if no response after a further 24–48h, consider adding a third daytime dose
  ▷ if necessary, consider increasing to a maximum of 30mg t.d.s.

Senna oral solution (7.5mg/5mL) can be used instead of tablets; it is tasteless, odourless and generally cheaper.

Rectal products

These are given either regularly and electively, or intermittently and p.r.n., generally in addition to laxatives PO. In practice, for soft faeces, a bisacodyl suppository is given on its own; and, for hard faeces, glycerol alone or glycerol plus bisacodyl (Table 32).

When treating a hard faecal impaction, a docusate sodium micro-enema will help to soften the faecal mass. This should be instilled into the rectum and retained overnight before giving a stimulant suppository (bisacodyl) or an osmotic enema (Table 32). High-dose macrogol 3350 is an alternative (see above). Digital evacuation is the ultimate approach to faecal impaction.

SKELETAL MUSCLE RELAXANTS

Skeletal muscle relaxants are used to relieve distressing recurrent cramp, painful chronic muscle spasm, and spasticity associated with neural injury, e.g. post-stroke, paraplegia, multiple sclerosis.

Cramp has many causes (see Chapter 11, Box J, p.208). Drug treatment of cramp and spasticity is essentially the same.

Drugs authorized for the treatment of spasticity include diazepam (see p.356) and baclofen. Baclofen is a chemical congener of the neurotransmitter GABA. It acts upon the GABA-receptor, inhibiting the release of the excitatory amino acids glutamate

Table 32 Rectal measures for the relief of constipation or faecal impaction[a]

Rectal laxative	Predominant mode of action	Time to effect
Suppositories[b] *(place in contact with rectal mucosa)*		
Bisacodyl 10mg	Stimulates propulsive activity after hydrolysis by enteric enzymes	20–45min
Glycerol 4g	Hygroscopic; softens and lubricates	15–30min
Enemas *(warm to room temperature before use)*		
Osmotic micro-enema (5mL volume)	Faecal softener and osmotic effect (see text below)	15min
Osmotic standard phosphate enema (118–128mL volume)[c]	Osmotic effect	2–5min
Docusate sodium micro-enema (120mg in 10g)	Faecal softener (surface-wetting agent), some direct stimulant action	5–20min
Arachis (peanut) oil retention enema (130mL volume)[d]	Faecal softener	Overnight retention enema

a. PR digital examination will indicate what is the most appropriate intervention
b. suppositories should be administered only if there are faeces in the rectum
c. use with caution in elderly patients because of a risk of serious electrolyte disturbances
d. do not use in patients with peanut allergy.

and aspartate, principally at spinal level, thereby decreasing skeletal muscle spasm. Baclofen also relieves hiccup, possibly by a direct effect on the diaphragm.

If there is no concurrent indication for a benzodiazepine, PO baclofen is the preferred first choice, particularly if long-term treatment is likely (Table 33). In severe spasticity, baclofen can be given IT.

For important cautions and undesirable effects, see Tables 34 and 35. Tolerance and dependence do not occur.

Dose optimization may be limited in patients who need spasticity to maintain ambulation, e.g. some patients with MND/ALS.

Table 33 PO skeletal muscle relaxants and spasticity

Drug	Starting dose	Maximum dose	Monitoring
Diazepam	2–5mg at bedtime	60mg/24h	Accumulation; prolongation of plasma halflife with cimetidine
Baclofen[a]	5mg once daily–t.d.s.	20mg q.d.s.	Periodic LFTs

a. requires dose reduction in renal impairment; see SPC.

Table 34 Important cautions with baclofen

Context	Danger
Abrupt discontinuation of PO or IT baclofen	Serious psychiatric reactions, e.g. agitation and insomnia, confusion, psychosis. Discontinue PO by gradual dose reduction over 1–2 weeks or longer if withdrawal symptoms occur
	Sudden withdrawal of IT baclofen can cause a potentially fatal withdrawal syndrome over the course of 1–3 days, including cardiovascular lability, hyperthermia, seizures, hepatic and renal failure
Epilepsy, Parkinson's disease or severe psychiatric disorders	May be exacerbated
Cerebrovascular disease or spastic states of cerebral origin	Undesirable effects more common
Peptic ulceration	PO baclofen is cautioned against in patients with a previous peptic ulcer and contra-indicated in those with an active peptic ulcer
Respiratory impairment	May cause respiratory depression
Hepatic impairment	May elevate LFTs
Renal impairment	Increased risk of undesirable effects. Dose reduction required (see SPC)
Hesitancy of micturition	May precipitate urinary retention
Drug interactions	Risk of hypotension increased with other hypotensive drugs

Table 35 Undesirable effects of baclofen

System	Undesirable effect
CNS	Sedation, dizziness, fatigue, hypotonia, weakness, muscle pain, ataxia, tremor, insomnia, headache, nystagmus, psychiatric disturbances, respiratory depression
Cardiovascular effects	Hypotension
GI	Nausea, vomiting, dry mouth, constipation, diarrhea
Miscellaneous	Urinary frequency or incontinence, dysuria, hyperhidrosis

FURTHER READING

Twycross R, Wilcock A, Howard P (2015) *Palliative Care Formulary 5th edition.* Palliativedrugs.com Ltd. Nottingham, UK. Available from www.palliativedrugs.com.

SYMPTOM MANAGEMENT DRUGS: SYNOPTIC TABLE

Introduction

Table 36 includes *typical* starting and *typical* effective doses for the drugs commonly used in the UK for pain and symptom management. Note: specific cautions should be observed, e.g. dose reduction in renal impairment. Indeed, in the elderly, frail, and with renal or hepatic impairment, for most drugs it is generally advisable to start at a low dose and tritrate upwards more slowly.

The *maximum* recommended doses may be higher; refer to the relevant sections for full details. However, when the *typical* effective dose has not helped, consider seeking specialist advice before titrating further.

With some symptoms, regular medication should be supplemented with rescue ('as needed', p.r.n.) medication. The frequency of p.r.n. drugs depends on the class and formulation of the drug in question and whether the patient is an inpatient or at home (see p.320).

For optimal relief, it is good practice to err on the side of generosity in relation to the frequency of p.r.n. drugs, typically q2h. If necessary, a maximum amount in mg/24h or number of additional doses can be specified. If the symptom fails to improve, the patient should be reviewed.

At the end of life, q1h p.r.n. may be preferable to facilitate rapid dose titration, should it be necessary (see p.274).

Table 36 Typical adult doses for common uses of main symptom management drugs. Use only *after* reading the introduction above and the respective sections

Drug	Use	Typical starting dose	Typical effective dose	Page
Amitriptyline	Neuropathic pain	10mg PO at bedtime	≤75mg PO at bedtime	339
Baclofen	Muscle spasm; hiccup	5mg PO once daily–t.d.s.	≤20mg PO q.d.s.	169,373
Bisacodyl	Laxative	5mg PO (prophylaxis) or 10mg PO (if constipated) at bedtime	≤20mg PO t.d.s.	127,372
Celecoxib	Analgesic	100mg PO b.d. or 200mg once daily	200mg PO b.d.	326
Codeine	Analgesic	30–60mg PO q4h	60mg PO q4h	326
	Antitussive	15–30mg PO t.d.s.	30mg PO q.d.s.	159
Cyclizine	Anti-emetic	50mg PO b.d.–t.d.s. & 50mg p.r.n. or 100–150mg/24h CSCI & 50mg SC p.r.n.	150mg/24h PO/CSCI	124,137, 333,345
Dexamethasone	Anorexia	2mg PO each morning	4mg PO each morning	107,367
	Anti-emetic; raised ICP	8–16mg PO each morning	16mg PO each morning	124,367
	GI obstruction	6.6–7.6mg SC each morning	15.2mg SC each morning	136,367
	Spinal cord compression	16mg PO each morning	16mg PO each morning	242,367
Diazepam	Anxiety/panic disorder; breathlessness	2mg PO at bedtime & 2mg p.r.n.	≤10mg PO at bedtime	154,187, 358
	Muscle spasm	2–5mg PO at bedtime & 2mg p.r.n.	≤30mg/24h PO	358,373
Diclofenac sodium	Analgesic	50mg PO b.d.–t.d.s.	150mg/24h PO	326
Docusate	Laxative	100mg PO b.d.	≤200mg PO t.d.s.	137,371
Domperidone	Anti-emetic	10mg PO b.d.	10mg PO t.d.s.	123,344

continued

Drug	Use	Typical starting dose	Typical effective dose	Page
Gabapentin	Neuropathic pain	100–300mg PO at bedtime	<1,200mg PO t.d.s.	347
Glycopyrronium	Death rattle	200microgram SC q1h p.r.n. ± 600microgram/24h CSCI	1,200microgram/24h CSCI	280, 351
	GI obstruction	600microgram/24h CSCI & 200microgram SC q2h p.r.n.	1,200microgram/24h CSCI	351
Granisetron	Anti-emetic	1–2mg SC once daily	2mg/24h SC	124, 137
Haloperidol	Anti-emetic	500microgram–1.5mg PO stat & at bedtime & q2h p.r.n. or 2.5–5mg/24h CSCI & 1mg SC q2h p.r.n.	≤10mg/24h PO/CSCI	123, 137, 355
	Delirium	500microgram PO stat & q2h p.r.n. (for severe distress, use 1.5–3mg PO)	≤5mg/24h PO	356
Hyoscine butylbromide	Bladder spasm	60–120mg/24h CSCI & 20mg SC q2h p.r.n.	120mg/24h CSCI	176
	Death rattle	20mg SC q1h p.r.n. ± 20–60mg/24h CSCI	120mg/24h CSCI	280, 351
	GI obstruction	60–120mg/24h CSCI & 20mg SC q2h p.r.n.	120mg/24h CSCI	124, 136, 351
Hyoscine hydrobromide	Death rattle	400microgram SC q1h p.r.n. ± 1,200microgram/24h CSCI	1,600microgram/24h CSCI	280, 351
Ibuprofen	Analgesic	400mg PO t.d.s.	400mg PO t.d.s.	251, 326
Lactulose	Laxative	15mL PO once daily–b.d.	<30mL PO t.d.s.	128, 371

continued

Table 36 Typical adult doses for common uses of main symptom management drugs. Use only *after* reading the introduction above and the respective sections (Continued)

Drug	Use	Typical starting dose	Typical effective dose	Page
Levomepromazine	Anti-emetic	6–6.25mg PO/SC at bedtime & q2h p.r.n.	≤50mg PO/SC at bedtime	124, 355
	Sedation	12.5–25mg SC q1h p.r.n. & 50–75mg/24h CSCI	≤100mg/24h CSCI	254, 274
Loperamide	Antidiarrhoeal	4mg PO stat and 2mg p.r.n. (after each loose stool)	<16mg/24h PO	341
Lorazepam	Acute psychotic agitation	2mg PO/IM p.r.n. every 30min		359
	Anxiety/panic disorder; anti-emetic	0.5–1mg PO/SL b.d. & 0.5mg p.r.n.	2–6mg/24h PO/SL	124, 154, 187, 358
Macrogol 3350	Laxative	1 sachet PO each morning	1 sachet PO t.d.s.	128, 371
Metoclopramide	Anti-emetic	10mg PO t.d.s.–q.d.s. & 10mg q2h p.r.n. or 30–40mg/24h CSCI & 10mg SC q2h p.r.n.	≤80mg/24h PO/CSCI	123, 136, 342
Midazolam	Breathlessness in EOLC (in conjunction with morphine)	2.5–5mg SC q1h p.r.n. & 10mg/24h CSCI	<60mg/24h CSCI	278
	Sedation	2.5–5mg SC q1h p.r.n. & 10mg/24h CSCI	≤60mg/24h CSCI	254
	Seizure (acute management)	10mg buccal/SC/IM/IV stat; repeat once after 10min p.r.n.	≤2 stat doses of 10mg, 10min apart	204, 205
	Seizures (in the imminently dying)	As above & 20–30mg/24h CSCI	≤60mg/24h CSCI	204, 205, 348

continued

Drug	Use	Typical starting dose	Typical effective dose	Page
Morphine (all opioid naive)	Analgesic	5mg PO q4h & q2–4h p.r.n.	≤120mg/24h PO	330
	Antitussive	2.5–5mg PO q.d.s.–q4h & p.r.n.	≤60mg/24h PO	159
	Breathlessness	2.5–5mg PO q1h p.r.n.	≤60mg/24h PO	153
	Breathlessness in EOLC (with midazolam)	2.5–5mg SC q1h p.r.n. & 10mg/24h CSCI	≤30mg/24h CSCI	278
Naloxone	Medicinal opioid overdose	100microgram IV stat & every 2min p.r.n.		238
Naproxen	Analgesic	250–500mg PO b.d.	500mg PO b.d.	251, 326
Nortriptyline	Neuropathic pain	10–25mg PO at bedtime	≤75mg PO at bedtime	339
Octreotide	GI obstruction	100microgram SC stat & 500microgram/24h CSCI	≤1,000microgram/24h CSCI	137
Ondansetron	Anti-emetic	16mg/24h CSCI	16mg/24h CSCI	124, 137
Paracetamol	Analgesic	500mg–1g PO q.d.s.	1g PO q.d.s.	323
Prednisolone	Anorexia	15mg PO each morning	30mg PO each morning	107, 367
Pregabalin	Neuropathic pain	25–75mg PO b.d.	<300mg PO b.d.	347
Senna	Laxative	15mg PO at bedtime (prophylaxis) or b.d. (if constipated)	<30mg PO t.d.s.	127, 372
Tramadol	Analgesic	50mg PO q.d.s.	400mg/24h PO	326
Tranexamic acid	Surface bleeding	1g PO q.d.s.	1g PO q.d.s.	226, 248
Valproate	Neuropathic pain	150–200mg PO m/r at bedtime	≤1g PO b.d.	347

Appendix 1: Curriculum for under-graduate medical education

Association for Palliative Medicine of Great Britain and Ireland 2014

INTRODUCTION

It is estimated that in the first year after qualification, a Foundation Year (FY) doctor will, on average, care for around 40 patients who die and an additional 120 patients in the final months of life. The care of patients approaching the end of life and the care of dying patients are thus core skills for all FY doctors, who in practice frequently use the knowledge, skills and attitudes outlined below in relatively unsupervised situations.

All UK Medical Schools include Palliative Medicine in their curricula, although the amount of time allocated is very variable. It is not envisaged that all elements of this curriculum will be taught by Palliative Medicine specialists or delivered within a Palliative Medicine course component: many of the learning outcomes can be achieved through integration with other course components. However, it is recommended that those responsible for coordinating Palliative Medicine teaching ensure that the learning outcomes outlined are covered in the curriculum of their Medical School.

In this document, learning outcomes are categorised as:

a) 'Demonstrate understanding of': knowledge to be shown.

b) 'Demonstrate ability to': skills to be shown.

c) 'Demonstrate appropriate attitudes towards': attitudes to be shown.

By the time of graduation and qualification as doctors, medical students should demonstrate the following learning outcomes.

BASIC PRINCIPLES

Demonstrate understanding of:
- terms 'palliative care', 'end-of-life care', 'life-limiting illness' and 'terminal illness'
- demographics of death, including causes and places of death
- range of palliative care patients with cancer and other conditions
- patient priorities and preferences at the end of life
- community services to enable patients to die at home
- frameworks to support end-of-life care provision
- range of palliative care services available
- when specialist palliative care services should be involved
- particular needs of children and young adults with life-limiting illnesses
- the potential need for palliative care concurrent with active disease management.

Demonstrate appropriate attitudes towards:
- palliative care as a generic skill and duty of all healthcare professionals, including themselves as future junior doctors.

PHYSICAL CARE

Disease processes

Demonstrate understanding of:
- the presentation, natural history and management of; cancer, dementia, progressive neurological, respiratory, cardiac, renal, chronic frailty and other life-limiting conditions
- the range of 'dying trajectories' and the significance of transition points
- the importance and limitations of prognostication and prognostic indicators.

Demonstrate appropriate attitudes towards:
- the benefits and burdens of investigations, treatments and non-intervention
- decision-making concerning ceilings of care and limits of treatment escalation
- recognition of a dying patient and accepting the refocusing of care provision
- the uncertainties in end-of-life care, particularly in non-malignant disease
- the concept of allowing 'natural death'.

Symptom management: general principles

Demonstrate understanding of:
- symptoms may be caused by the disease itself, the treatment or concurrent disorders
- importance of diagnosing the pathophysiology of a symptom for effective management
- range of drug and other options for symptom management
- role of anticipatory prescribing and the drugs commonly used.

Demonstrate ability to:
- formulate and review an appropriate personalised end-of-life care plan
- write a prescription for anticipatory symptom management
- write a prescription for a continuous subcutaneous infusion ('syringe driver').

Demonstrate appropriate attitudes towards:
- holistic care: identifying and addressing physical, psychological, social and spiritual needs of patients and their families.

Pain

Demonstrate understanding of:
- different types of pain: nociceptive, visceral, neuropathic and incident
- WHO ladder, including adjuvant analgesics
- factors influencing pain: physical, psychological, social and spiritual
- 'total pain'; the conflation of physical, psychological, social and spiritual suffering that patients may express as pain
- relative benefits / indications / contra-indications of a limited range of opioids
- principles of opioid conversions
- non-drug treatments: physical, psychological, complementary.

Demonstrate ability to:
- assess a patient's pain and formulate a management plan.

Other symptoms

Demonstrate understanding of the assessment and management of:

Gastrointestinal symptoms
- nausea, vomiting, constipation, ascites, dysphagia, diarrhoea, bowel obstruction, jaundice, hiccups and anorexia.

Cardiorespiratory symptoms
- breathlessness, cough, pleural effusion, haemoptysis.

Genitourinary symptoms
- catheter care, bladder spasm, urinary obstruction, urinary incontinence, sexual problems.

Neurological symptoms
- raised intracranial pressure, epileptic fits, muscle spasm.

Psychological symptoms
- depression, anxiety, fear, confusional states, delirium, insomnia.

Emergencies
- superior vena cava obstruction, spinal cord compression, hypercalcaemia, overwhelming pain / distress, severe haemorrhage.

Other symptoms
- fatigue, lymphoedema; care of fungating lesions, pressure area, wounds and mouth.

Care of the dying patient

Demonstrate understanding of
- signs indicating that a patient is dying
- stopping of drugs and the management of diabetes
- management of symptoms at the end of life
- ethical, legal and clinical issues of oral nutrition and hydration, clinically-assisted nutrition and hydration, sedation and use of opioids in the dying phase.

Demonstrate ability to:
- develop a personalized management plan for the care of a dying patient.

Demonstrate appropriate attitudes towards:
- recognition of a dying patient and acceptance of the refocusing of care provision.

PSYCHOSOCIAL CARE

Demonstrate understanding of:
- the difference between sadness and clinical depression
- the different responses and emotions expressed by patients and caregivers, including fear, guilt, anger, sadness, despair, collusion and denial
- the psychological impact of intractable symptoms

- other disciplines who could help patients to deal with psychological issues
- denial as a coping mechanism
- continuum of loss experienced by patients and caregivers throughout illnesses
- recognising unhelpful and potentially harmful psychological responses.

Demonstrate appropriate attitudes towards:
- fostering appropriate hope and achievement of goals other than cure.

COMMUNICATION WITH PATIENTS, RELATIVES AND OTHERS

Demonstrate understanding of:
- documents available to enable patients to record future care preferences
- importance of timely communication between primary and secondary care, particularly when transferring patients between settings
- methods for sharing clinical information between services while maintaining patient confidentiality, including: patient held records, e-mail, fax, shared electronic records and Electronic Palliative Care Co-ordination Systems (EPaCCS).

Demonstrate ability to:
- use communication skills in empathic listening
- elicit a patient's physical, psychological, social and spiritual concerns
- respond appropriately to patient and lay caregiver concerns
- deliver bad news sensitively and at an appropriate pace for the individual
- deal with difficult questions and challenging conversations
- enable those patients who wish to do so to formulate advance care plans
- discuss DNACPR with patients and lay caregivers
- communicate risk and prognostic uncertainty with patients and lay caregivers
- document care and communicate well between team members to ensure patients receive a consistent message.

Demonstrate appropriate attitudes towards:
- respecting that some patients may not wish to know or talk about their prognosis
- maintaining patient confidentiality.

SOCIAL AND FAMILY RELATIONSHIPS

Demonstrate understanding of:
- social impact of life-limiting illnesses in relation to a person's family, friends, work and other social circumstances
- needs of partners, families and other carers
- impact of illnesses on body image, sexuality and role.

Demonstrate ability to:
- take a narrative family history in order to elicit family myths and scripts in terminal illness
- communicate with and support family members as a group and individually.

GRIEF AND BEREAVEMENT

Demonstrate understanding of:
- importance of identifying those who are bereaved
- models of bereavement, the process of grieving and adjustment to loss
- ways to support a bereaved person both before and after the bereavement
- features of abnormal or complicated bereavement requiring intervention
- impact of bereavement on children and others with special needs.

Demonstrate ability to:
- communicate with and support bereaved people.

Demonstrate appropriate attitudes towards:
- integral role of doctors as part of the wider team in caring for bereaved people.

PERSONAL AND PROFESSIONAL ISSUES

Demonstrate appropriate attitudes towards:
- personal emotional impact of palliative care on themselves and colleagues
- personal limitations and asking for help and support
- sources of help in dealing with personal and professional issues.

CULTURE, LANGUAGE, RELIGIOUS AND SPIRITUAL ISSUES

Demonstrate understanding of:
- major cultural and religious practices in relation to care at the end of life and after death
- distinction between an individual's spiritual and religious needs
- role of the hospital chaplain.

Demonstrate ability to:
- elicit and respond to spiritual concerns, seeking help if necessary.

Demonstrate appropriate attitudes towards:
- doctors' personal values and belief systems and how these may influence professional judgements and behaviours.

ETHICAL AND LEGAL ISSUES

Demonstrate understanding of:
- GMC ethical guidance including 'Treatment and Care Towards the End of Life'.

Demonstrate ability to:
- apply ethical frameworks (Beneficence, Non-Maleficence, Autonomy, Justice) to ethical issues at the end of life, including:
  ▷ Double effect
  ▷ requests for euthanasia and assisted dying
  ▷ DNACPR decisions
  ▷ withholding/withdrawing treatment
  ▷ withholding/withdrawing clinically-assisted nutrition and hydration.

LEGAL FRAMEWORKS

Demonstrate understanding of:
- the law in relation to end-of-life care
- guidelines produced by the GMC, BMA and Royal Colleges
- capacity to give consent
- the Mental Capacity Act (2005) and the role of IMCAs
- deprivation of Liberty Safeguards
- the procedures involved in death verification and certification and cremation
- the situations when liaison with the Coroner's office or Procurator Fiscal's office is required
- the procedures for relatives following a death
- the law concerning Advance Statements of Wishes, Advance Decisions to Refuse Treatment, Power of Attorney for Health and Welfare.

Demonstrate ability to:
- complete a medical certificate of cause of death
- complete a cremation certificate.

Appendix 2: Certifying death

This Appendix supplements information about death certification in Chapter 6 (p.72).

VERIFICATION OF DEATH

Anyone, such as a family member, can declare a person dead and note the date and time of death. However, in hospital or hospice, confirmation of death is carried out by a doctor or registered nurse (extended role). In the community, this is generally done by the GP.

Unlike with brain stem death, there are no standardized criteria for confirmation of death in other circumstances. Death is confirmed when there is unconsciousness, irreversible apnoea and no circulation:
- observe patient for a *minimum of five minutes* to ensure that cessation of cardiorespiratory function is irreversible
- confirm absence of a carotid pulse on palpation
- auscultate to confirm absence of heart sounds
- confirm the absence of pupillary response to light (or absence of corneal reflex or any motor response to supra-orbital pressure).[1]

MEDICAL CERTIFICATE OF CAUSE OF DEATH (MCCD)

England and Wales

Information from MCCDs are collected to measure the contribution of different disorders to mortality and are used in medical research.[2]

MCCDs are supplied in books, and have notes on how to complete the certificate (and when to refer deaths to the coroner). Doctors are expected to state the cause of death to the best of their belief. It is advisable for junior doctors to discuss the cause of death with a senior doctor before completing the MCCD.

The cause of death section on the MCCD is divided into two parts:
- Part I: the immediate or direct cause of death is written first, and the fatal sequence of conditions or events that led to this is written in reverse order on subsequent lines. If the certificate is properly completed, the condition on the lowest line on part I will have caused all the conditions listed on the lines above it. This condition is known as the underlying cause of death.
- Part II: significant conditions contributing to the death but not related to the disorder causing it are given.

It is important to give as much detail about the cause of death as possible, e.g. histological type and anatomical site of cancer, the infecting organism and site of an infection. Approximate time intervals should also be given.

If a post-mortem has been done, include information from this. If the cause of death is known but further detailed information will be available later (e.g. from a post-mortem), the MCCD can still be issued but the Registrar General will contact the doctor for the additional information later.

Terms to avoid include:
- *old age*: this should be given as the sole cause of death only if the person is >80 and was not known to suffer from any potentially fatal conditions
- *organ failure* as the underlying cause of death: the disease responsible for the organ failure must be given
- *vague terms* or modes of death, e.g. cardiovascular event
- *abbreviations*: but HIV/AIDS and MRSA are acceptable.

The cause of death should also be written in the patient's notes.

Northern Ireland

Principles governing the issuing of an MCCD in Northern Ireland are broadly similar to those in England and Wales. However, provided the doctor had seen the person within 28 days of their death (cf. 14 days in England and Wales), an MCCD can be issued if the death was from natural causes.[3]

Scotland

Principles governing issuing of an MCCD in Scotland are broadly similar to those elsewhere in the UK. However, the Certification of Death Scotland Act 2011 which came into force in 2015 has made several changes.[4]

There is now a new review process of MCCDs to improve accuracy:
- 10% of deaths not reported to the Procurator Fiscal will be randomly selected for Level 1 review (expected to be completed in one working day) and a medical reviewer will speak to the certifying doctor
- 2% of deaths will be subject to both Level 1 and Level 2 review (expected to be completed in three working days); this is more in-depth and includes an examination of patient records.

Other changes include:
- an Advance Registration process (to allow funerals to go ahead before a review is completed, e.g. for religious, cultural, compassionate or practical reasons)
- electronic completion of MCCDs (although a paper copy will need to be printed off for the next of kin)
- the same level of scrutiny of the cause of death for both burials and cremations
- abolition of cremation fees and Crematoria Medical Referees
- feeding information from MCCDs to Health Boards to improve public health information.

REPORTING A DEATH TO THE CORONER OR PROCURATOR FISCAL

England and Wales

If there is any uncertainty about the cause of death or whether to refer a death to the Coroner, it should be discussed with the Coroner's office. Refer to the coroner if:

- the cause of death appears to be unknown
- no doctor attended the deceased during his or her last illness
- although a doctor attended the person during the last illness, the deceased was not seen by the certifying doctor *either* within 14 days before death *or* after death
- the death was/may be:
  - ▷ violent or unnatural or suspicious
  - ▷ due to an accident (whenever it occurred, including falls)
  - ▷ due to an industrial disease or related to the deceased's employment
  - ▷ due to self-neglect or neglect by others
  - ▷ related to a medical mishap or equipment failure
  - ▷ related to an operation or before recovery from the anaesthetic
  - ▷ related to drugs (including adverse drug reactions)
  - ▷ due to an abortion
  - ▷ suicide.

Further rules cover notification of deaths of people detained under the Mental Health Act, in police custody, for infants and children, and children in care.

Scotland

These are broadly similar to the criteria for notifying a coroner in England and Wales. However there are some differences.[5] The Procurator Fiscal must be notified of:

- a death which pose an acute and serious risk to public health due to either a Notifiable Infectious Disease or Organism in terms of Schedule 1 of the Public Heath (Scotland) Act 2008 (see http://www.legislation.gov.uk/asp/2008/5/schedule/1) or any other infectious disease or syndrome
- when the relatives of the deceased are concerned or if there has been a complaint about the care received
- withdrawal of life-sustaining treatment or other medical treatment of a patient in persistent vegetative state.

In Scotland, the following are *not* automatic reasons for rendering a death reportable:

- death within 24h (or any other timescale) of admission to hospital
- death within 24h (or any other timescale) of an operation
- someone with a known terminal illness who died earlier than expected
- someone who had *not* been seen by a doctor for some time (cf. <14 or <28 days in other parts of the UK).

CREMATION REGULATIONS

In the UK, the majority of people are cremated rather than buried. Permission to cremate the body must be applied for by the patient's close relatives or executors (the applicants). Doctors will be requested to complete a cremation form.

England and Wales[6,7]

The first part (cremation form 4) gives additional detail and evidence about the circumstances surrounding the death and is completed by a doctor who:

- is registered and holds a licence to practice with the GMC (including temporary or provisional registration)
- treated the patient during their last illness
- has seen the patient within 14 days preceding the death.

The second part (cremation form 5, the confirmatory medical certificate) is completed by a doctor who:

- is fully registered for at least five years and hold a licence to practice
- is not a colleague or partner of the doctor completing form 4.

The role of this doctor is to check the circumstances surrounding the death. Doctors completing forms 4 and 5 are entitled to be paid a fee by the funeral director.

The Crematoria Medical Referee then checks the form to ensure sound clinical grounds are given for the cause of death, that the death has been registered, and all certificates completed before authorizing cremation. The applicants for cremation have a right to inspect the cremation forms.

Northern Ireland

The process is similar to that in England and Wales (forms 4 and 5 are numbered B and C).

Scotland

Information required for cremation is now included in the MCCD and no additional medical checks or forms are needed.

REFERENCES

1 Colleges AoMR (2008) *A code of practice for the diagnosis and confirmation of death.* www.bts.org.uk/Documents/A%20CODE%20OF%20PRACTICE%20FOR%20THE%20DIAGNOSIS%20AND%20CONFIRMATION%20OF%20DEATH.pdf

2 Office for National Statitics Death Certification Advisory Group (2010) *Guidance for doctors: completing medical certificates of the cause of death and its quality assurance.* www.gro.gov.uk/images/medcert_july_2010_pdf

3 Births and Deaths Registration (Northern Ireland) Order 1976. www.legislation.gov.uk/nisi/1976/1041/contents

4 Chief Medical Officer and National Records of Scotland (2014) *Guidance for doctors: completing medical certificates of the cause of death and its quality assurance.* www.sehd.scot.nhs.uk/cmo(2014)2027.pdf

5 Crown Office and Procurator Fiscal Service (2015) *Reporting Deaths to the Procurator Fiscal 2015 Information and guidance for Medical Practitioners.* www.copfs.gov.uk/publications/deaths

6 The Cremation (England and Wales) Regulations (2008) www.legislation.gov.uk/uksi/2008/2841/pdfs/uksi_20082841_en.pdf

7 Guidance on completion of cremation certificates (2012) www.gov.uk/government/uploads/system/uploads/attachment_data/file/325750/cremation-doctors-guidance.pdf

Appendix 3: Essential drugs

Both the World Health Organization (WHO) and the International Association for Hospice and Palliative Care (IAHPC) have produced lists of essential drugs for palliative care (Table 1).[1,2] The WHO list contains 20 items, and is extracted from the *WHO Model Drug List*. The latter is based on the needs of economically poorer countries and widespread generic availability.

For the IAHPC, the starting point was a list of the more common symptoms seen in palliative care practice. Twenty one symptoms were identified, for which 33 drugs were eventually included in the *List of Essential Medicines for Palliative Care*. Methodology was a Delphi survey involving 112 doctors and pharmacologists (77 from developing countries), followed by a consensus meeting of representatives from 26 pain and palliative care organizations.[3]

The Essential Palliative Care Formulary (EPCF) in IPC features more drugs than either essential drugs list (noted by page number in Table 1) although some receive minor mention only. In practice, choice of drug depends foremost on availability coupled with efficacy and cost, together with local custom. Fourteen drugs are common to both Lists and to IPC (highlighted in Table 1).

Table 1 Comparison of Essential Drugs Lists

Drug	WHO	IAHPC	EPCF
Amitriptyline	+	+	339
Acetylsalicylic acid (aspirin)	+		−
Baclofen			373
Bisacodyl		+	372
Buprenorphine			334
Carbamazepine		+	347
Celecoxib			325
Codeine	+	+	326
Cyclizine	+		344
Denosumab			364
Dexamethasone	+	+	367
Diamorphine (UK only)			331
Diazepam	+	+	358
Diclofenac		+	325
Dihydrocodeine			326
Diphenhydramine		+	−
Docusate	+		371
Domperidone			344
Fentanyl		+	334
Gabapentin		+	347
Glycopyrronium			351
Haloperidol	+	+	355
Hydromorphone			334
Hyoscine *butylbromide*	+	+	351

Drug	WHO	IAHPC	EPCF
Hyoscine *hydrobromide*	+		351
Ibandronic acid			359
Ibuprofen	+	+	325
Lactulose	+		371
Levetiracetam		+	348
Levomepromazine			355
Loperamide	+	+	341
Lorazepam		+	358
Macrogols			371
Megestrol acetate		+	–
Methadone		+	334
Methylphenidate			340
Metoclopramide	+	+	342
Midazolam	+	+	358
Mineral oil enema		+	–
Mirtazapine		+	340
Morphine	+	+	329
Naproxen			325
Nortriptyline			339
Octreotide		+	342
Olanzapine			355
Ondansetron	+		342
Oral rehydration salts		+	–
Oxcarbazepine			348
Oxycodone		+	334
Pamidronate disodium			363
Paracetamol (acetaminophen)	+	+	323
Prednisolone		+	366
Pregabalin			347
Risperidone			356
Senna	+	+	372
SSRI (choice differs)	+	+	338
Sodium picosulfate			370
Tramadol		+	326
Trazodone		+	–
Valproate			347
Zoledronic acid			363
Z-drugs (choice differs)		+	358

REFERENCES

1 WHO (2013) Essential medicines in palliative care. www.who.int
2 IAHPC (2015) Essential medicines for palliative care. www.hospicecare.com
3 De Lima L (2012) Key concepts in palliative care: the IAHPC List of Essential Medicines in Palliative Care. *European Journal of Hospital Pharmacy* 19: 34–37.

Drug Index

Topic Index